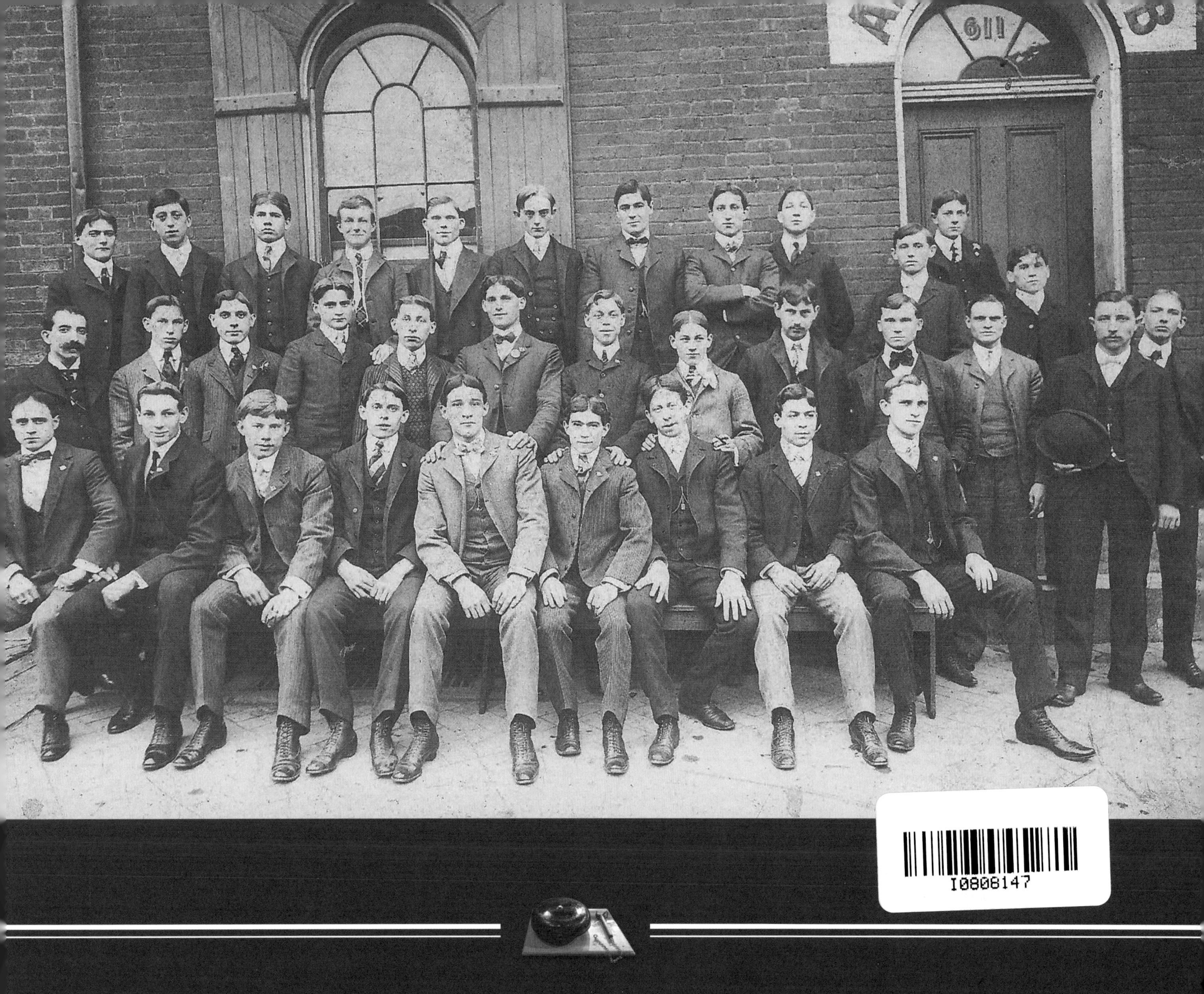

South Broadway ATHLETIC CLUB

St. Louis's Home for Boxing, Wrestling, and Cheap Beer Since 1899

By Miriam Moynihan and Ryan Buckley

Introduction by NiNi Harris

REEDY PRESS

Reedy Press
PO Box 5131
St. Louis, MO 63139, USA
www.reedypress.com

Unless otherwise noted, all photos are courtesy of the authors, South Broadway Athletic Club members, or believed to be in the public domain.

Library of Congress Control Number: 2024948778

ISBN: 9781681065878

Design by Eric Marquard

Front cover photo: Courtesy of the St. Louis Mercantile Library at the University of Missouri–St. Louis
Back cover photo: South Broadway Athletic Club

Printed in Canada
25 26 27 28 29 5 4 3 2 1

Dedication

For the members—past, present, and future.

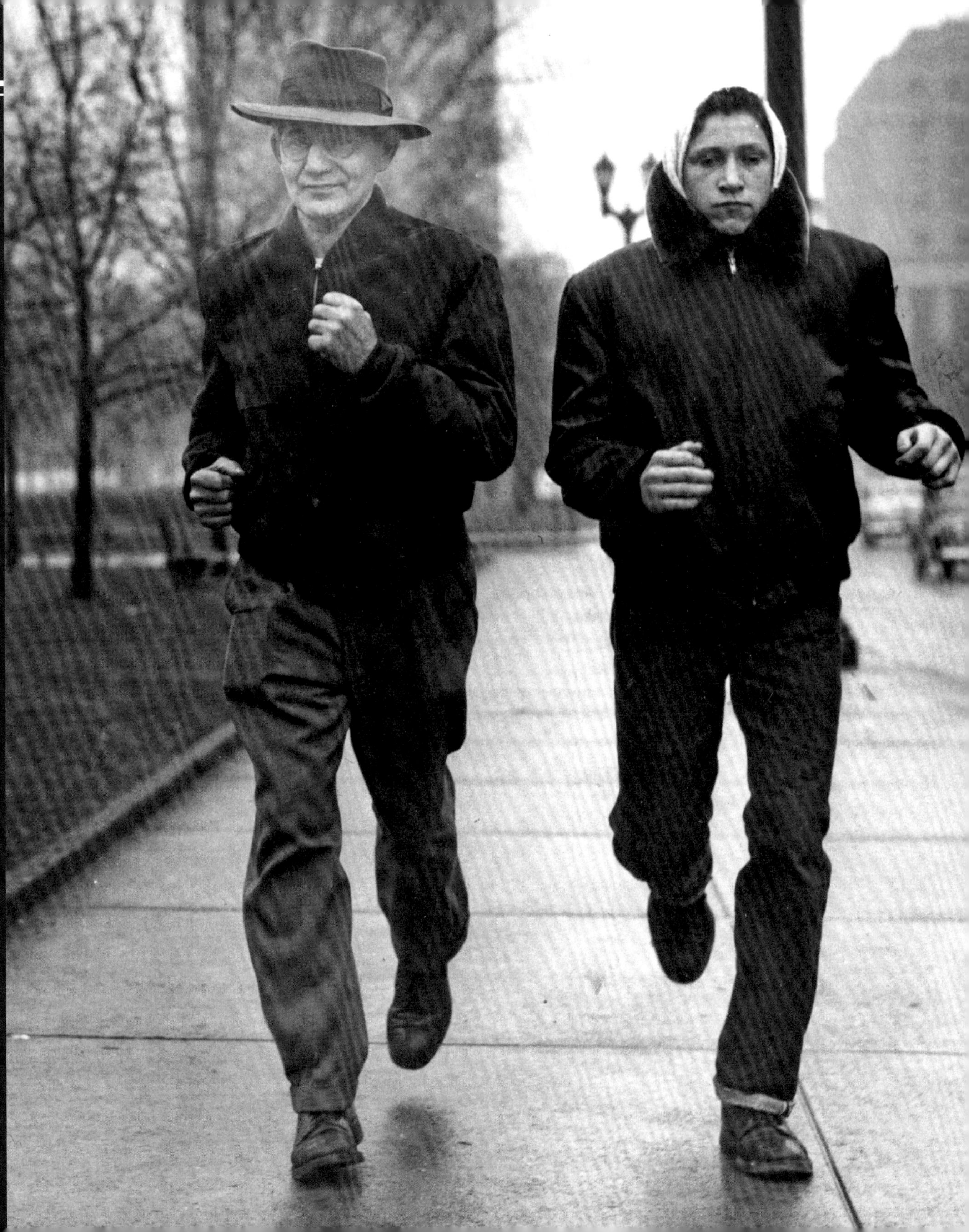

SBAC boxing coach Joe Weber (left) taking a jog around the plaza on Market Street to help his fighter Jerry Mikes, 118-pound novice, trim off two pounds in order to hit his required weight for a 1952 match

Courtesy of the St. Louis Mercantile Library at the University of Missouri–St. Louis

Contents

SOULARD IN 1899

When the South Broadway Athletic Club Was Founded

By NiNi Harris

EVERYWHERE YOU LOOKED there was brick. The streets were brick. The sidewalks were brick. The buildings standing shoulder to shoulder, mostly along the sidewalks' edges—houses, tenements, stores, factories—they were brick. Scattered, larger brick homes were set back from the street, with small front gardens framed by ornamental iron fences. The larger homes were built by immigrant families who had prospered as quarry operators, wholesalers, physicians, and brewers. These successful businessmen stayed in their old immigrant communities, in their churches, and in their clubs. Even the Busch family lived in a grand home in the midst of their growing brewery. The street views of humble row houses and tall townhouses reminded people of the German fatherland, even though much of the neighborhood was still called Frenchtown in honor of its original French settlers.

People—speaking a dozen languages—crowded the sidewalks and streets. Large families lived in three-room dwellings. Everywhere people walked to work, to school, to the market, to church, and to the corner tavern. Soulard had grown into one of the most crowded neighborhoods in the city, and maybe in the nation, by 1899, and community life spilled beyond the streets and sidewalks.

Narrow, iron-gated passageways led between the buildings to courtyards that were enclosed by more brick houses. Networks of wooden, two-story porches framed these courtyards, and their stairs led to the doors of second- and third-floor apartments. Children played in the yards. Women used the manure left by horses pulling coal wagons to fertilize their small gardens. In these kitchen gardens, they grew herbs and vegetables. On wash day, laundry lines heavy with sheets, diapers, and work clothes crisscrossed the courtyards. On the hottest summer nights, people tried to cool off by sleeping on their back porches around their courtyards.

Church steeples towered over the blocks of homes. Instead of clocks, the ringing of bells marked the hour. The center of life for many Soulard families was the churches, and hymns of church choirs brought music into daily life.

In this crowded neighborhood, medieval-style walled convents

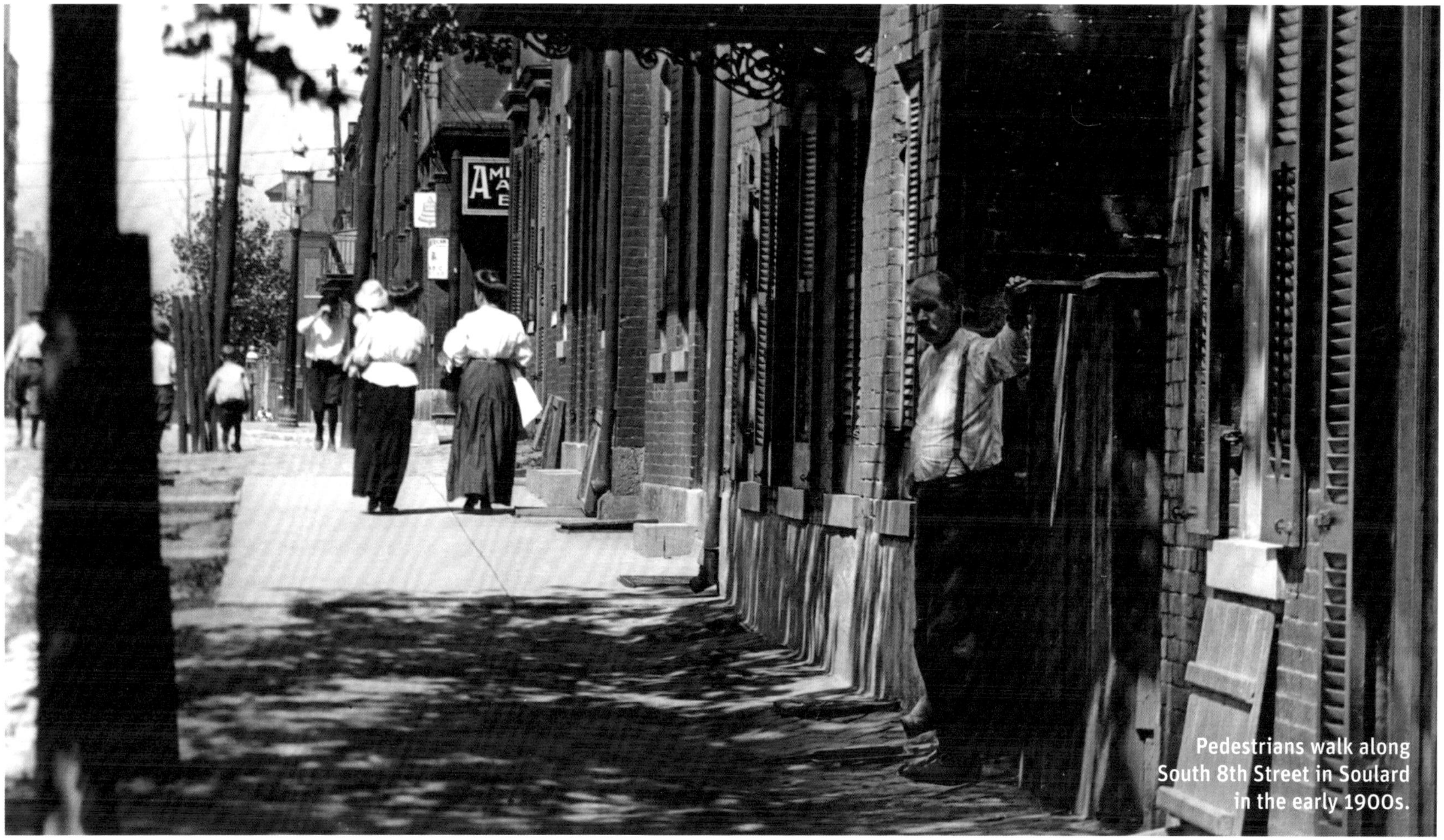

Pedestrians walk along South 8th Street in Soulard in the early 1900s.

gave a unique rhythm to the streetscapes. The Ursuline Sisters from the Austro-Hungarian Empire lived at their convent and school at Russell Avenue and 12th Street. Their block-sized grounds were planted and walled. The Carmelite Sisters pursued their cloistered life on a brick-walled block with convent and prayer gardens on 13th Street.

Large factories filled more and more of the riverfront and lined the railroad tracks that followed the river. Here, immigrants and their adult children worked at American Car Foundry, at the Bemis Bag factory, or at Hager Hinge Company. At other factories, the immigrant work force made rope or cast iron. At the southern tip of the neighborhood, Anheuser-Busch Brewery bustled with activity as the workers filled refrigerated railcars with their brews and shipped them all over the southwest.

The hours doing hard, physical work were long. The factories, mills, and foundries were cold in winter and miserably hot in summer.

While the men labored in factories, the women scrubbed. They rubbed the laundry on wood and brass scrubboards until their knuckles were raw. The battle against the clouds of coal dust that spewed from the mills required constant cleaning. They scrubbed the stone steps at their front doors and the pine floors of their flats. When the women were not cleaning, they schlepped fruits and vegetables, particularly potatoes and cabbages, from the farmers' stalls at Soulard Market. They shredded the cabbages to make sauerkraut, German style sweetened with apples or Bohemian style with caraway seeds.

For most people in Soulard in 1899, the amenities were few. Even indoor plumbing was rare.

Life in Soulard was not just hard, it was also exotic. The most common language in businesses and in churches was German. There were still descendants of the French in Soulard, some who attended St. Vincent DePaul Church. The large Bohemian community spoke the Czech language in their homes, at their clubs, and at St. John Nepomuk Church. The Poles spoke Polish in their community and at their boardinghouses. There were the seeds of other, newer communities—Lebanese, Croatian, Ruthenian, Serbian, Russian, Slovak—in the neighborhood.

English was heard and taught to the children of immigrants attending the public schools. The fortunate children were able to finish grade school before they went to work in factories or workshops to help pay family bills.

At the turn of the century, the neighborhood was packed with immigrant families working backbreaking jobs with minimal pay, depending on their young children to translate the English language and American culture for them. These immigrant Americans faced their challenges by forming fraternal societies and clubs around their ethnic groups and ethnic churches. They participated in Sunday afternoon religious processions through the streets. Their churches offered theater troupes and socials. They formed singing societies like the Liederkranz and the Saengerbund. Athletic clubs like the Turnverein (German gymnastic clubs) and a Sokol (Bohemian gymnastic club) offered dances, concerts, libraries, and political discussions.

This network of associations, clubs, and camaraderie gave the neighborhood resiliency. That strength was demonstrated after the tornado of 1896 ripped through Soulard. It tore the roofs off houses, leveled walls, and knocked church steeples to the street. It reduced some buildings to piles of bricks. Yet the residents rebuilt the neighborhood—with its characteristic row houses and church steeples. In a couple of years, Soulard was again thriving, picturesque, and quaint.

In this setting, five young men saw a need for a club that focused on what was then called "physical culture." As Soulard residents, organizing was not a theory or treatise in a textbook. These young men had witnessed Soulard being built, and rebuilt. When they envisioned a club that encouraged sports competitions, debate, discussion, and camaraderie, they formed the South Broadway Athletic Club (SBAC).

Through the decades, SBAC's sporting competitions and social events evolved and changed, but they continued. The SBAC programs became a focus of life through two world wars, the Great Depression, social unrest, and the physical destruction wrought by highways. The Club provided stability both as the neighborhood suffered neglect and then later as a new generation of residents restored Soulard's architecture and reinvigorated its community life. Today, the neighborhood has rediscovered its picturesque, now iconic, character, and the SBAC is reengergized.

Lehnbeuter-Deichman Manufacturing, on the southeast corner of 14th and Soulard Streets

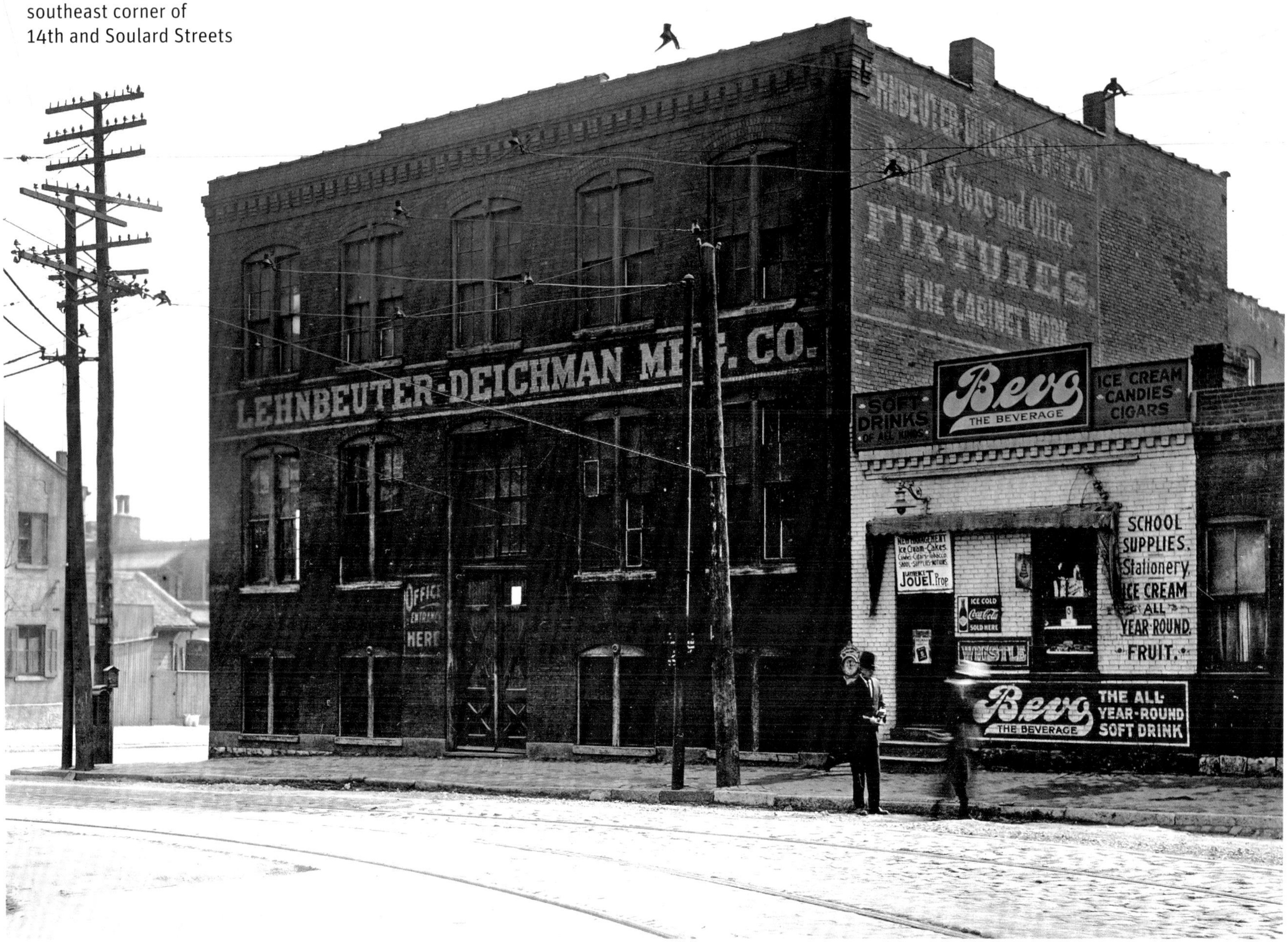

Foreword

AS PRESIDENT of the South Broadway Athletic Club (SBAC), it is my honor and privilege to commemorate this remarkable milestone: our 125th anniversary. Reaching such a significant landmark is no small feat. It's a testament to the dedication, resilience, and shared values of our members, volunteers, and supporters throughout the years. This anniversary is more than just a celebration of longevity; it is a recognition of the countless individuals who have contributed to making the SBAC a pillar of our community.

This commemorative book aims to capture the stories of our past and the vibrant community we have today. Throughout its pages, you will find memories of pivotal moments, triumphs, and tales of perseverance that reflect the very fabric of our club's identity. It is a tribute to all who have contributed to our legacy and an inspiration for the future generations who will carry it forward.

Founded in 1899, the SBAC was established with a vision of promoting physical fitness, camaraderie, and community spirit. The story of the SBAC is one of perseverance. Our founders were immigrants and working-class citizens who understood the value of community and the importance of providing opportunities for youths to engage in positive, healthy activities. They laid the foundation upon which we still stand today. They couldn't have known then how far their vision would reach, but their legacy has endured, inspiring each generation to carry the torch forward.

Boxing has been at the heart of the SBAC since its inception. It is a sport that mirrors the very spirit of our club—one of grit, determination, and the willingness to face challenges head-on.

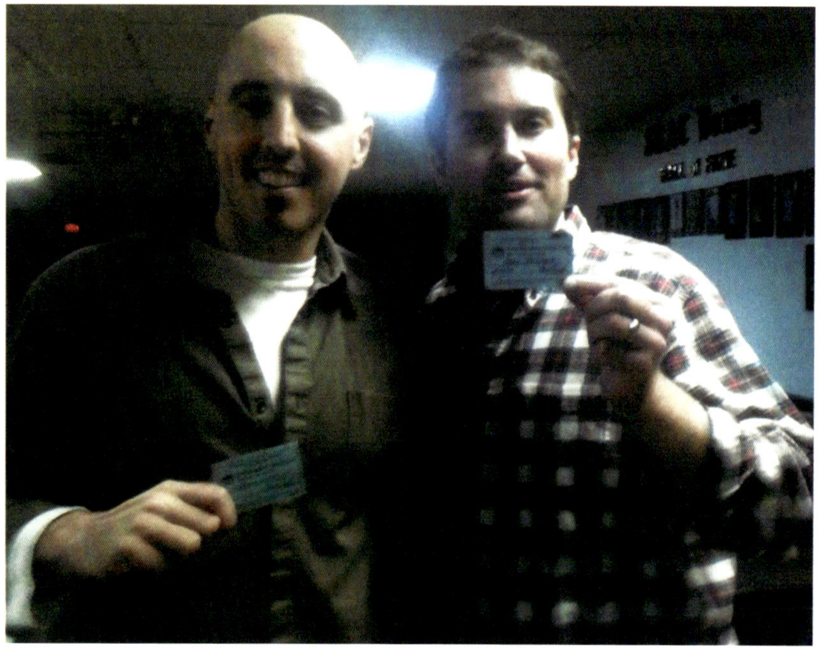

SBAC President Kevin Wilkins with Evan Bolesta on the night they joined the club in 2015

For many, the club has been a sanctuary, a place to escape the pressures of daily life and focus on self-improvement. The stories of our fighters, both in the ring and in life, reflect the perseverance that defines the SBAC.

Beyond boxing, the SBAC has always been a social hub, a place where friendships are formed and memories are made. From our numerous social events to our community outreach programs, the SBAC has been a constant source of support and connection for the Soulard neighborhood. It's a place where people come to celebrate life's moments, big and small, and where the bonds of friendship and family are strengthened.

Our commitment to the community has remained a cornerstone of the SBAC's mission. We have always believed in giving back, whether through youth programs, charitable events, or by simply providing a safe and welcoming environment for all. We are proud to have positively impacted the lives of so many individuals, offering a place for fellowship, growth, and personal development. Our community partnerships have also been instrumental in helping us achieve our goals, as local businesses, sponsors, and volunteers have generously supported our efforts over the years.

As we celebrate 125 years of history, we also look forward to the future. The world continues to change rapidly, and so must we. The challenges we face today are different from those faced by our founders, but the spirit of resilience and adaptability that has defined the SBAC for more than a century remains as strong as ever. Our commitment to fostering an inclusive, supportive environment is unwavering. We are continually seeking new ways to grow and evolve, ensuring that SBAC remains a vibrant and relevant part of the community for the next 125 years.

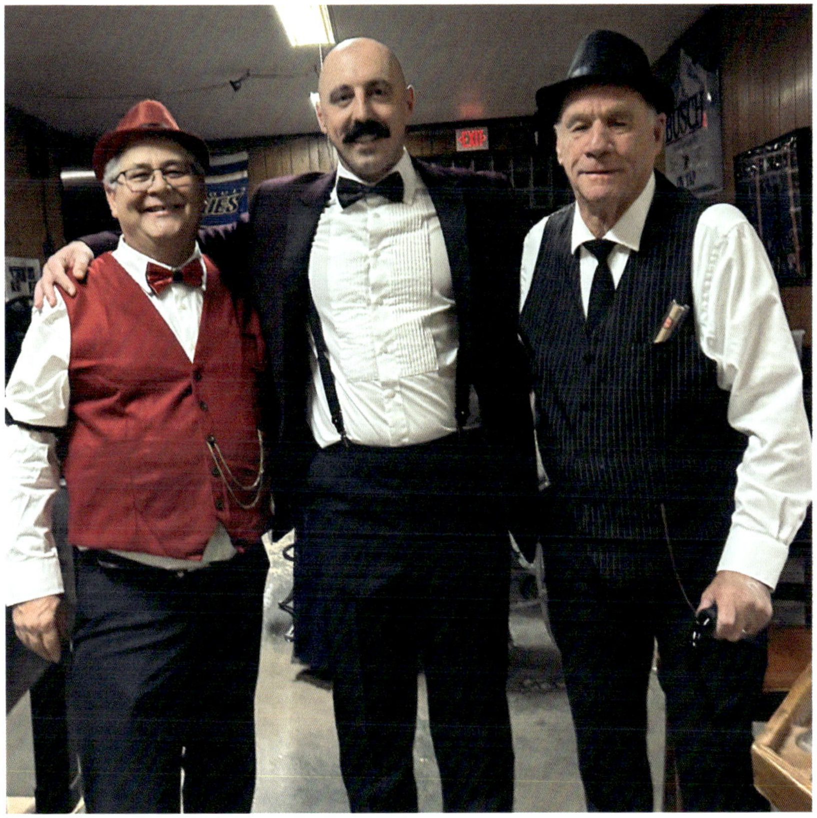

The three living presidents: Mike Button (left) Kevin Wilkins, and Al Bauman

This book serves as a tribute to everyone who has been a part of the SBAC's journey. It is a collection of memories, achievements, and stories that reflect the heart and soul of our organization. As you read through these pages, I hope you feel the same sense of pride and nostalgia that I do. The history of the SBAC is not just about the milestones we've achieved or the events we've hosted; it's about the people who have walked through our doors, the relationships that have been formed, and the lives that have been touched.

To our current members, thank you for your ongoing commitment and for carrying on the values that make the SBAC so special. To those members who have passed on before us, your legacy lives on in these pages and in every new member who finds community and connection within our organization.

As we reflect on our past and celebrate this significant anniversary, we also embrace the opportunities that lie ahead. The SBAC has withstood the test of time, not because of any one individual, but because of the collective effort of everyone who has been a part of this incredible journey. Through it all, the SBAC has remained steadfast, continuing to serve as a second home to generations of our members. Here's to 125 years of camaraderie, resilience, and community—and to many more to come.

With sincere gratitude and excitement for the future,

Kevin Wilkins
President of the South Broadway Athletic Club

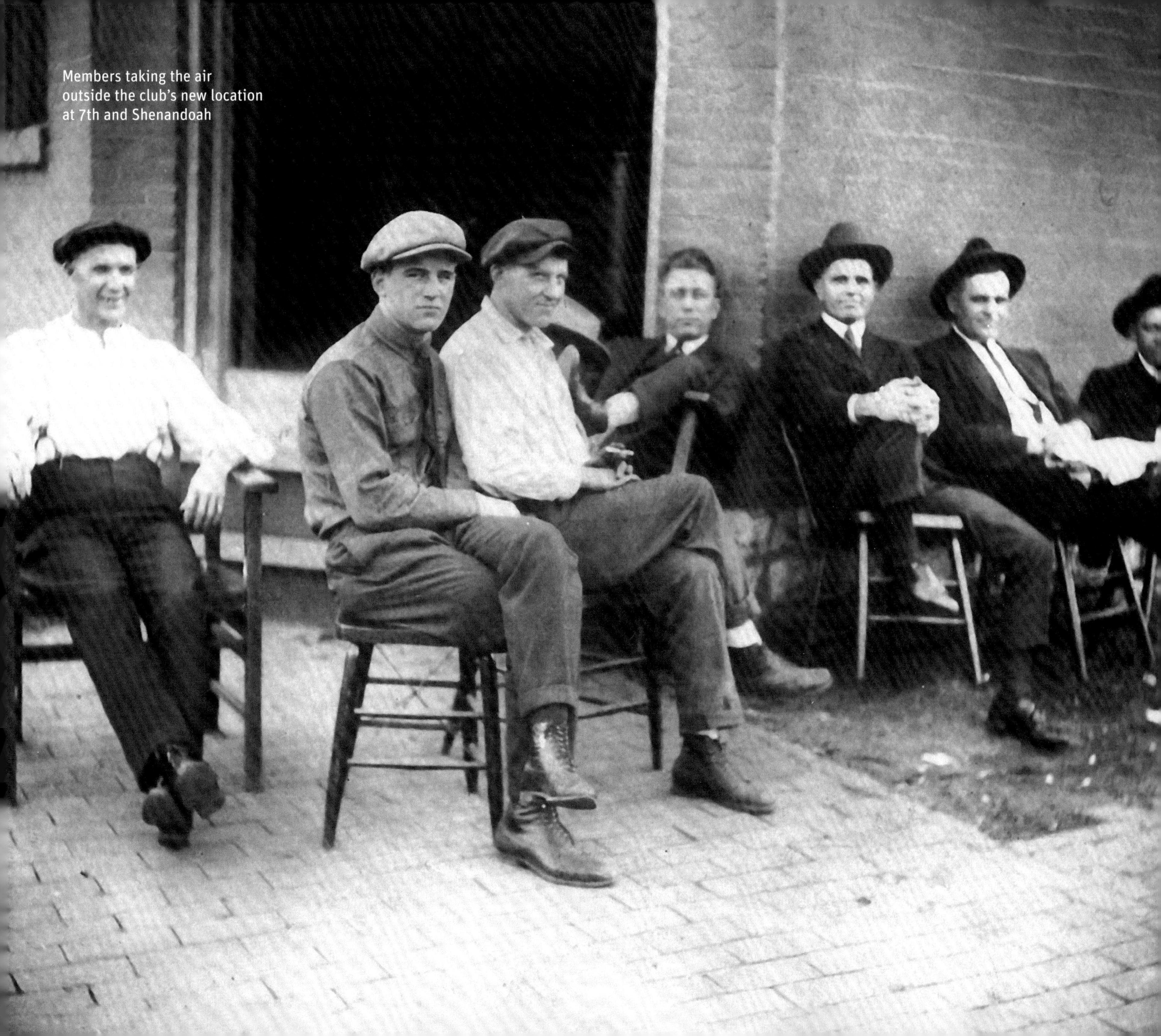

Members taking the air
outside the club's new location
at 7th and Shenandoah

Chapter 1

The Founding

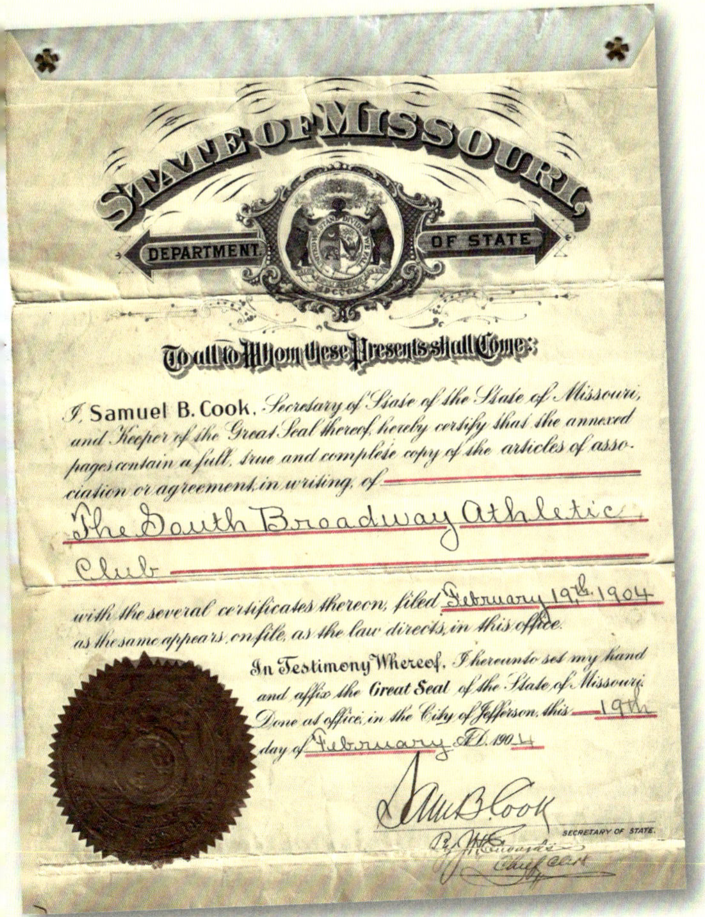
State of Missouri

Department of State

To all to Whom these Presents shall Come:

I, Samuel B. Cook, Secretary of State of the State of Missouri, and Keeper of the Great Seal thereof, hereby certify that the annexed pages contain a full, true and complete copy of the articles of association or agreement, in writing, of The South Broadway Athletic Club with the several certificates thereon, filed February 19th 1904 as the same appears on file, as the law directs, in this office.

In Testimony Whereof, I hereunto set my hand and affix the Great Seal of the State of Missouri. Done at office, in the City of Jefferson, this 19th day of February A.D. 1904

Sam B. Cook

Secretary of State.

State of Missouri articles of association officially recognizing the organization of the South Broadway Athletic Club (1904)

> "It shall be the object and purpose of this club to encourage debating, reading and the study of literature, to promote the science of physical culture by special systematic, athletic training. To develop and strengthen the young men of the community and advance the commercial interest and prosperity of the City by the mutual exchange of ideas and frequent associations."
>
> —South Broadway Athletic Club 1904 Charter

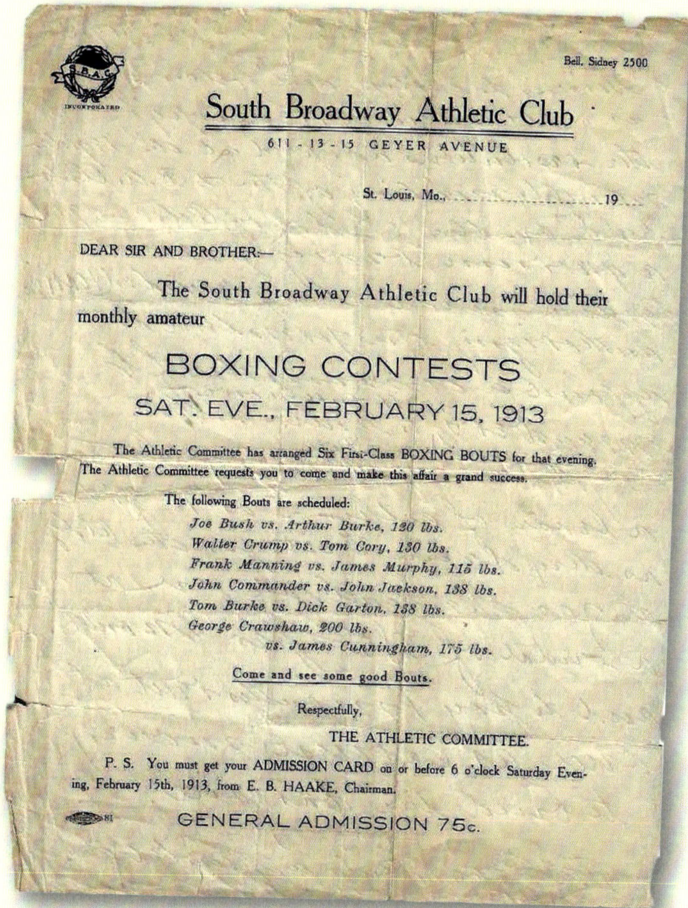
Bell, Sidney 2500

S.B.A.C. Incorporated

South Broadway Athletic Club

611-13-15 GEYER AVENUE

St. Louis, Mo., ...19....

DEAR SIR AND BROTHER:—

The South Broadway Athletic Club will hold their monthly amateur

BOXING CONTESTS

SAT. EVE., FEBRUARY 15, 1913

The Athletic Committee has arranged Six First-Class BOXING BOUTS for that evening. The Athletic Committee requests you to come and make this affair a grand success.

The following Bouts are scheduled:

Joe Bush vs. Arthur Burke, 120 lbs.
Walter Crump vs. Tom Cory, 130 lbs.
Frank Manning vs. James Murphy, 115 lbs.
John Commander vs. John Jackson, 138 lbs.
Tom Burke vs. Dick Garton, 138 lbs.
George Crawshaw, 200 lbs.
vs. James Cunningham, 175 lbs.

Come and see some good Bouts.

Respectfully,

THE ATHLETIC COMMITTEE.

P. S. You must get your ADMISSION CARD on or before 6 o'clock Saturday Evening, February 15th, 1913, from E. B. HAAKE, Chairman.

GENERAL ADMISSION 75c.

Flier from the 1913 slate of boxing matches with a 75-cent entrance fee

THE 1904 OLYMPICS

IT WAS 1904, the third Olympics of the modern era, and the five-year-old SBAC was there to wrestle.

As part of the World's Fair in St. Louis, the 1904 Olympics featured a new division: the Department of Physical Culture. The goal was to highlight the best athletes and the latest methods of physical fitness. It would be the first year that gold, silver, and bronze medals were awarded at the Olympics, and the SBAC would bring home some hardware.

To invite athletes to take part and to promote the upcoming competitions, the committee mailed around 250,000 entry forms to newspapers, athletic clubs, schools, international groups, YMCAs, military associations, and Turner groups. About 650 athletes competed in 95 events.

It wasn't just sports. The exhibition was intended to educate the public with lectures on the physiology of exercise and through exhibits

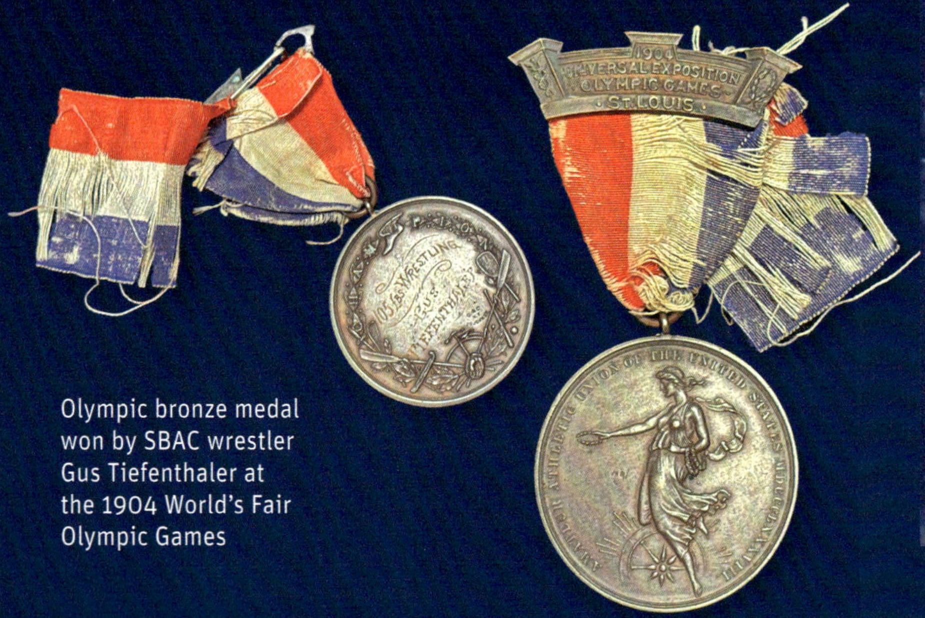

Olympic bronze medal won by SBAC wrestler Gus Tiefenthaler at the 1904 World's Fair Olympic Games

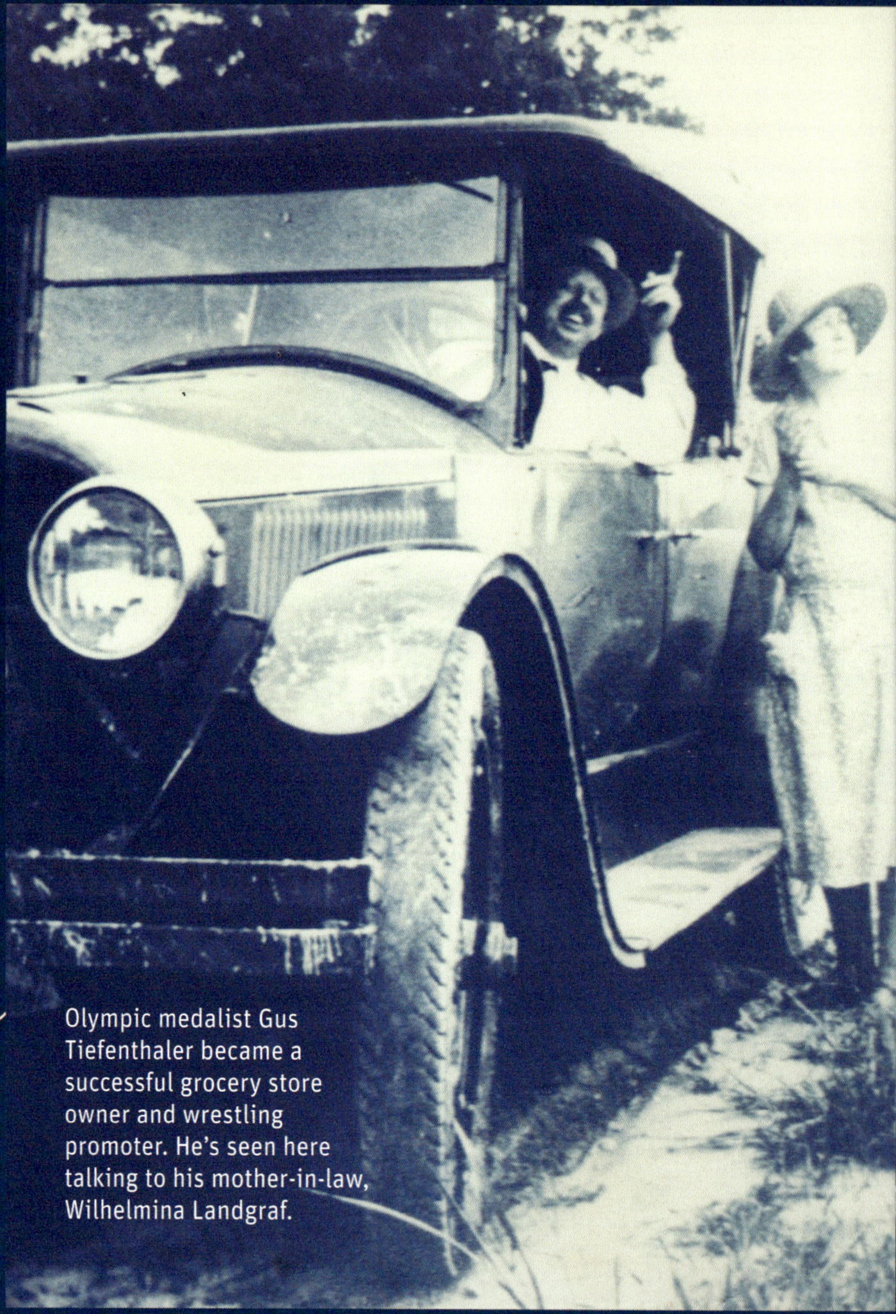

Olympic medalist Gus Tiefenthaler became a successful grocery store owner and wrestling promoter. He's seen here talking to his mother-in-law, Wilhelmina Landgraf.

including a fully equipped gym with the latest equipment and playground models for schools. There was also a display on orthopedic surgery and physical rehabilitation.

That year, the SBAC sent two men to compete in freestyle wrestling, Gustav Tiefenthaler and Louis Strebler, and each brought home a bronze medal. Tiefenthaler was 18 and a featherweight wrestler at 105 pounds. Strebler was a bantamweight at 125 pounds.

Wrestling was a popular event at the Olympics. "Freestyle wrestling caught people's attention," Gustav's grandson Randy Tiefenthaler said. "It was so dynamic."

Gus Tiefenthaler, who had emigrated from Switzerland as a child, became a businessman and wrestling promoter in St. Louis. He owned a group of grocery stores called Wisconsin Creamery Stores, and he became a prominent wrestling promoter, spending his time finding wrestlers and promoting matches. News stories from the era repeatedly mention Gus Tiefenthaler's latest show and wrestlers at Battery A or Sportsman's Park, and how he used some of his take to donate to the Olympics and to help athletes.

"I came into the wrestling promotion business with the flat declaration that I didn't care whether I made anything out of it or not, so long as I could get an even break," he told the *Post-Dispatch* in 1924. The Wisconsin Creamery Stores were lucrative until the Great Depression. He went bankrupt in 1933.

Louis Strebler became a furniture mover. He lost an arm in a streetcar accident after his foot got caught in the rail and the streetcar hit him. He carried on moving furniture using straps, and eventually opened his own company.

Louis was SBAC member Steve Strebler's distant cousin. "He shook my right hand with his left hand, and even though he was 80 years old, he had an extremely strong grip," Steve remembers.

Now, 120 years later, the stories of these men are still told in the hallowed halls of the SBAC.

—Miriam Moynihan

ON DECEMBER 5, 1899, five men met in South St. Louis and planted a firm stake in historic Soulard. They gathered to form a new club that has become a hub of sport, social activity, and community in the city. The South Broadway Athletic Club (SBAC) founders—Gus Holt, Herman Kempf, Ed Boehm, Joe Kern, and Frank Doran—met at the home of Gus Holt, who became the first president.

Folklore has it that our founding initially started as a debate club and naturally transitioned into a boxing and wrestling organization. The men launched into the club's mission right away, holding its first official boxing match, in which SBAC founder Herman "Kid" Kempf stopped Buddy Morgan of the Newsboy Home in two rounds.

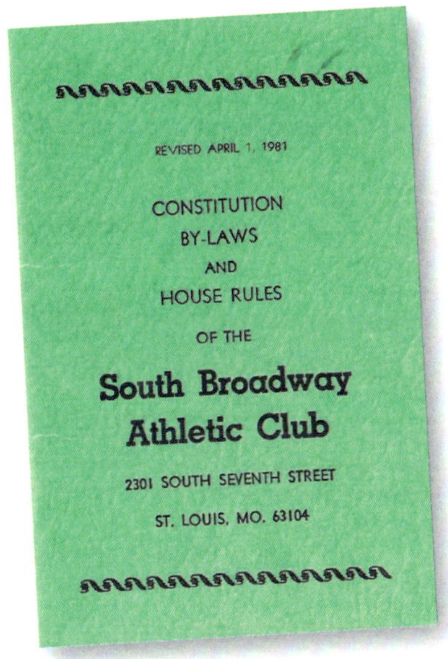

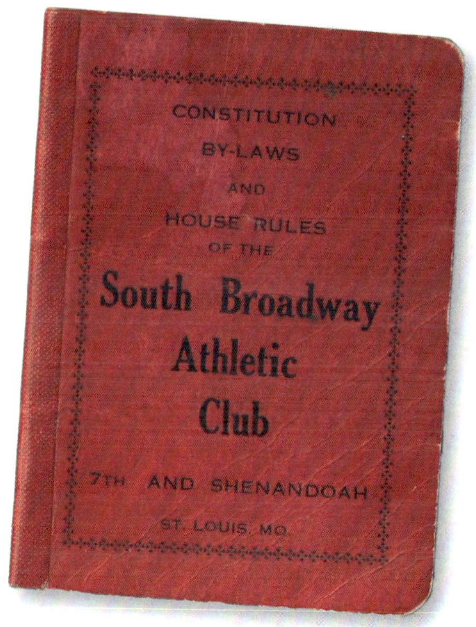

Early constitution, bylaws, and house rules

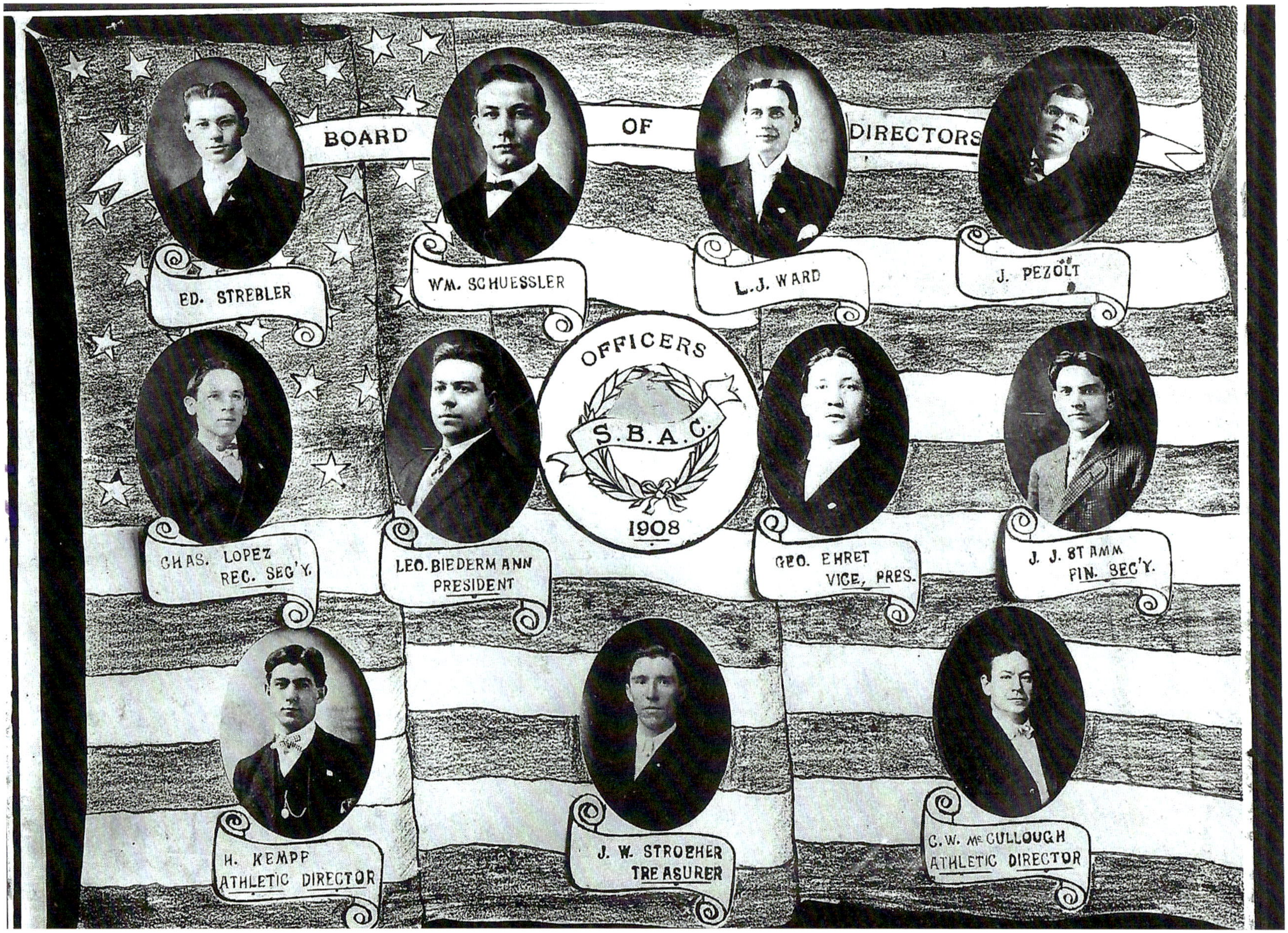

Portraits of the 11 SBAC officers in 1908. The officers were, from left to right, Edward Strebler, William Schuesller, L. J. Ward, J. Pezolt, Charles Lopez (recording secretary), Leo Bidermann (president), George Ehret (vice president), J. J. Stamm (financial secretary), H. Kempp (athletic director), J. W. Stroeher (treasurer), C. W. McCullough (athletic director).

In the generations since that first meeting, the club has grown and prospered. For years, it produced the city's best boxing talent and dominated local competitions. The SBAC sent freestyle wrestlers from its ranks to the 1904 Olympics, where two of its athletes brought home bronze medals.

The objectives for the club's founding—focused on "the development of physical culture" and "social activities"—have always been at its heart.

Five years after its founding—on February 14, 1904—the SBAC incorporated under Missouri laws. The club made 611 Geyer Avenue its first home, using only the first floor and basement. Four years later, the club took over the second floor.

As it continued to grow, the SBAC prospered enough to move to its present headquarters at 7th and Shenandoah in 1914. In 1923, SBAC members marked off another important milestone when they purchased the building.

The 1904 charter was set to last for 50 years. In 1954, a charter amendment was revised to state "that this association shall have perpetual existence."

By 1949, the club had grown to 400

M. A. C. BOXERS LOATH TO MEET S. BROADWAY BOYS

Boxing Team of the Big Club is in a Demoralized and Disorganized Condition and Objects to Facing South Side Athletes in Inter-Club Meeting.

There is an active revolution brewing in M. A. C. boxing circles because the governing board insists that the fistic representatives of the club shall meet the South Broadway Athletic Club, and it appears at the present time as if the board will have to recede from its action and ask for a postponement of the dual meet, which is scheduled for Dec. 23, or suffer the ignominy of seeing their boxers walloped by the husky Germans of the South Side.

The boxers are being backed in their attitude by the Athletic Committe, which feels that it is unjust to ask them to train and box on such short notice. The boxers did not like this hasty notice. On Tuesday the only member of the M. A. C. boxing squad who has answered the call of the Athletic Committee was Morris Snyder, the Post-Dispatch newsboy.

Gresham, who was to have met Herman Kempf in the 105 group, has not reported for work. Charley Stevens, the 125-pound champion, has retired from active participation in boxing events, and will not meet William Pausbach. O. L. Kirk is angry at the club members for what he claims was unjust criticism and discrimination evinced toward him in his last appearance at a tournament.

Joe Lydon is still nursing his hand, injured some time ago, and he will be unable to meet Gruppe.

Hussman, the M. A. C. 145-pound representative, has not been seen around the club for the past month. It is said that he feels roe because the club did not discipline Joe Lydon for the load incident. Hussman has forsaken the M. A. C. and will not be in the ring the night of Dec. 23 to meet Gruppe in the 145-pound class. John Sauter, who was recently suspended by the M. A. C., is anxious and willing to meet Senf.

A 1905 *St. Louis Post-Dispatch* article emphasizes the rivalry between the MAC and the SBAC.

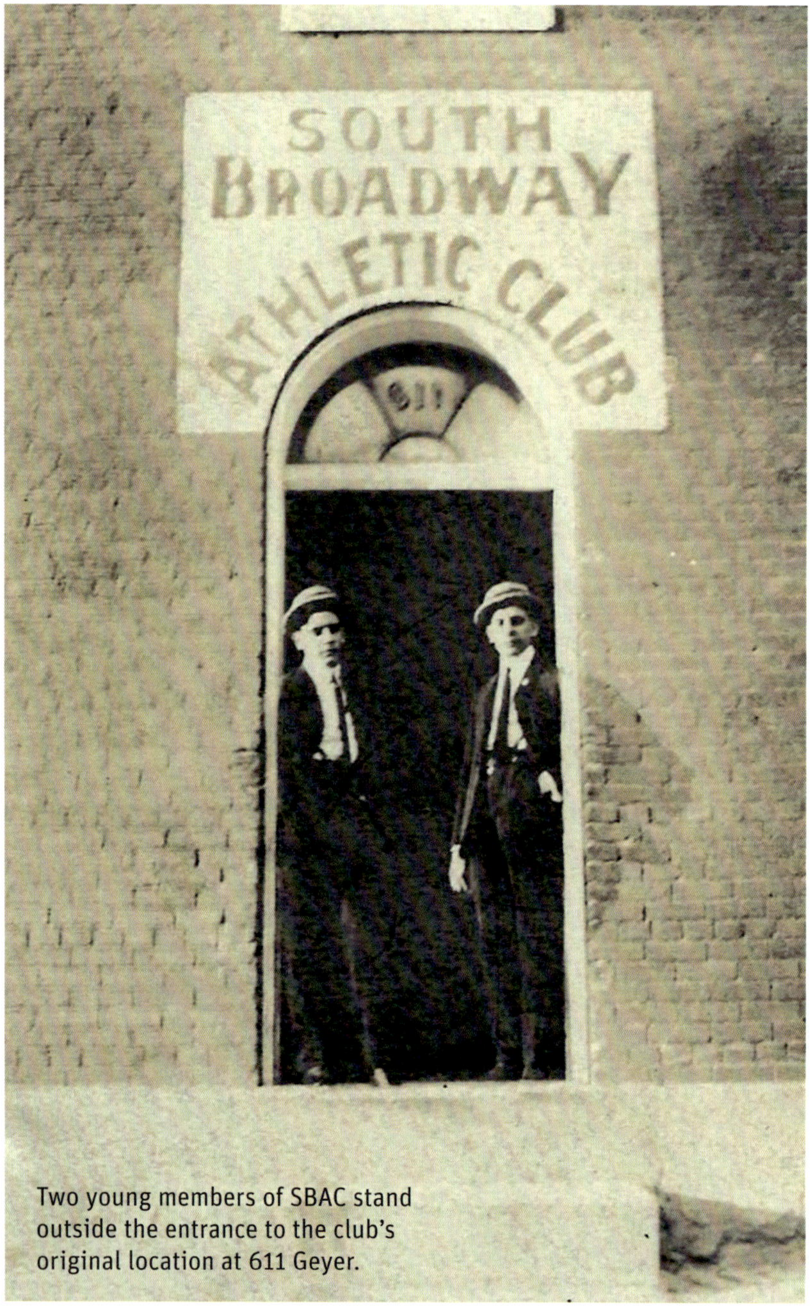

Two young members of SBAC stand outside the entrance to the club's original location at 611 Geyer.

members. It celebrated its golden jubilee with a gala and a "smoker"—a boxing program with drinks, camaraderie, and plenty of smoking. Media articles and notes of congratulation were glowing with praise for the club's accomplishments and boxing domination.

It was no accident, wrote *Globe-Democrat* sports editor Robert L. Burns, that the "blue-trunked boys" of the SBAC had won more Golden Gloves team titles than any other organization. He continued, "all the other coaches in the area have as their rallying cry 'Stop South Broadway!'

"Literally scores of such clubs flourished before World War I,

Historical Note

Our First Home

The first location of SBAC was a two-story brick building at 611 Geyer, a stone's throw from South Broadway. At first the club used only the first floor and basement, then expanded to the upper floor. The basement was used for refreshments, lockers, and baths. The gymnasium was on the main floor. The top floor had a boxing arena and hosted sporting competitions and social entertainments.

By its 10th anniversary in 1909, the club had grown into a mecca for pugilists and other athletes. The roster of SBAC included 42 boxers, 6 wrestlers, "15 or 16 minor league ball tossers" who wintered in St. Louis, 5 swimmers, 9 teams of handball players, and a few track athletes.

(*St. Louis Post-Dispatch*, December 5, 1909, p. 1S)

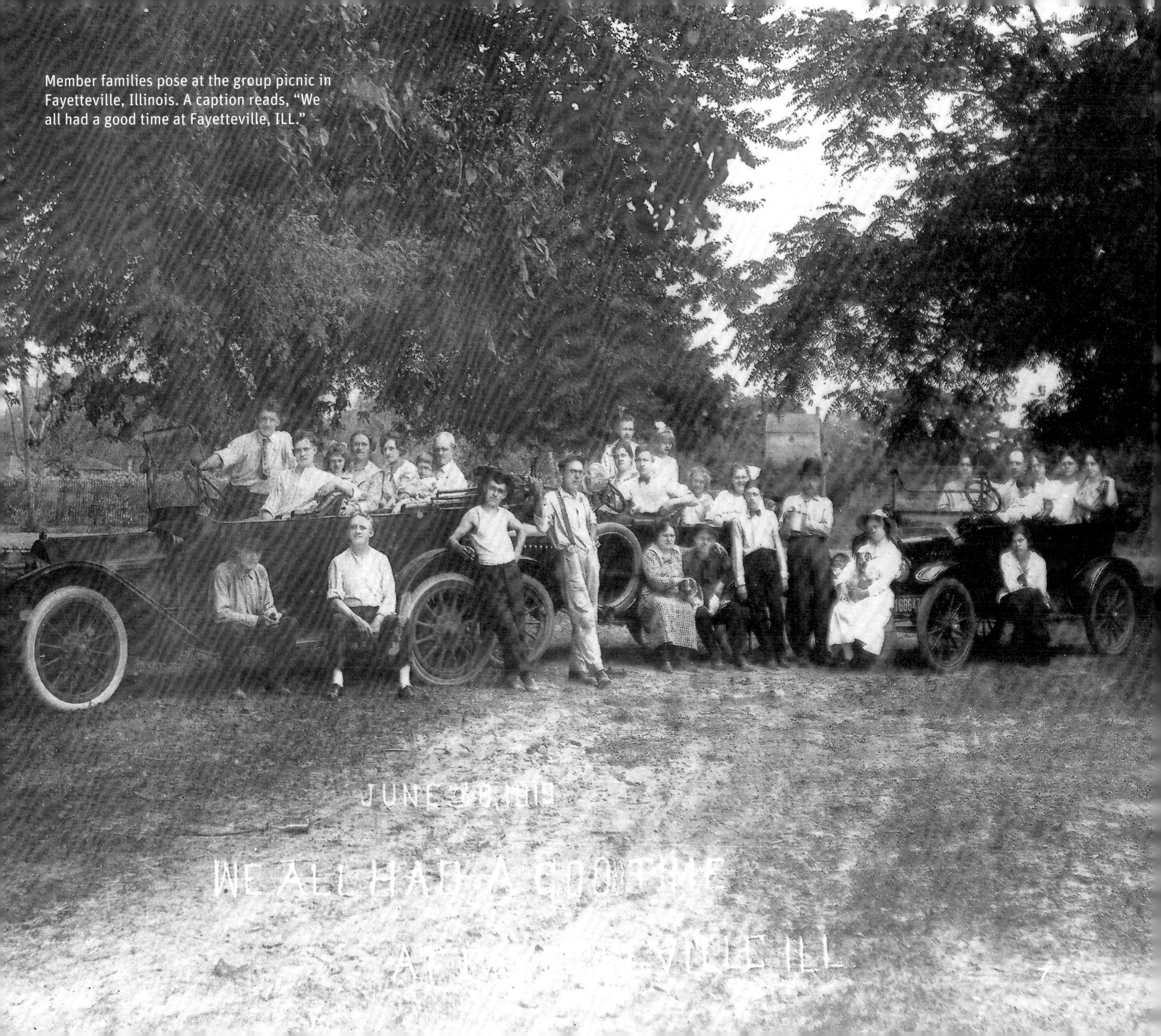

Member families pose at the group picnic in Fayetteville, Illinois. A caption reads, "We all had a good time at Fayetteville, ILL."

MORE THAN BRICKS

IN 1914, the SBAC decided to move from its first home at 611 Geyer to its new and current home, on the corner of 7th and Shenandoah. The history of that land goes back a long time. At the city's founding, the plot of land that would eventually become the club's new headquarters was part of La Petite Prairie, a swath of grassland that ran from modern-day Russell to Arsenal.

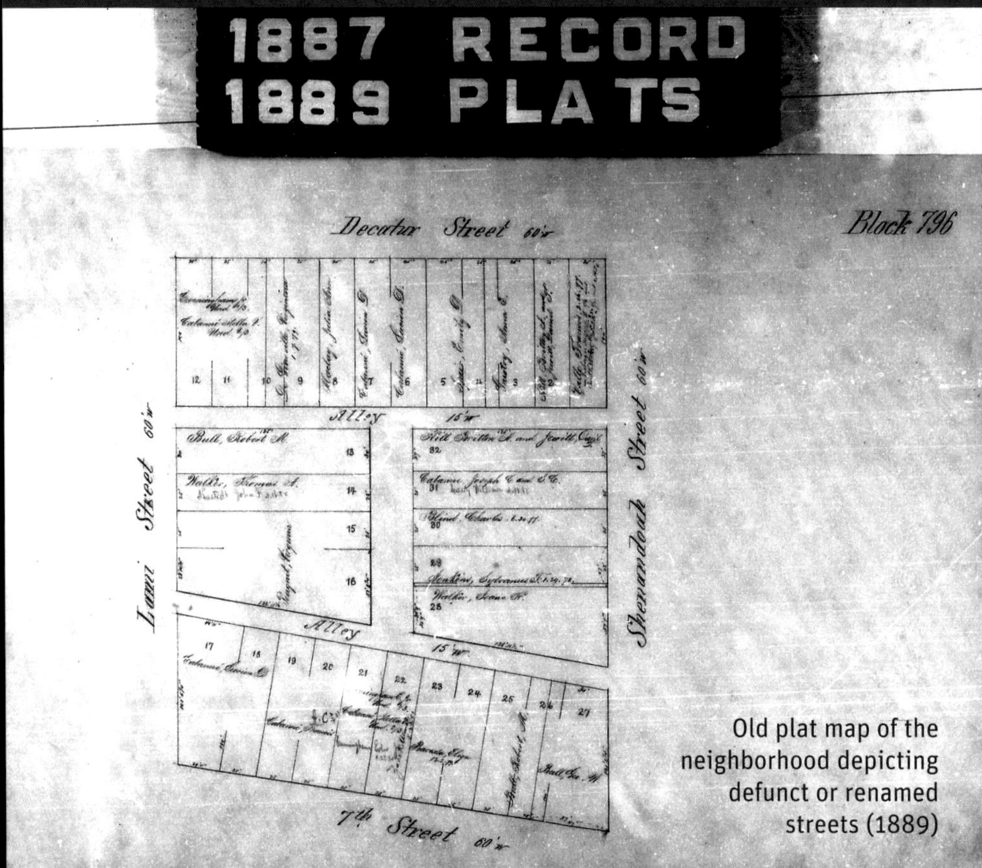

Old plat map of the neighborhood depicting defunct or renamed streets (1889)

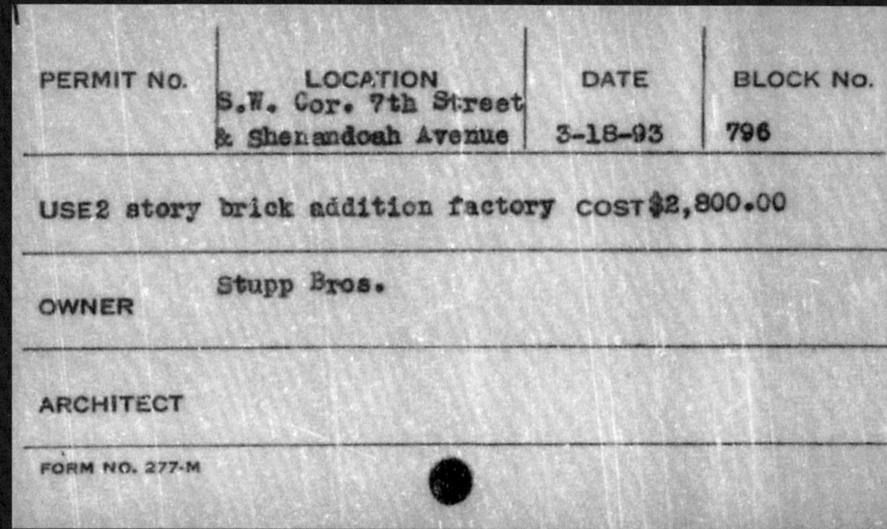

PERMIT NO.	LOCATION	DATE	BLOCK No.
	S.W. Cor. 7th Street & Shenandoah Avenue	3-18-93	796

USE 2 story brick addition factory COST $2,800.00

OWNER Stupp Bros.

ARCHITECT

FORM NO. 277-M

An 1893 permit to add an addition to the club's current location at 7th and Shenandoah by its original occupants, the Stupp Bros., who were in the iron works business

As the city grew, the land was acquired by Jean Pierre Cabanne and Julia Gratiot. Cabanne was a fur trader who split time between his trading post in Nebraska and his country home in what is now Forest Park. Beginning with the wave of German immigration in the late 1840s, Soulard started to be built up. Eventually the block on 7th between Shenandoah and Ann was bought by the Stupp Brothers Bridge and Iron Company.

Johann Stupp began his career assisting James Eads in constructing ironclads during the Civil War. In 1890 he formed a partnership with his brother Peter, a machinist. They shifted their enterprise to bridge-making to take advantage of the boom in railroad construction, and they moved their operations to their newly constructed building on 7th Street.

While structural brick dominated South St. Louis, the new building was a unique structure for the time, using steel trusses to create a large open space. The steel was supplied by Carnegie Steel, which had facilities on the east side of the river and was heavily involved in the bridge building trade, including supplying the steel for Eads Bridge, which opened in 1874.

The company expanded rapidly, and by the 1900s it had offices in Kansas and Iowa. It soon grew too large for its facility on 7th and vacated the building. The building was subdivided, with part rented out to the Western Mineral Water Company and the other to the Third Tabernacle Baptist Church. Neither of these enterprises lasted long, and in 1914 SBAC moved into the property, which it has occupied ever since. Additions were made periodically, and the two-story building's space is now 99 feet by 175 feet.

While the board entertained the notion of moving the club in the 1960s, the motion was rejected in favor of investing and modernizing the building, doubling down on the club's commitment to the neighborhood at a time when many groups were leaving the city.

—Mitchell Goist

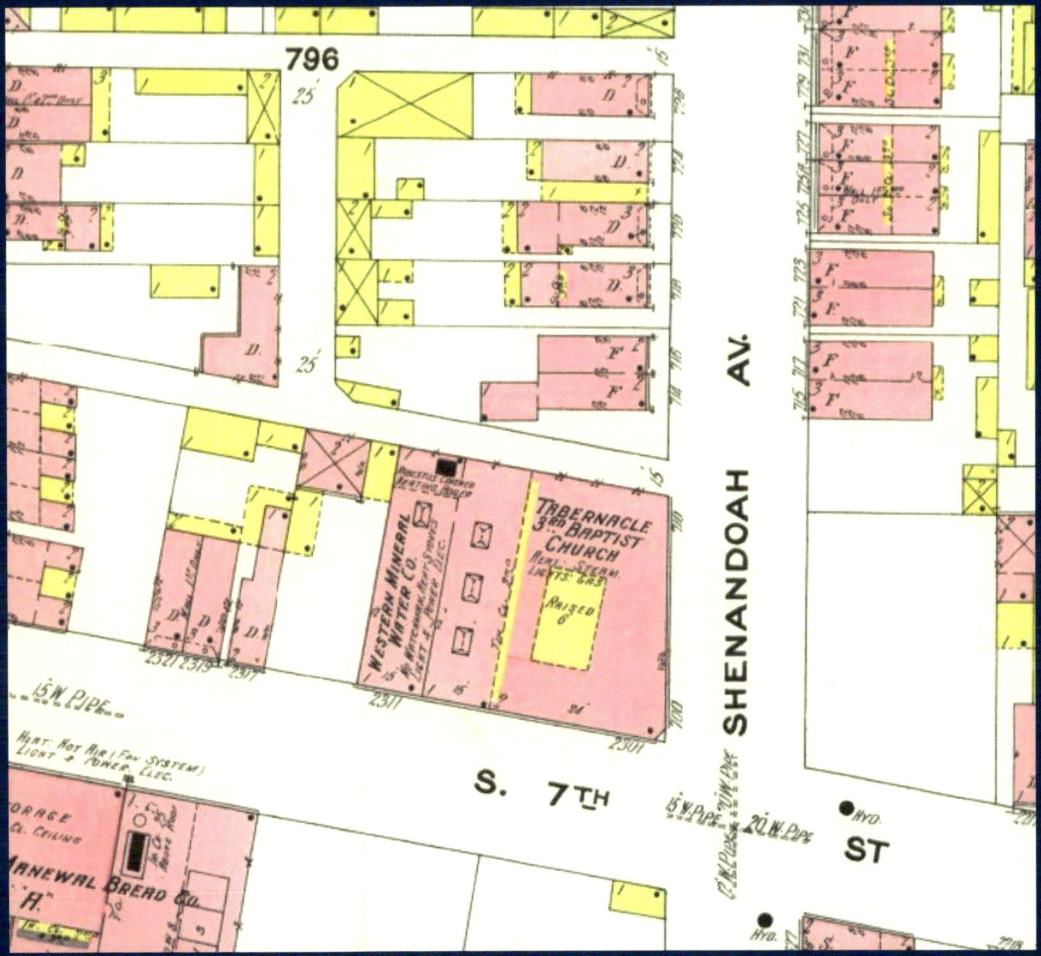

1909 Sanborn Fire Insurance Map showing the current South Broadway Athletic Club occupied by the 3rd Tabernacle Baptist Church, with the Western Mineral Water Company directly to the south

1896 Whipple Fire Insurance Map showing the Russell Avenue Mission in the building currently occupied by the South Broadway Athletic Club, attached to a bottling plant

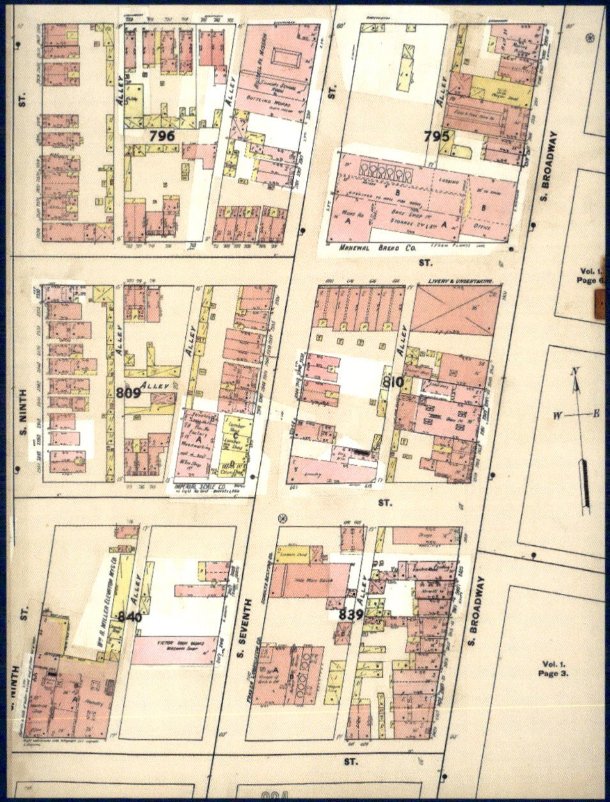

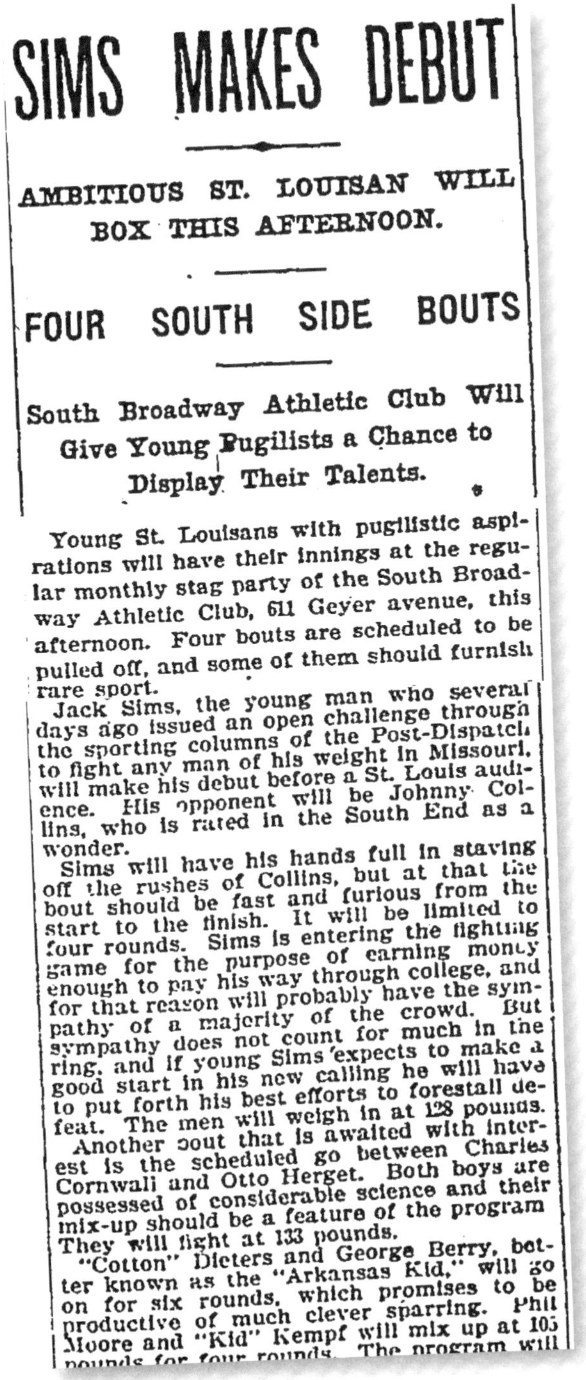

SIMS MAKES DEBUT

AMBITIOUS ST. LOUISAN WILL BOX THIS AFTERNOON.

FOUR SOUTH SIDE BOUTS

South Broadway Athletic Club Will Give Young Pugilists a Chance to Display Their Talents.

Young St. Louisans with pugilistic aspirations will have their innings at the regular monthly stag party of the South Broadway Athletic Club, 611 Geyer avenue, this afternoon. Four bouts are scheduled to be pulled off, and some of them should furnish rare sport.

Jack Sims, the young man who several days ago issued an open challenge through the sporting columns of the Post-Dispatch to fight any man of his weight in Missouri, will make his debut before a St. Louis audience. His opponent will be Johnny Collins, who is rated in the South End as a wonder.

Sims will have his hands full in staving off the rushes of Collins, but at that the bout should be fast and furious from the start to the finish. It will be limited to four rounds. Sims is entering the fighting game for the purpose of earning money enough to pay his way through college, and for that reason will probably have the sympathy of a majority of the crowd. But sympathy does not count for much in the ring, and if young Sims expects to make a good start in his new calling he will have to put forth his best efforts to forestall defeat. The men will weigh in at 128 pounds.

Another bout that is awaited with interest is the scheduled go between Charles Cornwall and Otto Herget. Both boys are possessed of considerable science and their mix-up should be a feature of the program. They will fight at 133 pounds.

"Cotton" Dieters and George Berry, better known as the "Arkansas Kid," will go on for six rounds, which promises to be productive of much clever sparring. Phil Moore and "Kid" Kempf will mix up at 105 pounds for four rounds. The program will

St. Louis Post-Dispatch article from December 2, 1900, describes an afternoon "stag party" of boxing.

but changing times have resulted in the disappearance of most of them . . . The South Broadway club today is the only important active member of that group," Ed Wray wrote in the *St. Louis Post-Dispatch* about the jubilee. "It isn't an overstatement to say that today the SBAC and its fine staff of coaches is still a most potent factor in developing boxers in this area."

In the decades since, there have been good years—and some difficult ones. And the South Broadway Athletic Club is still here—older than the Missouri Athletic Club and the IRS, and accessible to regular St. Louisans.

"There is no doubt that the South Broadway is rich with tradition," wrote *St. Louis Star-Times* sports editor Sid Keener in 1949. "To its club members and friends, the little brick building on the South Side was more important than any huge multi-million-dollar palace of its era."

—Miriam Moynihan

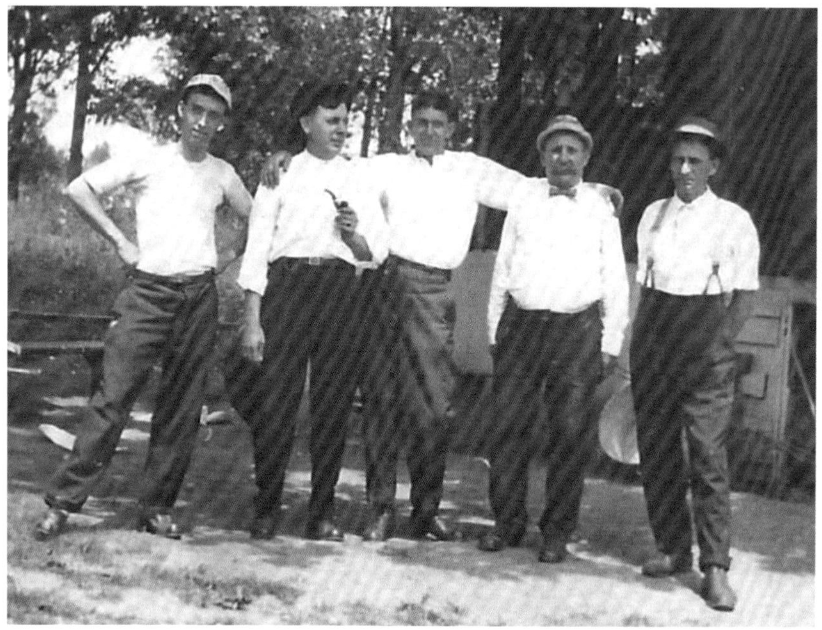

A photo from the collection of Edward Messmer, an early member and leader of the SBAC

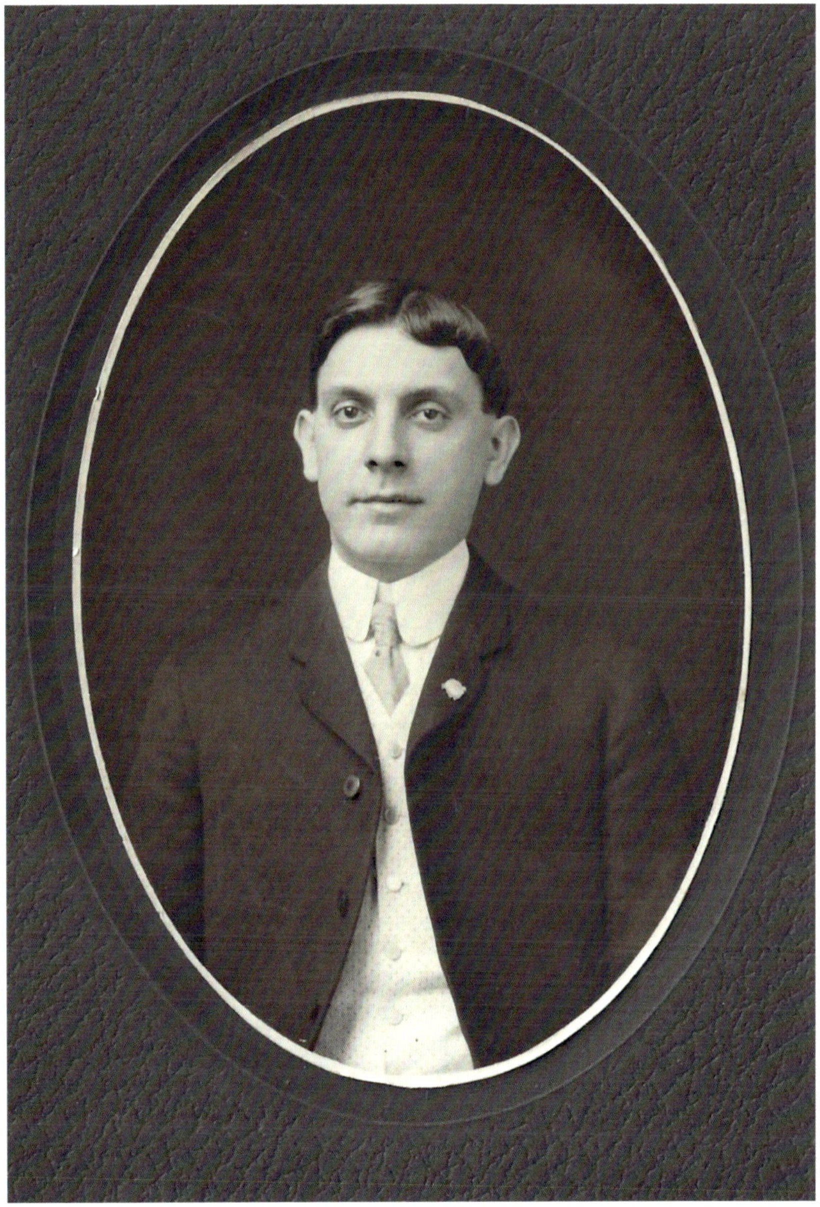

A professional photo of one of the SBAC founders, Edward Messmer, taken by Meier St. Louis at 1406 South Broadway

Historical Note

Husky Germans

The headline read, "MAC Boxers Loath to meet S. Broadway Boys" in the *Post-Dispatch* sports section on December 12, 1905. "There is an active revolution brewing in M.A.C. Boxing circles because the governing board insists that the fistic representatives of the club shall meet the South Broadway Athletic Club, and it appears at the present time as if the board will have to recede from its action and ask for a postponement of the dual meet . . . or suffer the ignominy of seeing their boxers walloped by the husky Germans of the South Side."

(*St. Louis Post-Dispatch*, December 12, 1905, p. 14)

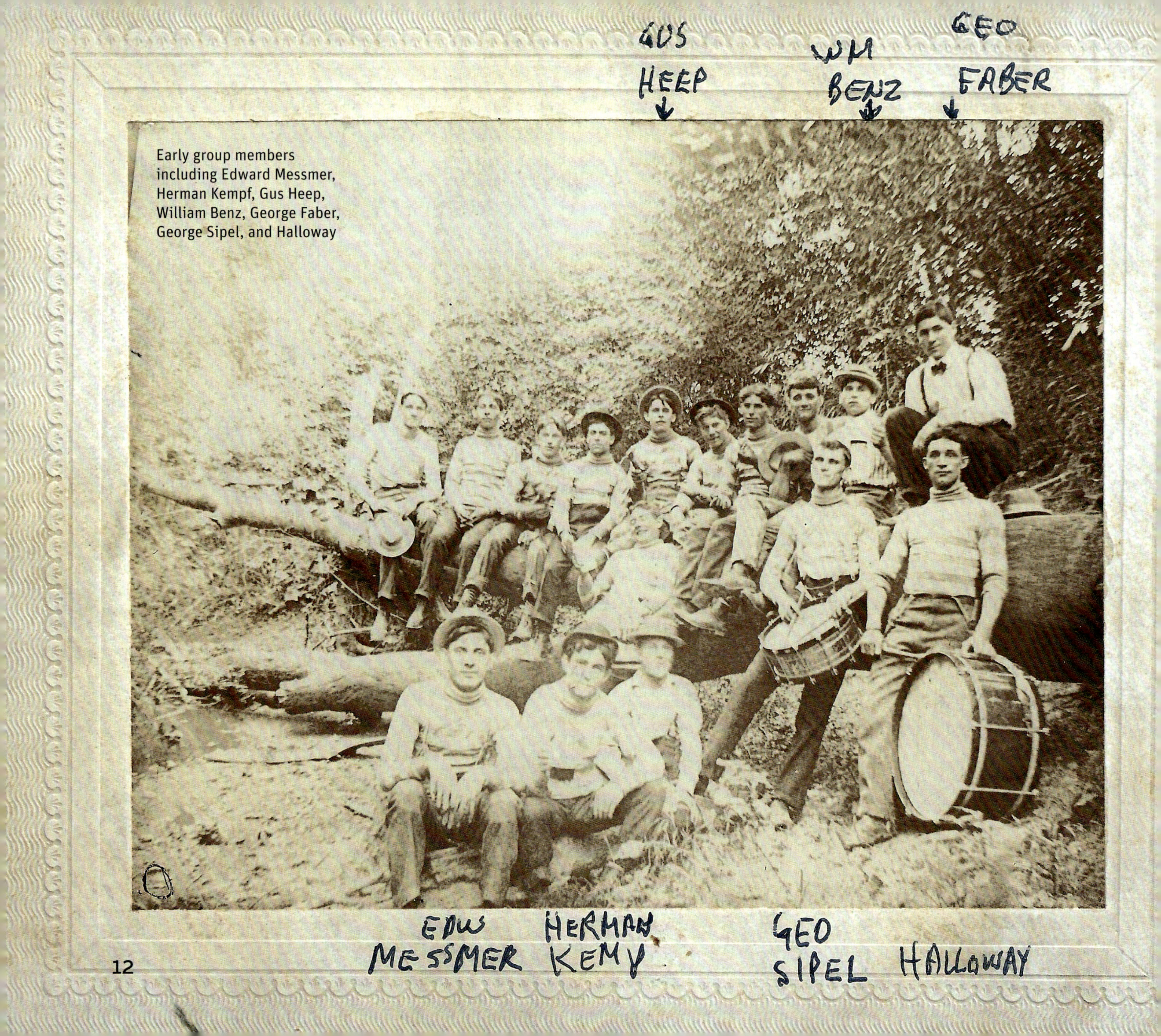

Early group members including Edward Messmer, Herman Kempf, Gus Heep, William Benz, George Faber, George Sipel, and Halloway

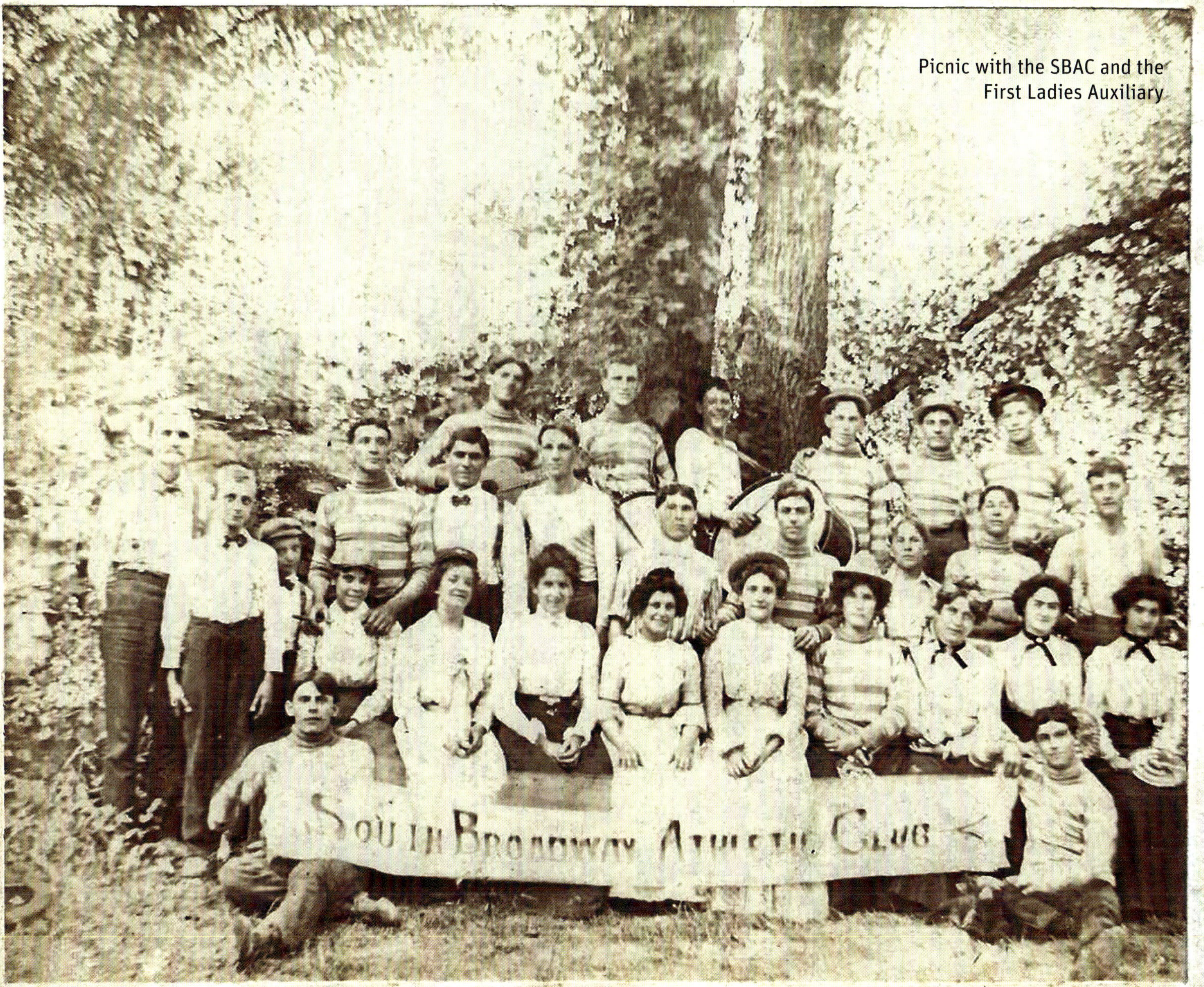

Picnic with the SBAC and the First Ladies Auxiliary

A young SBAC boxer stands tall after dropping his rival.

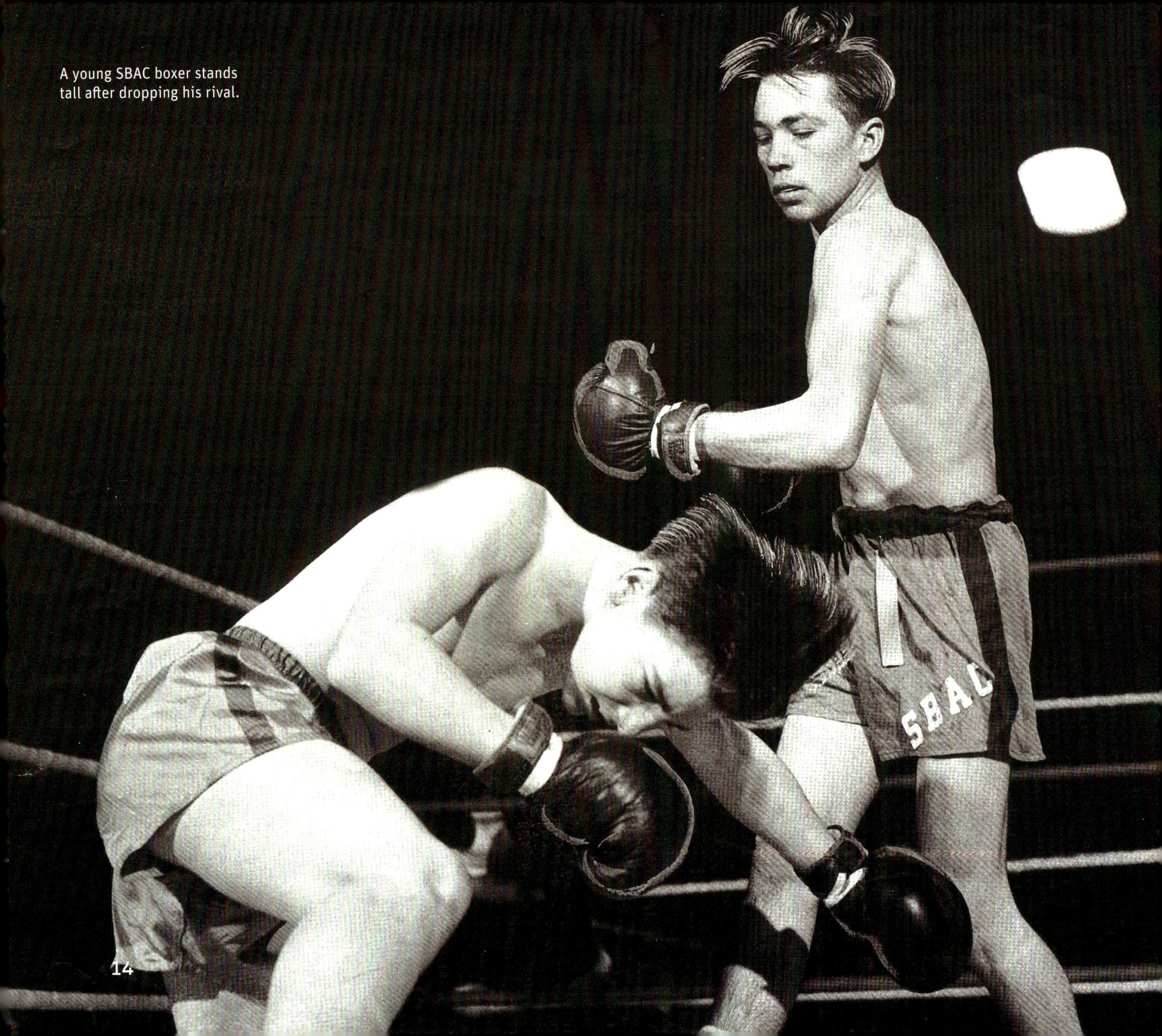

Chapter 2

An Athletic Club

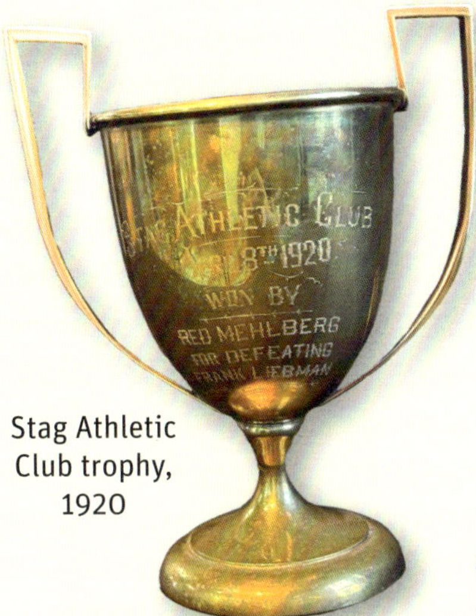

Stag Athletic Club trophy, 1920

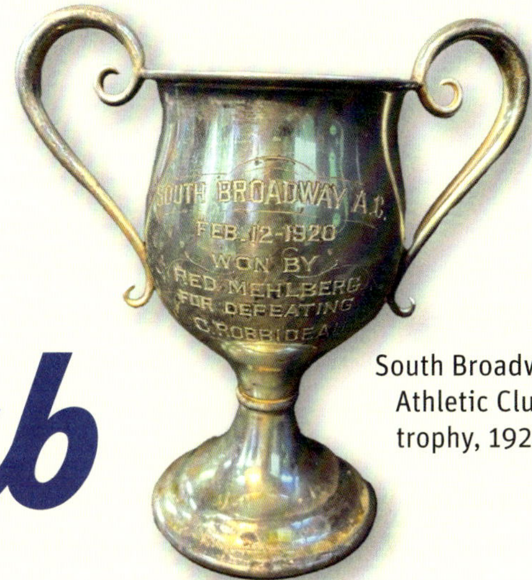

South Broadway Athletic Club trophy, 1920

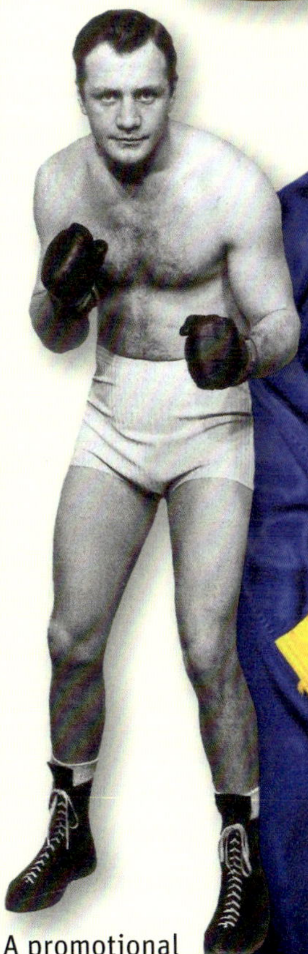
A promotional photo of heavyweight contender Mike Buha

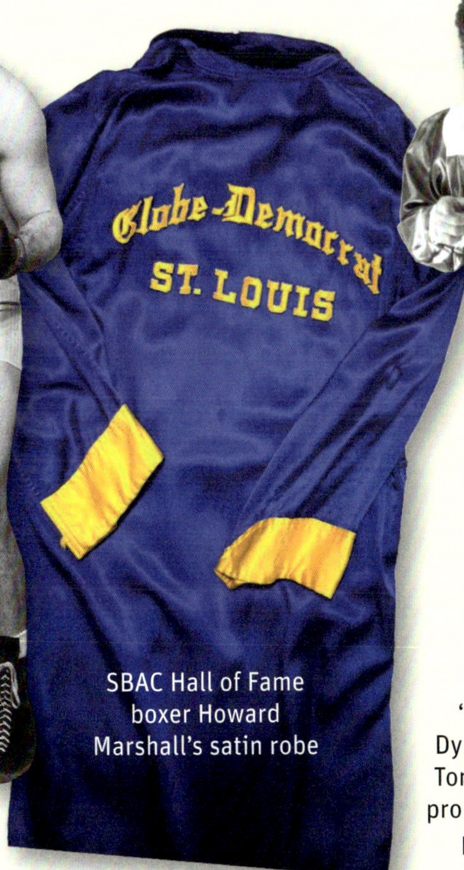

SBAC Hall of Fame boxer Howard Marshall's satin robe

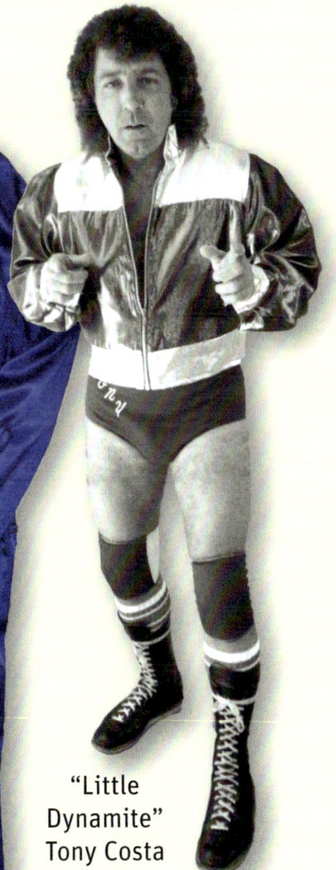
"Little Dynamite" Tony Costa promotional photo

IT'S SAID that there's a bar or church on every corner in South St. Louis, and when the familiar sounds of church bells ring, the faithful gather. At the SBAC, loyal adherents gather to the sound of a different bell: the ringside bell.

Boxing and wrestling are written into the 125-year-old club's founding documents, and they're still the cornerstones that have structured the club as much as the red bricks with which it was built.

By the 1890s, with the introduction of timed rounds and boxing gloves, organized boxing and wrestling were rapidly gaining popularity across the country, particularly with immigrant groups. As boxing gyms sprang up around St. Louis, every neighborhood had its hero.

The SBAC joined this tradition enthusiastically; a December 1900 *St. Louis Post-Dispatch* story described the club's monthly "stag parties" as occasions when young men could display talents at both sports. In the early 1900s, the SBAC developed a reputation

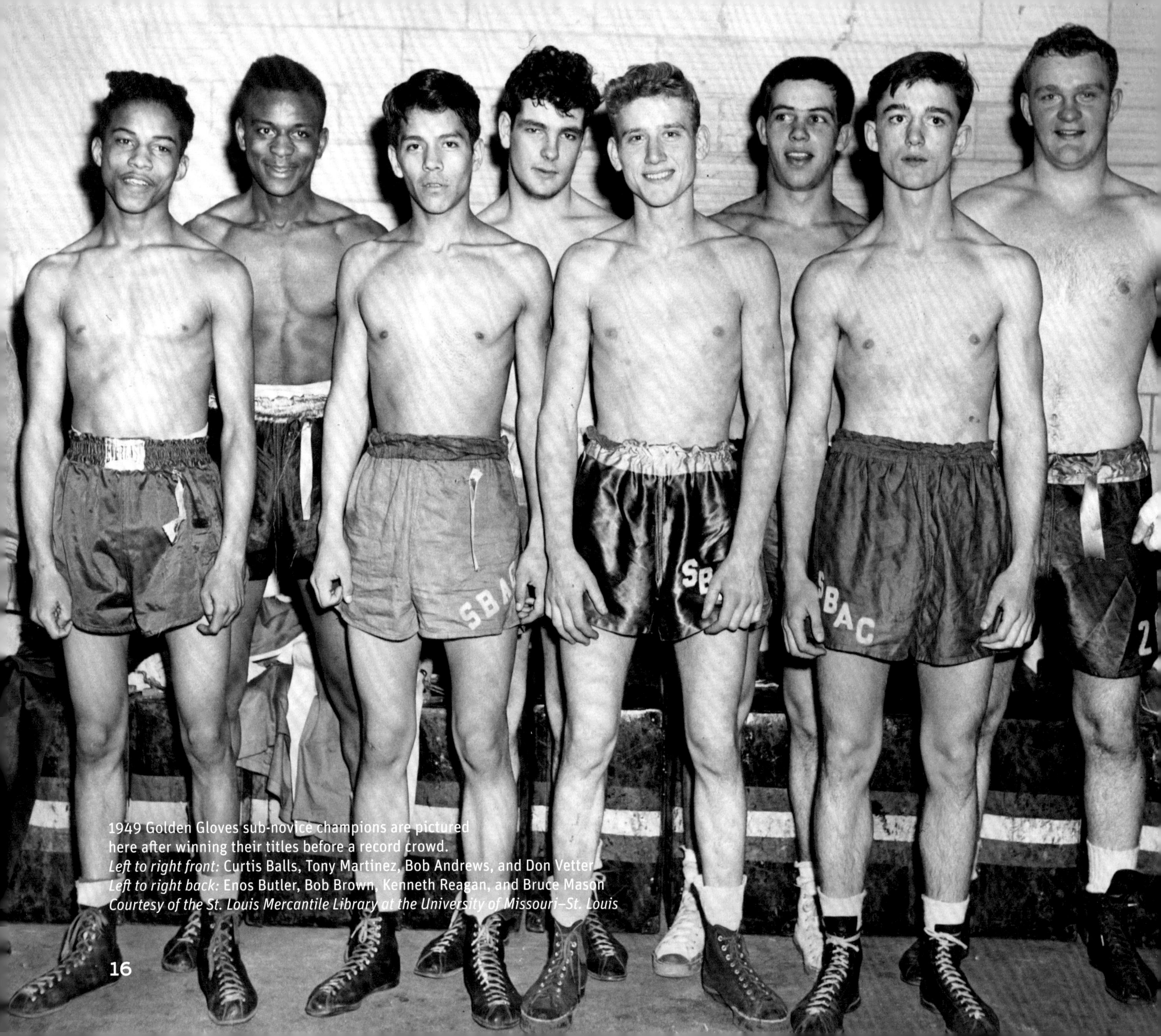

1949 Golden Gloves sub-novice champions are pictured here after winning their titles before a record crowd.
Left to right front: Curtis Balls, Tony Martinez, Bob Andrews, and Don Vetter
Left to right back: Enos Butler, Bob Brown, Kenneth Reagan, and Bruce Mason
Courtesy of the St. Louis Mercantile Library at the University of Missouri–St. Louis

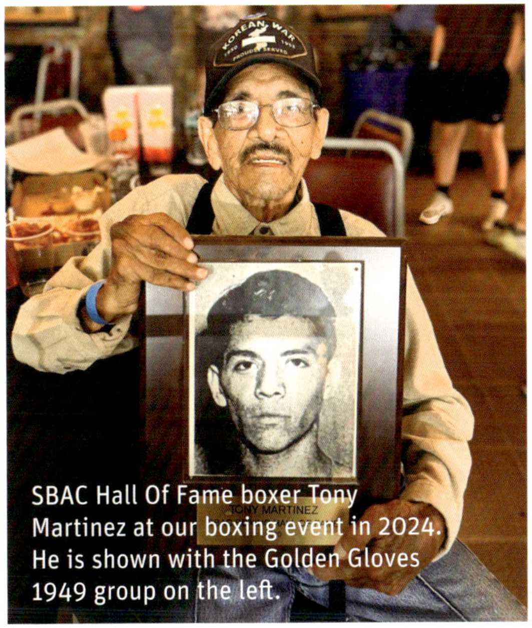

SBAC Hall Of Fame boxer Tony Martinez at our boxing event in 2024. He is shown with the Golden Gloves 1949 group on the left.

for producing fierce fighters at all weight classes. First battling against fighters from other local clubs, then fighting their way out of St. Louis, Billy Grupp, George Kirkwood, and Fred Gillmaster brought the SBAC early fame with their out-of-town victories. In the early 1920s the club sent Johnny (Peewee) Kaiser to Madison Square Garden, where he was beaten by Irish Johnny Curtain.

Into the 1940s and '50s, boxers became coaches, sharing their wisdom with the

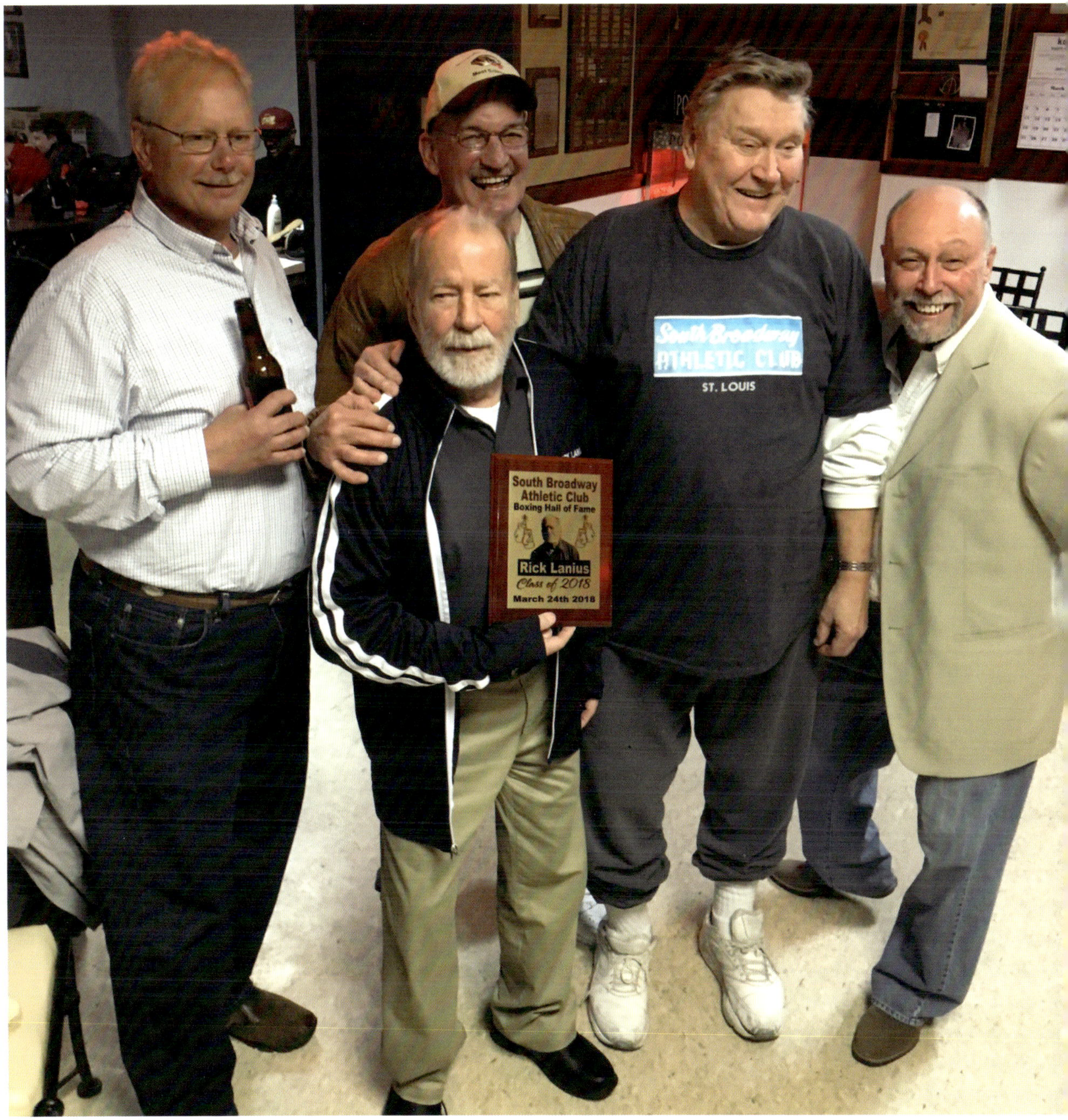

Rick Lanius holding his Boxing Hall of Fame placard with friends Craig Neumeister (left), Al Dobernic, "Cadillac" Rich Brady, and Rex Bridges.

next generation. Two legendary coaches were Joe Herbst and Joe Weber. As they began training young fighters, the *St. Louis Globe Democrat* began its Golden Gloves amateur boxing tournament, which the SBAC dominated throughout the 1940s. In March 1946, the SBAC once again sent fighters to Madison Square Garden, with Eddie Dames and Mike Buha winning Golden Gloves National Championships. "What the Yanks are to baseball, South Broadway A.C. is to the Golden Gloves," the *Globe-Democrat* wrote in 1953.

The 1960s saw boxing fade at the club. Cultural shifts and changing demographics saw "The Sweet Science" of boxing exit the ring. Though it hasn't made a return to those glory days, those whose lives it touched found a way to bring it back to center ring. In 1990, the club purchased the Stag Athletic Club gym, set up rings and equipment, and once again began training fighters. The gym was popular and packed every night. George Foreman made a commercial there, and Polish Olympic bronze medalist Andrew Golota trained there.

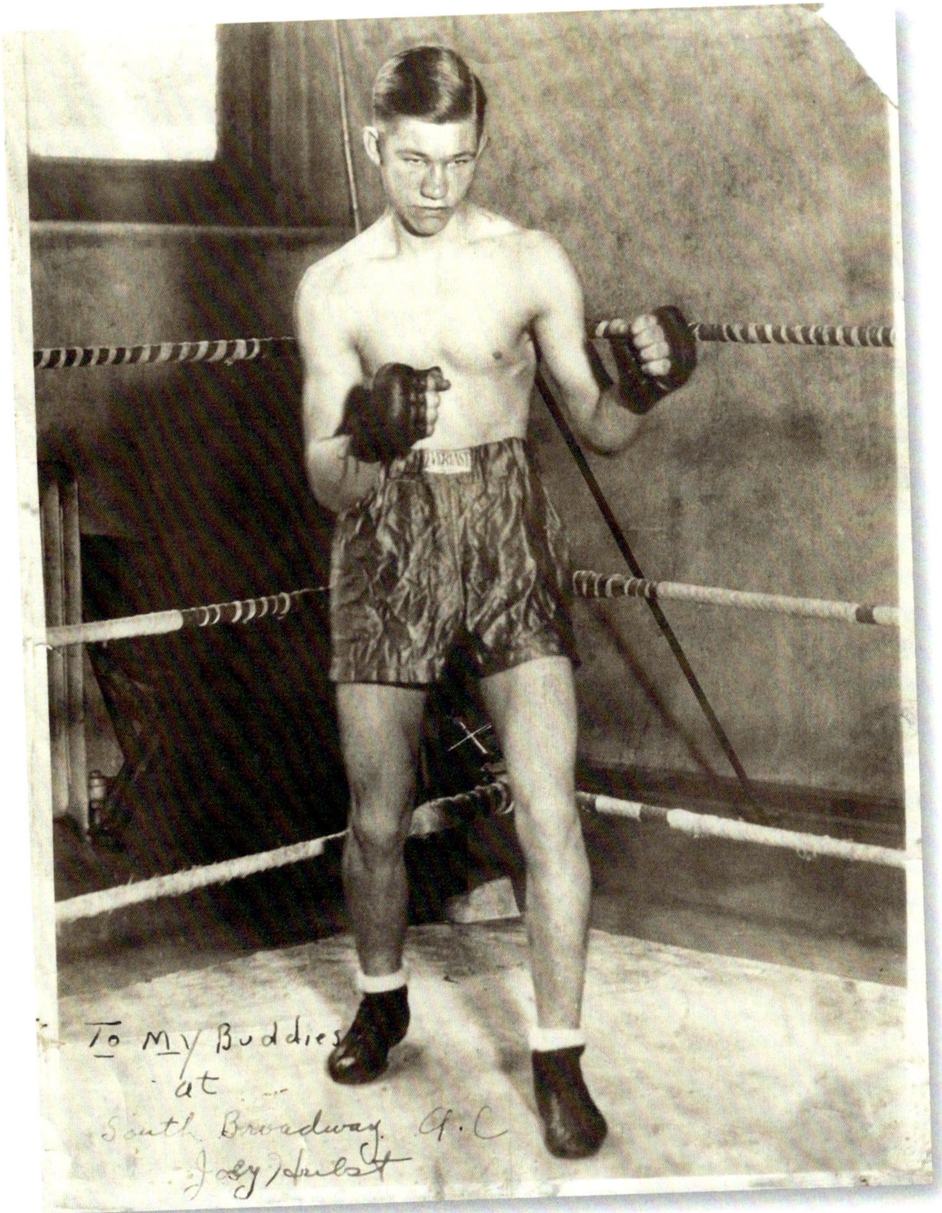

SBAC boxer and former president Joe Herbst in the ring. He wrote on the photo: "To my buddies at South Broadway A.C.—Joey Herbst."

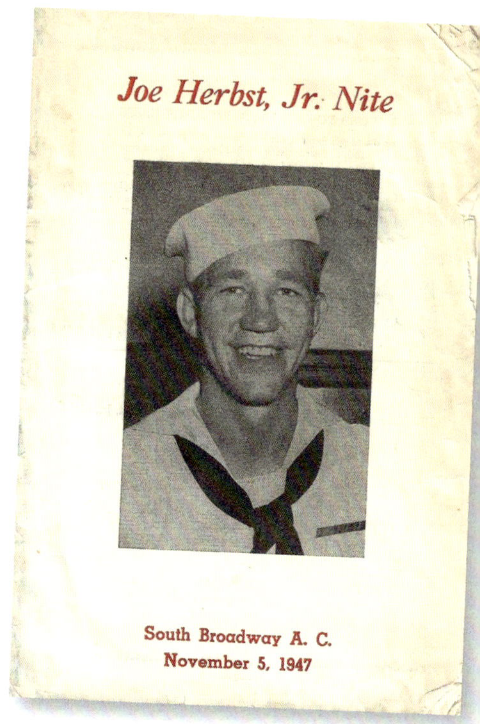

Joe Herbst Jr. Nite was a celebrated event at the SBAC.

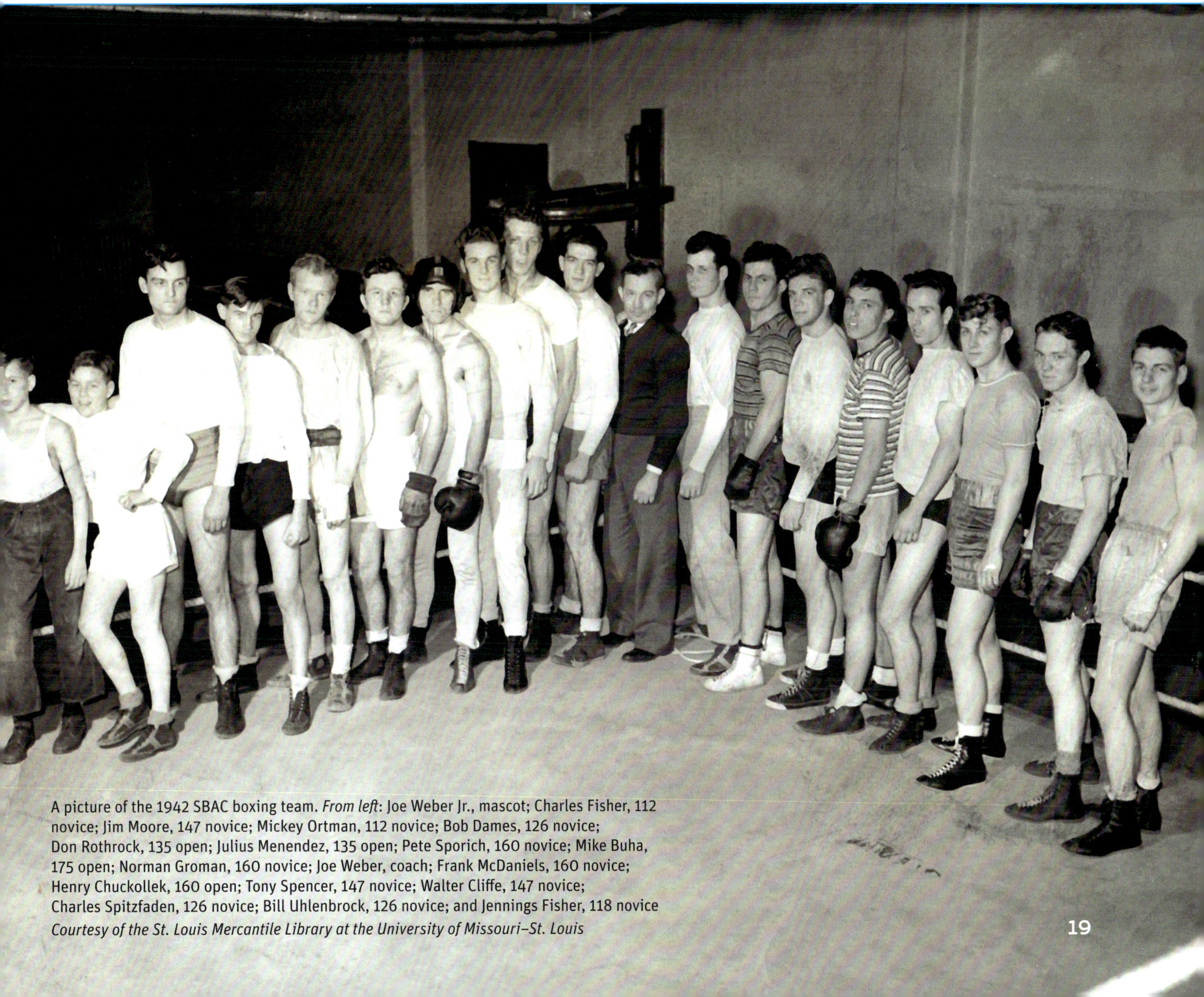

A picture of the 1942 SBAC boxing team. *From left*: Joe Weber Jr., mascot; Charles Fisher, 112 novice; Jim Moore, 147 novice; Mickey Ortman, 112 novice; Bob Dames, 126 novice; Don Rothrock, 135 open; Julius Menendez, 135 open; Pete Sporich, 160 novice; Mike Buha, 175 open; Norman Groman, 160 novice; Joe Weber, coach; Frank McDaniels, 160 novice; Henry Chuckollek, 160 open; Tony Spencer, 147 novice; Walter Cliffe, 147 novice; Charles Spitzfaden, 126 novice; Bill Uhlenbrock, 126 novice; and Jennings Fisher, 118 novice
Courtesy of the St. Louis Mercantile Library at the University of Missouri–St. Louis

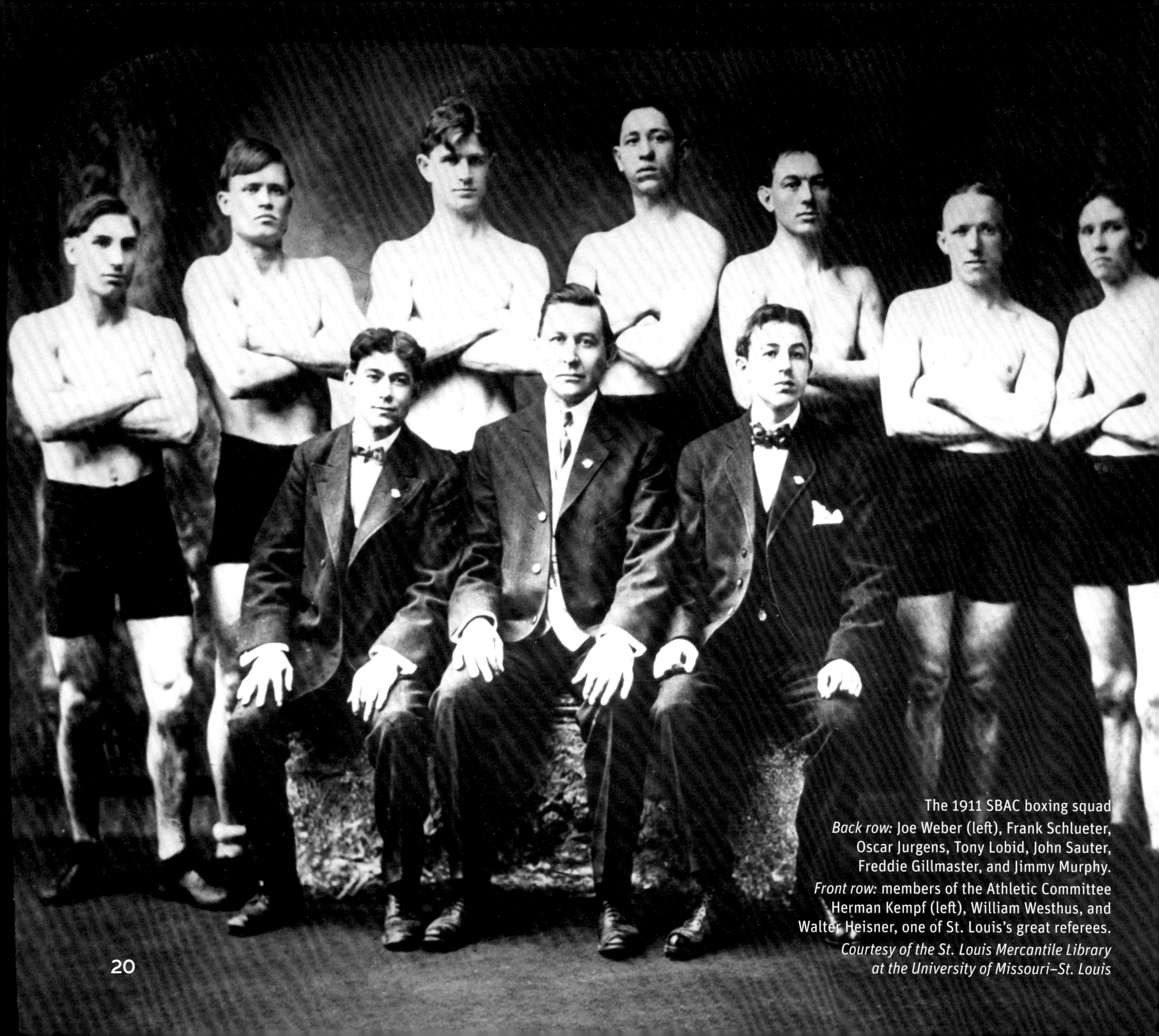

The 1911 SBAC boxing squad
Back row: Joe Weber (left), Frank Schlueter, Oscar Jurgens, Tony Lobid, John Sauter, Freddie Gillmaster, and Jimmy Murphy.
Front row: members of the Athletic Committee Herman Kempf (left), William Westhus, and Walter Heisner, one of St. Louis's great referees.
Courtesy of the St. Louis Mercantile Library at the University of Missouri–St. Louis

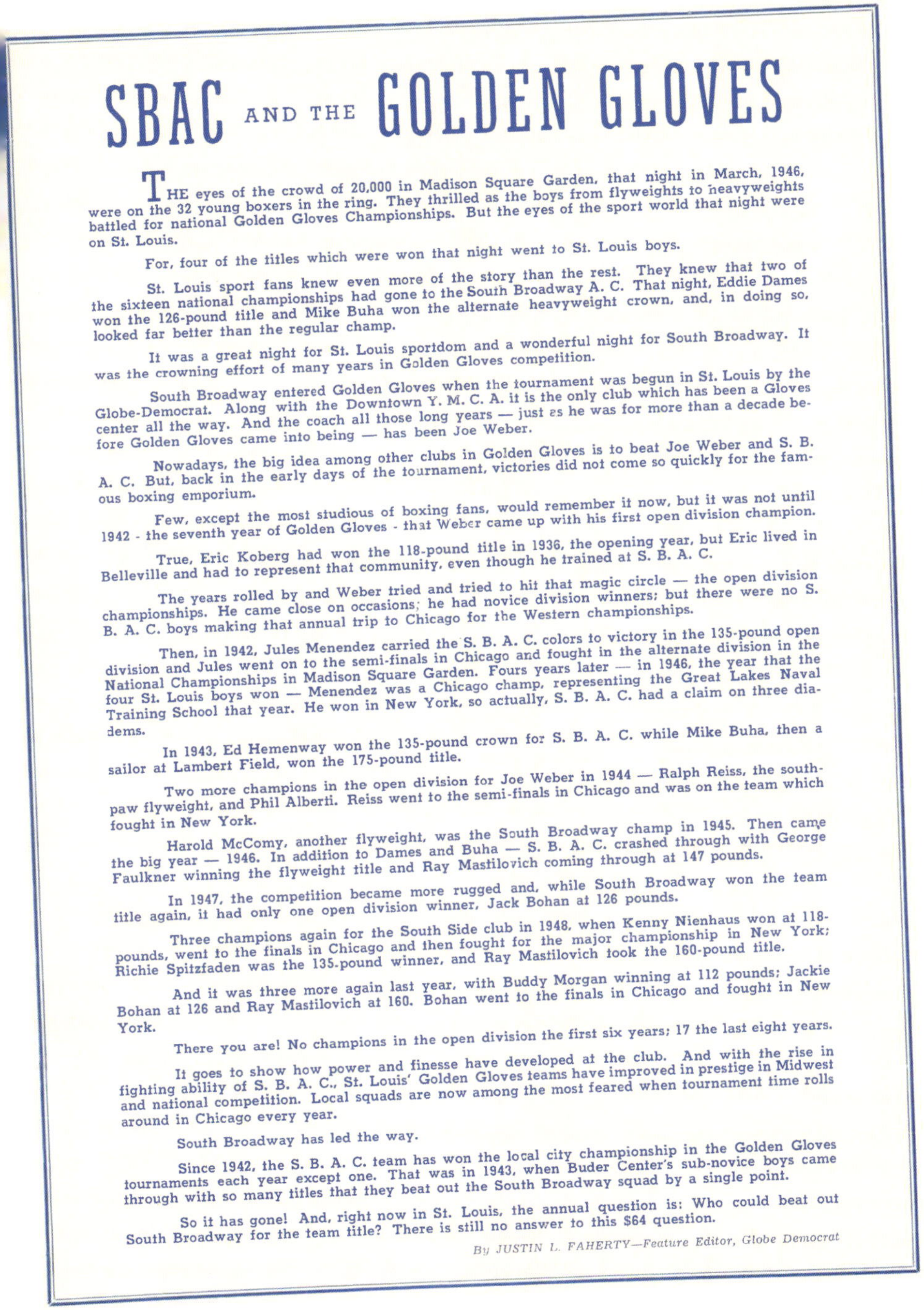

SBAC AND THE GOLDEN GLOVES

THE eyes of the crowd of 20,000 in Madison Square Garden, that night in March, 1946, were on the 32 young boxers in the ring. They thrilled as the boys from flyweights to heavyweights battled for national Golden Gloves Championships. But the eyes of the sport world that night were on St. Louis.

For, four of the titles which were won that night went to St. Louis boys.

St. Louis sport fans knew even more of the story than the rest. They knew that two of the sixteen national championships had gone to the South Broadway A. C. That night, Eddie Dames won the 126-pound title and Mike Buha won the alternate heavyweight crown, and, in doing so, looked far better than the regular champ.

It was a great night for St. Louis sportdom and a wonderful night for South Broadway. It was the crowning effort of many years in Golden Gloves competition.

South Broadway entered Golden Gloves when the tournament was begun in St. Louis by the Globe-Democrat. Along with the Downtown Y. M. C. A. it is the only club which has been a Gloves center all the way. And the coach all those long years — just as he was for more than a decade before Golden Gloves came into being — has been Joe Weber.

Nowadays, the big idea among other clubs in Golden Gloves is to beat Joe Weber and S. B. A. C. But, back in the early days of the tournament, victories did not come so quickly for the famous boxing emporium.

Few, except the most studious of boxing fans, would remember it now, but it was not until 1942 - the seventh year of Golden Gloves - that Weber came up with his first open division champion.

True, Eric Koberg had won the 118-pound title in 1936, the opening year, but Eric lived in Belleville and had to represent that community, even though he trained at S. B. A. C.

The years rolled by and Weber tried and tried to hit that magic circle — the open division championships. He came close on occasions; he had novice division winners; but there were no S. B. A. C. boys making that annual trip to Chicago for the Western championships.

Then, in 1942, Jules Menendez carried the S. B. A. C. colors to victory in the 135-pound open division and Jules went on to the semi-finals in Chicago and fought in the alternate division in the National Championships in Madison Square Garden. Fours years later — in 1946, the year that the four St. Louis boys won — Menendez was a Chicago champ, representing the Great Lakes Naval Training School that year. He won in New York, so actually, S. B. A. C. had a claim on three diadems.

In 1943, Ed Hemenway won the 135-pound crown for S. B. A. C. while Mike Buha, then a sailor at Lambert Field, won the 175-pound title.

Two more champions in the open division for Joe Weber in 1944 — Ralph Reiss, the southpaw flyweight, and Phil Alberti. Reiss went to the semi-finals in Chicago and was on the team which fought in New York.

Harold McComy, another flyweight, was the South Broadway champ in 1945. Then came the big year — 1946. In addition to Dames and Buha — S. B. A. C. crashed through with George Faulkner winning the flyweight title and Ray Mastilovich coming through at 147 pounds.

In 1947, the competition became more rugged and, while South Broadway won the team title again, it had only one open division winner, Jack Bohan at 126 pounds.

Three champions again for the South Side club in 1948, when Kenny Nienhaus won at 118-pounds, went to the finals in Chicago and then fought for the major championship in New York; Richie Spitzfaden was the 135-pound winner, and Ray Mastilovich took the 160-pound title.

And it was three more again last year, with Buddy Morgan winning at 112 pounds; Jackie Bohan at 126 and Ray Mastilovich at 160. Bohan went to the finals in Chicago and fought in New York.

There you are! No champions in the open division the first six years; 17 the last eight years.

It goes to show how power and finesse have developed at the club. And with the rise in fighting ability of S. B. A. C., St. Louis' Golden Gloves teams have improved in prestige in Midwest and national competition. Local squads are now among the most feared when tournament time rolls around in Chicago every year.

South Broadway has led the way.

Since 1942, the S. B. A. C. team has won the local city championship in the Golden Gloves tournaments each year except one. That was in 1943, when Buder Center's sub-novice boys came through with so many titles that they beat out the South Broadway squad by a single point.

So it has gone! And, right now in St. Louis, the annual question is: Who could beat out South Broadway for the team title? There is still no answer to this $64 question.

By JUSTIN L. FAHERTY—Feature Editor, Globe Democrat

An article describing South Broadway Athletic Club's showing in the March 1946 Golden Gloves National Championship held at Madison Square Garden. Two SBAC members, Eddie Dames (126 pounds) and Mike Buha (Heavyweight), won national titles during the competition.

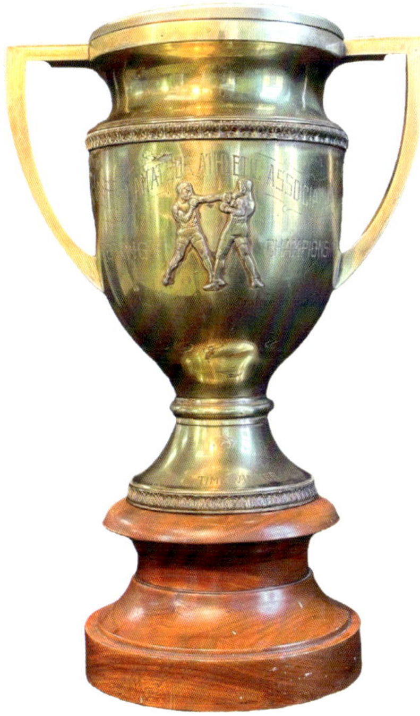

Western Amateur Athletic Association boxing trophy—three-time winners, 1925, 1926, and 1928

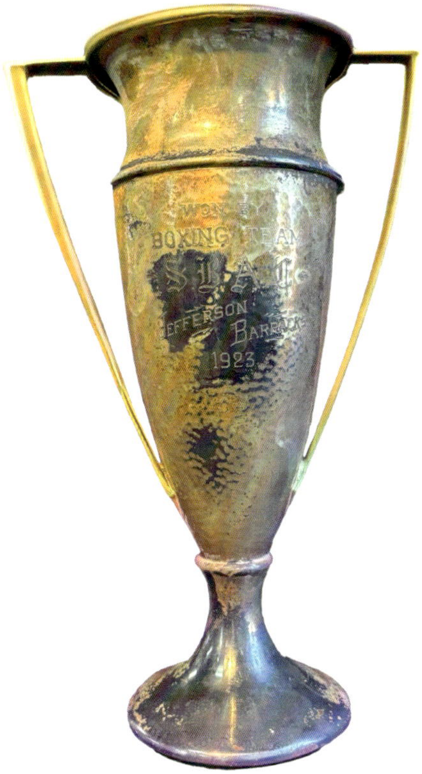

Boxing trophy won by SBAC at Jefferson Barracks, 1923

A TALE OF TWO BOXERS

AT 24 YEARS OLD, Tammy Dyer weighed in between 106 and 110 pounds and stood only 4 feet 11 inches tall—and she wanted to box.

She learned to fight the hard way. As one of five girls, she lived with her single mother and four sisters in the tough Forest Park Southeast neighborhood. She also spent time in foster care and living with relatives in Florida and Oklahoma. It was rough, and she learned to defend herself.

She eventually found herself at the South Broadway Athletic Club gym, working hard as she knew how to do. On April 2, 1994, Dyer became Missouri's first female Golden Gloves champion when she knocked out her opponent in 28 seconds.

"I thrive on boxing," she told the *Post-Dispatch* the next year. "I read up on boxing. I watch boxing. I go to boxing all the time. It's good for fitness, and it builds your confidence."

Female boxing had only been sanctioned for two years at the time, and it wasn't easy to find competitors, especially in the St. Louis area. But SBAC legend Myrl Taylor—known in St. Louis as the godfather of amateur boxing for reviving the sport in the region—was willing to give Dyer a shot, and she rose to the occasion.

"These girls are superbly conditioned athletes who compete hard," Taylor told the *Post-Dispatch*. He would know. Taylor had his own glory days in the ring during his 145 wins in 156 amateur fights and 18–0 pro bouts. His father, Earl Taylor Sr., was also a boxer who wanted to see his twin sons, Earl Jr. and Myrl, follow his path. Earl Jr. boxed a little; Myrl went hard.

"When we got good, we all went to South Broadway. When you got to be a top guy, you got your own locker. It was like *Rocky*. When they gave you that key, that was like king stuff," Taylor said.

He later became a union official and turned his attention to coaching a new generation of talent at the SBAC.

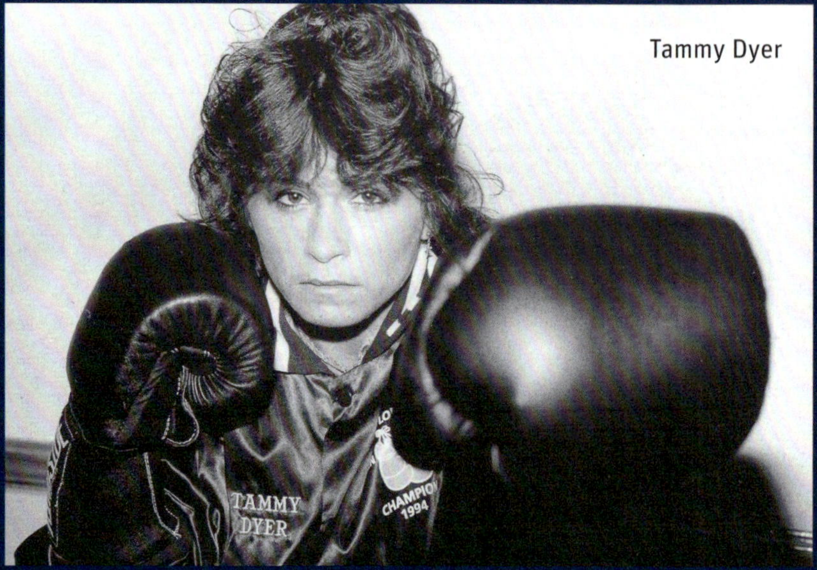

Tammy Dyer

"Our coaches . . . are a special breed. Most of them have given of their time almost every night for years. Many people have worked very hard training kids, tying gloves, escorting boxers, selling ads, tickets, concessions, begging donations, learning to officiate, wrap hands, and even just putting an arm around a boy who needs somebody," one parent wrote in a program.

With Grey Eagle Distributors's Jerry Clinton, Taylor founded the Guns 'N Hoses event that raises money for Backstoppers. To celebrate the club's return to boxing, he started the Reunion Rumbles and invited past champions and supporters from near and far to come to the club. The events lasted until 2012.

Taylor was inducted into the National Golden Gloves Hall of Fame in 1994. He served as president of the St. Louis Amateur Boxing Association, was vice president of the National Golden Gloves Association, and at the time of his death in 2004 was one of six lifetime members of the National Golden Gloves Board of Directors.

—Miriam Moynihan

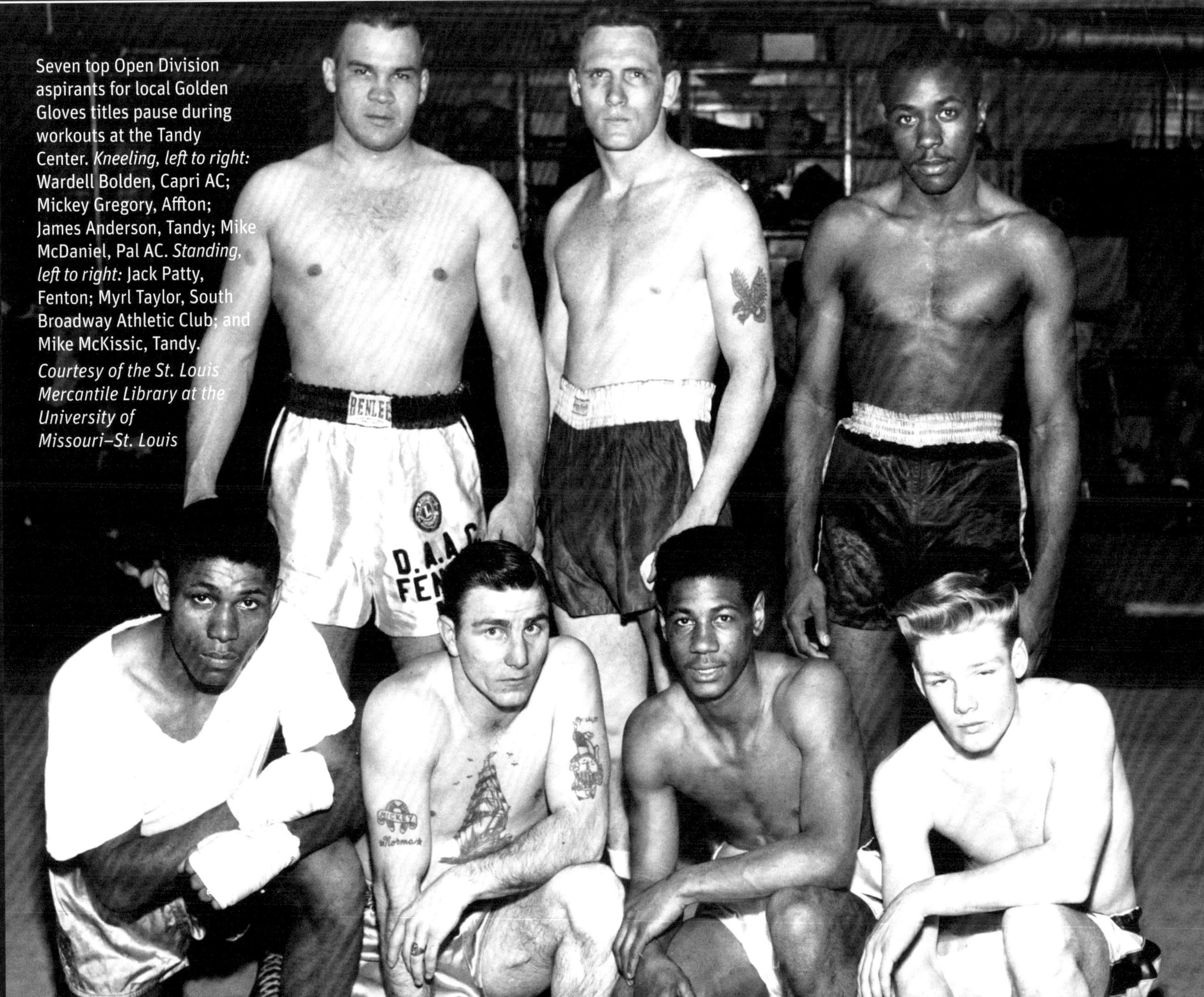

Seven top Open Division aspirants for local Golden Gloves titles pause during workouts at the Tandy Center. *Kneeling, left to right:* Wardell Bolden, Capri AC; Mickey Gregory, Affton; James Anderson, Tandy; Mike McDaniel, Pal AC. *Standing, left to right:* Jack Patty, Fenton; Myrl Taylor, South Broadway Athletic Club; and Mike McKissic, Tandy.

Courtesy of the St. Louis Mercantile Library at the University of Missouri–St. Louis

The Reunion Rumble, started in 1993 by former SBAC fighter Myrl Taylor, was part of a boxing revival. The events were well attended and brought in names such as Stan Musial, Jack Buck, Joe Buck, Red Schoendienst, Whitey Herzog, Cory Spinks, George Foreman, and Butterbean to sit ringside.

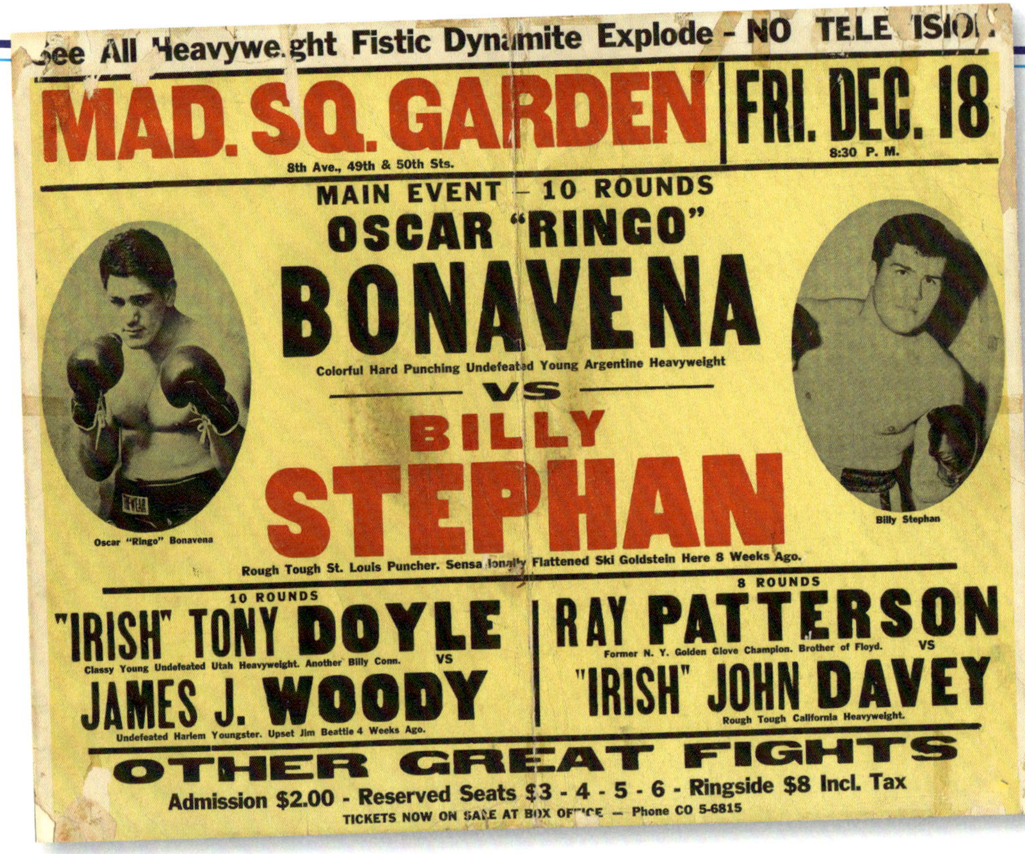
See All Heavyweight Fistic Dynamite Explode - NO TELE
MAD. SQ. GARDEN
8th Ave., 49th & 50th Sts.
FRI. DEC. 18
8:30 P. M.
MAIN EVENT – 10 ROUNDS
OSCAR "RINGO"
BONAVENA
Colorful Hard Punching Undefeated Young Argentine Heavyweight
VS
BILLY
STEPHAN
Rough Tough St. Louis Puncher. Sensationally Flattened Ski Goldstein Here 8 Weeks Ago.
Oscar "Ringo" Bonavena
Billy Stephan
10 ROUNDS
"IRISH" TONY DOYLE
Classy Young Undefeated Utah Heavyweight. Another Billy Conn.
VS
JAMES J. WOODY
Undefeated Harlem Youngster. Upset Jim Beattie 4 Weeks Ago.
8 ROUNDS
RAY PATTERSON
Former N. Y. Golden Glove Champion. Brother of Floyd.
VS
"IRISH" JOHN DAVEY
Rough Tough California Heavyweight.
OTHER GREAT FIGHTS
Admission $2.00 - Reserved Seats $3 - 4 - 5 - 6 - Ringside $8 Incl. Tax
TICKETS NOW ON SALE AT BOX OFFICE – Phone CO 5-6815

Fight poster promoting 1964 match between SBAC boxer Billy Stephan and Oscar "Ringo" Bonavena at Madison Square Garden

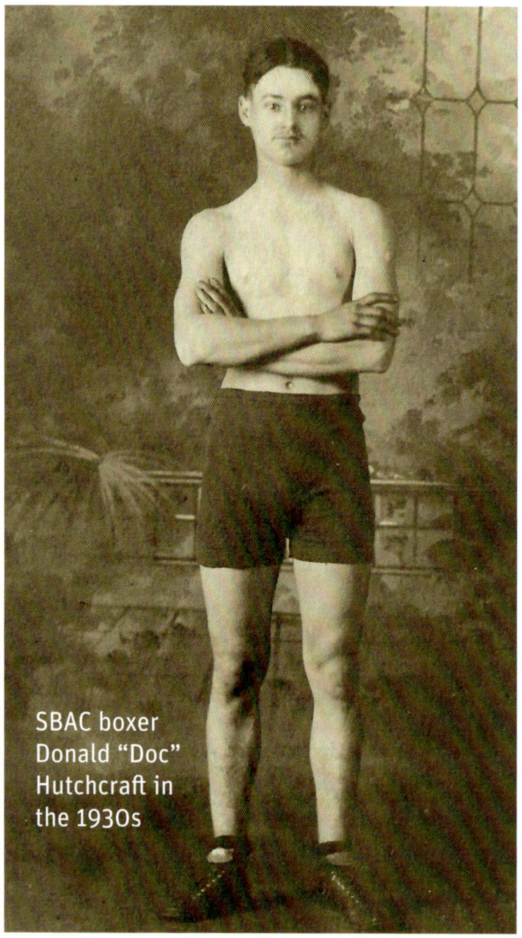

SBAC boxer Donald "Doc" Hutchcraft in the 1930s

Historical Note

The Fighters

The fighters were called pugilists or fistics. The SBAC was described during its early years as "a concentrated amateur fight foundry." During the eight years leading up to the club's 50th anniversary, representatives of SBAC won 17 individual Golden Gloves Open championships.

The ranks of the SBAC old-time fighters include Kid Bandy, Happy Jackson, Sailor Jerabec, Pewee Kaiser, Red Roland, and Larrupin Lou Terry.

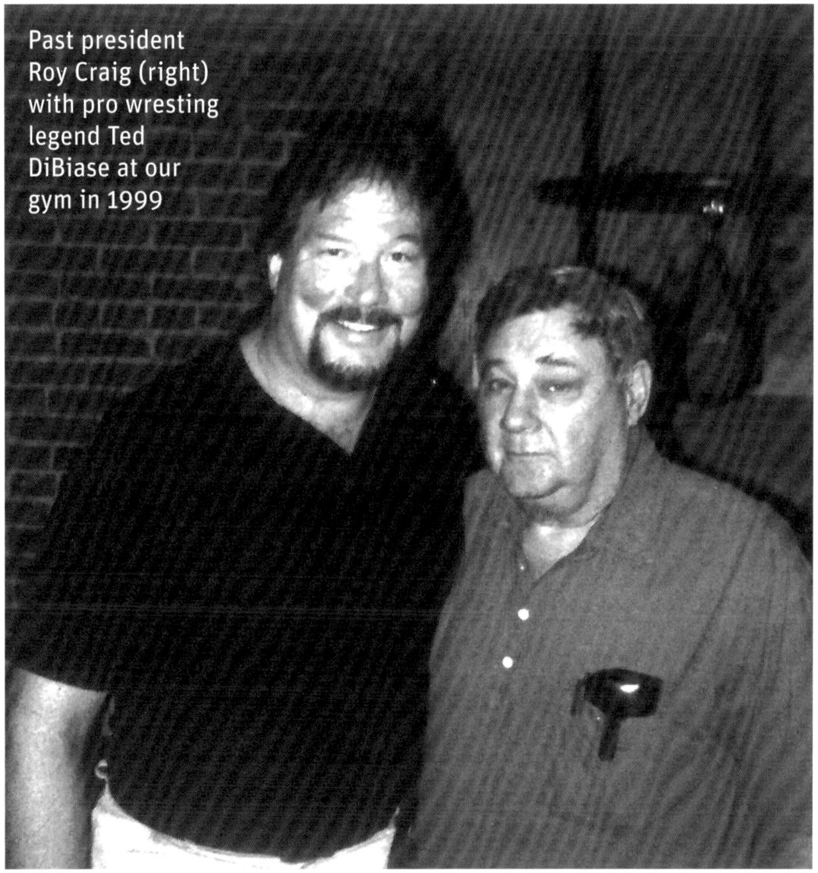

Past president Roy Craig (right) with pro wrestling legend Ted DiBiase at our gym in 1999

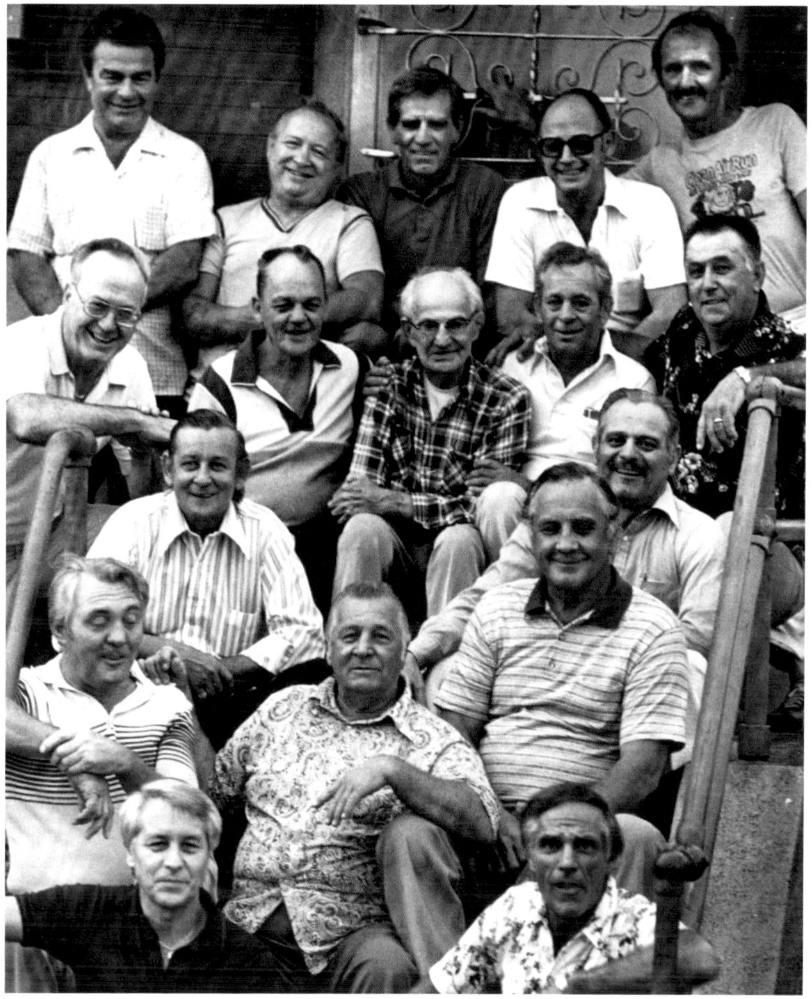

Coach Joe Weber's "boys"—his SBAC boxing stars—paid him a visit in his later years.
Front row: Emil Brcic (left) and Earl Johnson; *second row:* Tom Vetter, Ed Hemenwey, and Mike Buha; *third row:* Harold Bonenberg and Steve Souris; *fourth row:* Steve Spitzfaden, Jack Bohan, Joe Weber, Buddy Morgan, and Ray Hemenway; *fifth row*: Nate Tolie, George Huskey, Kenny Niehaus, Lefty Barton, and Don Vetter.
Courtesy of the St. Louis Mercantile Library at the University of Missouri–St. Louis

Boxing gave the SBAC its first notoriety and filled the trophy cases, but when the gloves came off, wrestling stepped up. The club trained and sent its wrestlers as far as the Olympics, bringing home two bronze medals in 1904. By 1907 the club had a 20-man wrestling team and took to pinning wrestlers from every athletic club in St. Louis.

Olympic-style wrestling was eventually surpassed by a new style of "professional wrestling," as much theater as it was fighting. These wrestlers and promoters learned that putting on a show put people in the seats. As wrestlers taunted and dazzled the crowds,

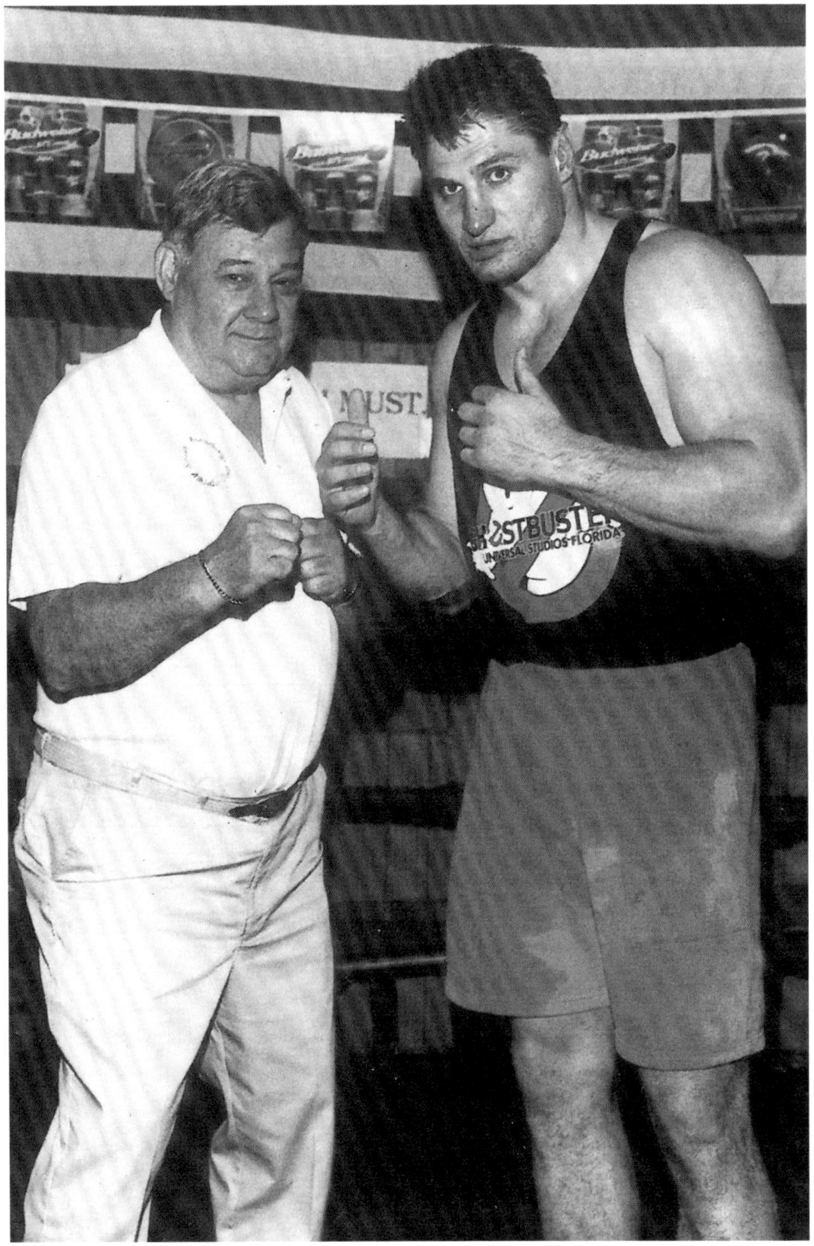

Past president Roy Craig posing with pro boxer Andrew Golota at a Reunion Rumble event

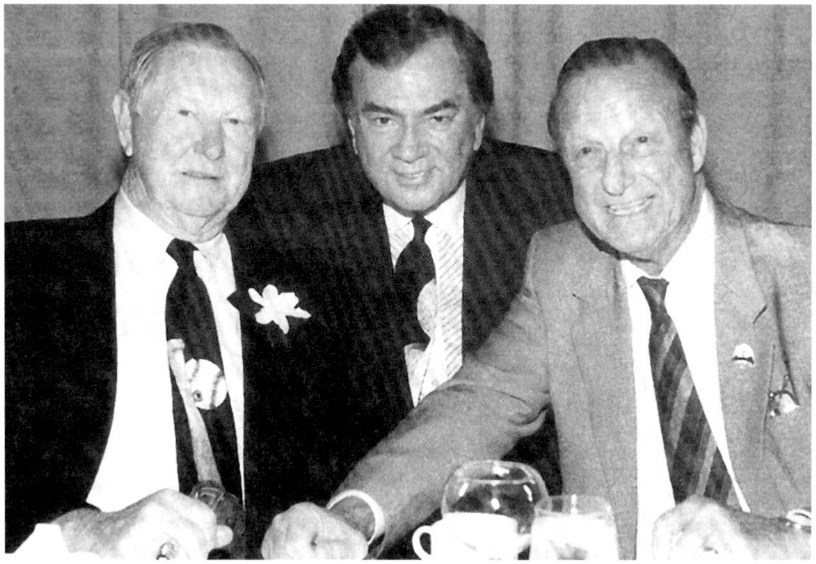

Member Jerry Clinton (center) posing with Red Schoendienst (left) and Stan Musial (right)

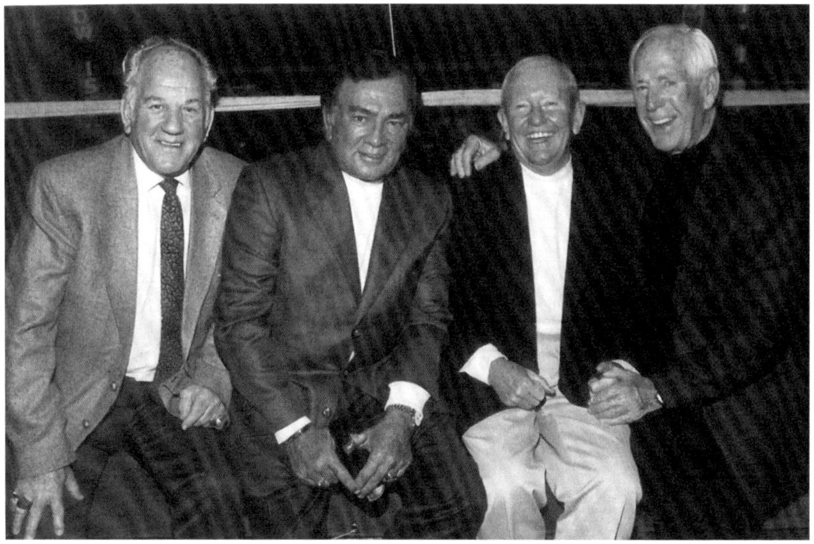

"Johnny Mac" McArthur (left), Jerry Clinton, Charlie Spoonhour, and Jack Buck pose ringside at the SBAC

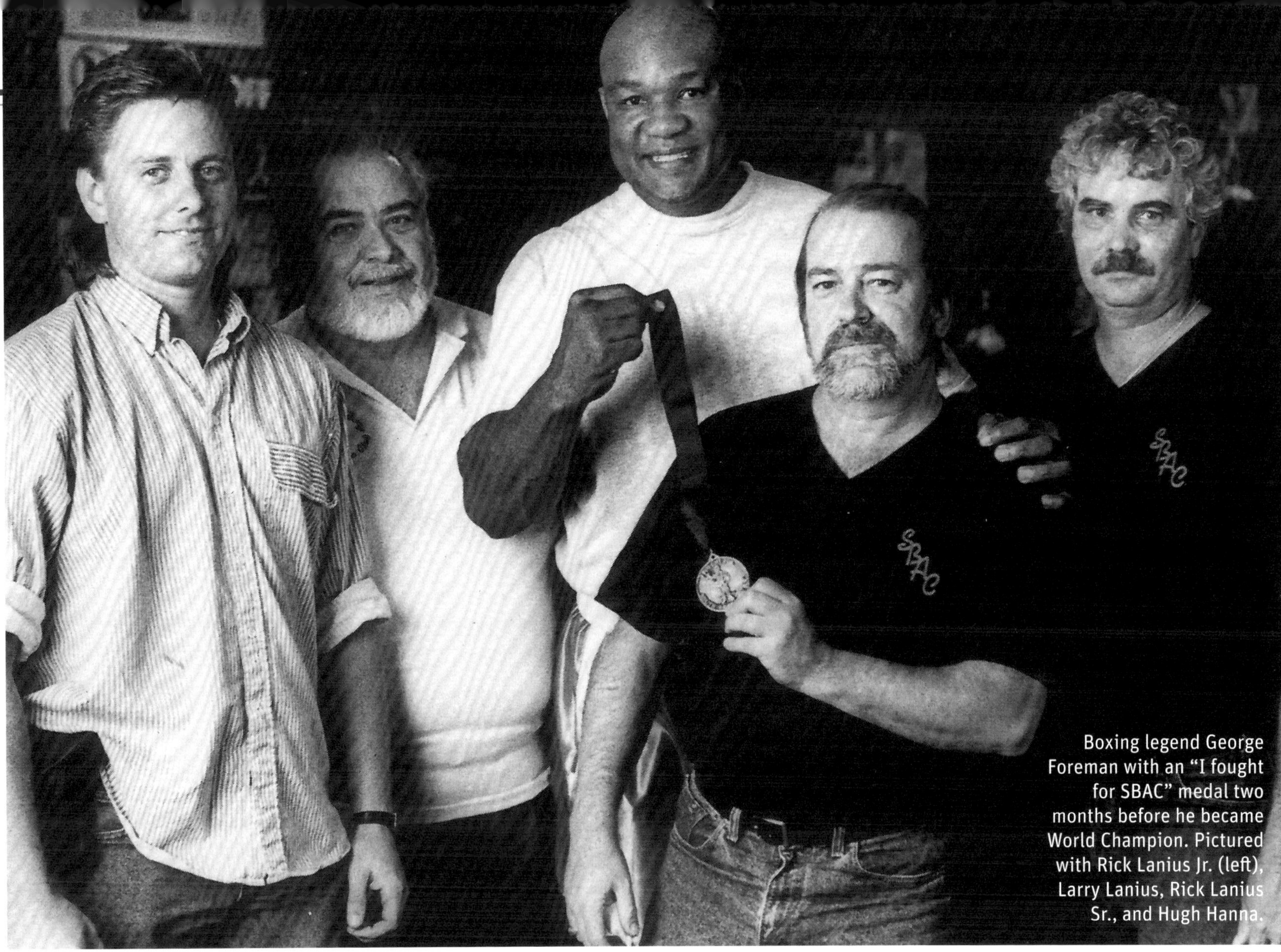

Boxing legend George Foreman with an "I fought for SBAC" medal two months before he became World Champion. Pictured with Rick Lanius Jr. (left), Larry Lanius, Rick Lanius Sr., and Hugh Hanna.

a new style emerged that would eventually become a multibillion-dollar entertainment industry.

What began as a network of regional territories eventually combined to become the behemoth that is the WWE today. St. Louis was an important hub in the National Wrestling Alliance, with *Wrestling at the Chase* being one of the first televised wrestling shows, running from 1959 to 1983. Wrestling's biggest names came there, putting St. Louis on the map. With an avid fanbase and a ring in place, the Mid-Missouri Wrestling Alliance began shows at the club in the early 1980s. Led by Tony "Little Dynamite" Costa, a wrestler-turned-promoter, the MMWA has put on matches the second Saturday of every month for more

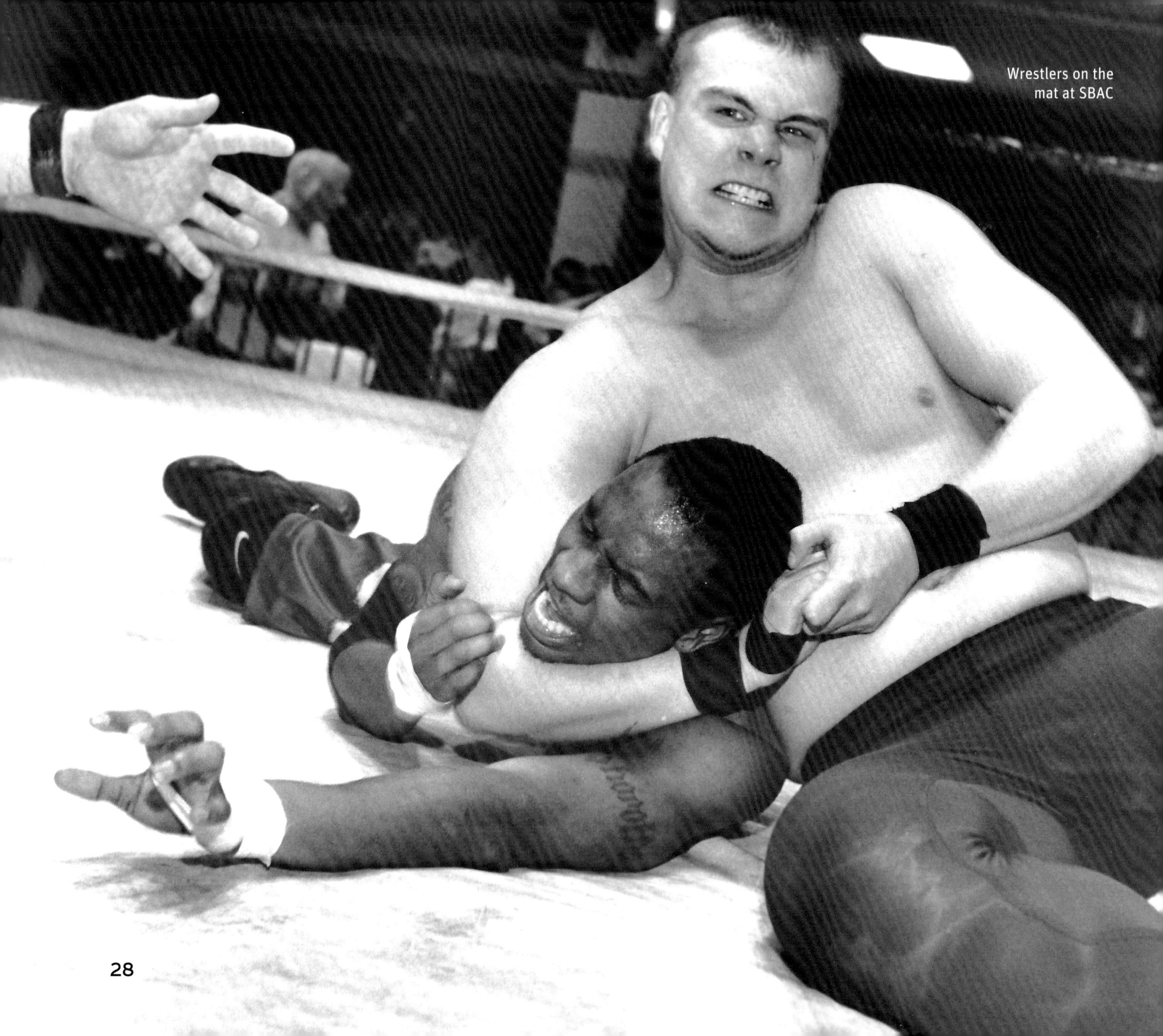

Wrestlers on the mat at SBAC

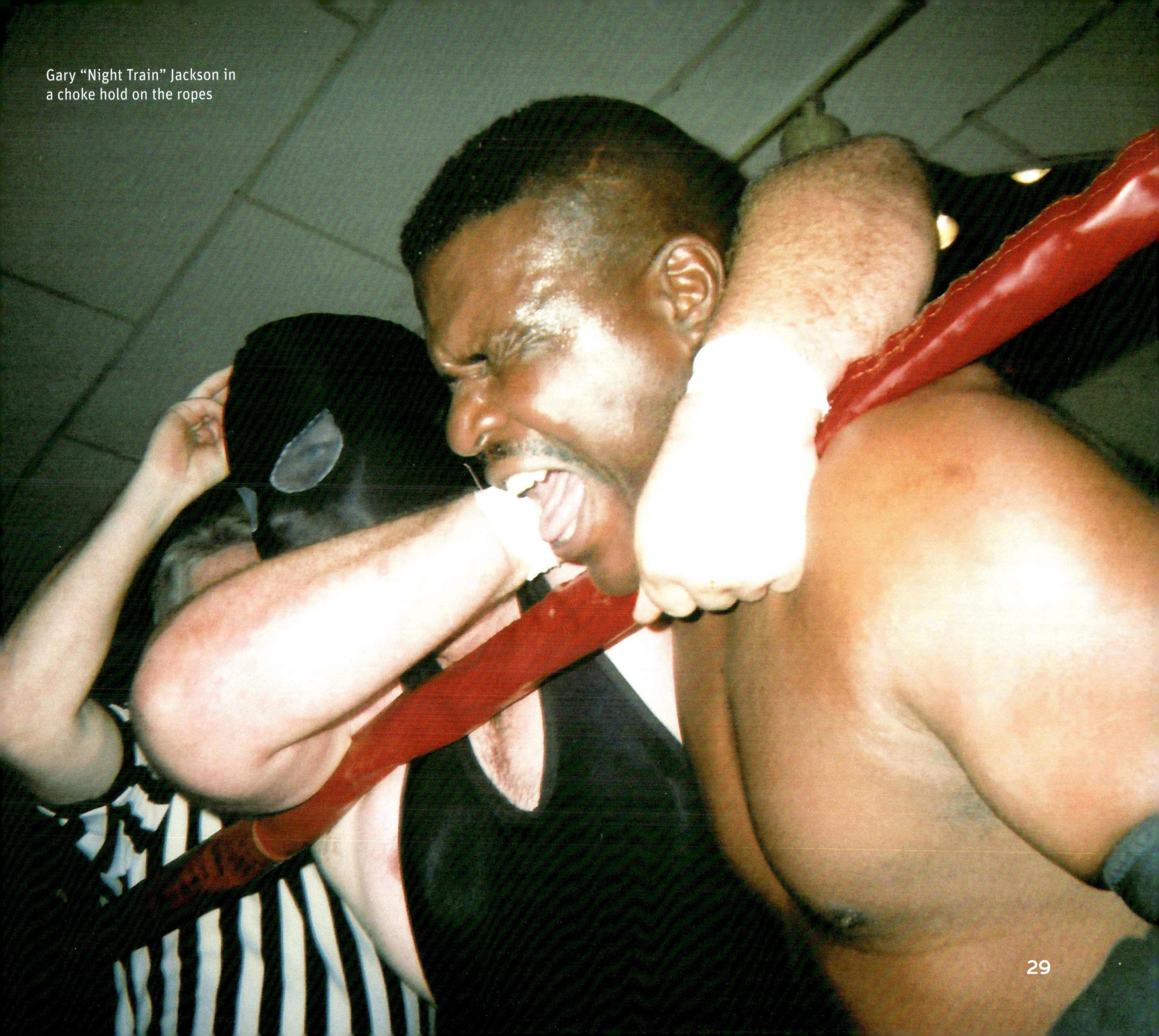

Gary "Night Train" Jackson in a choke hold on the ropes

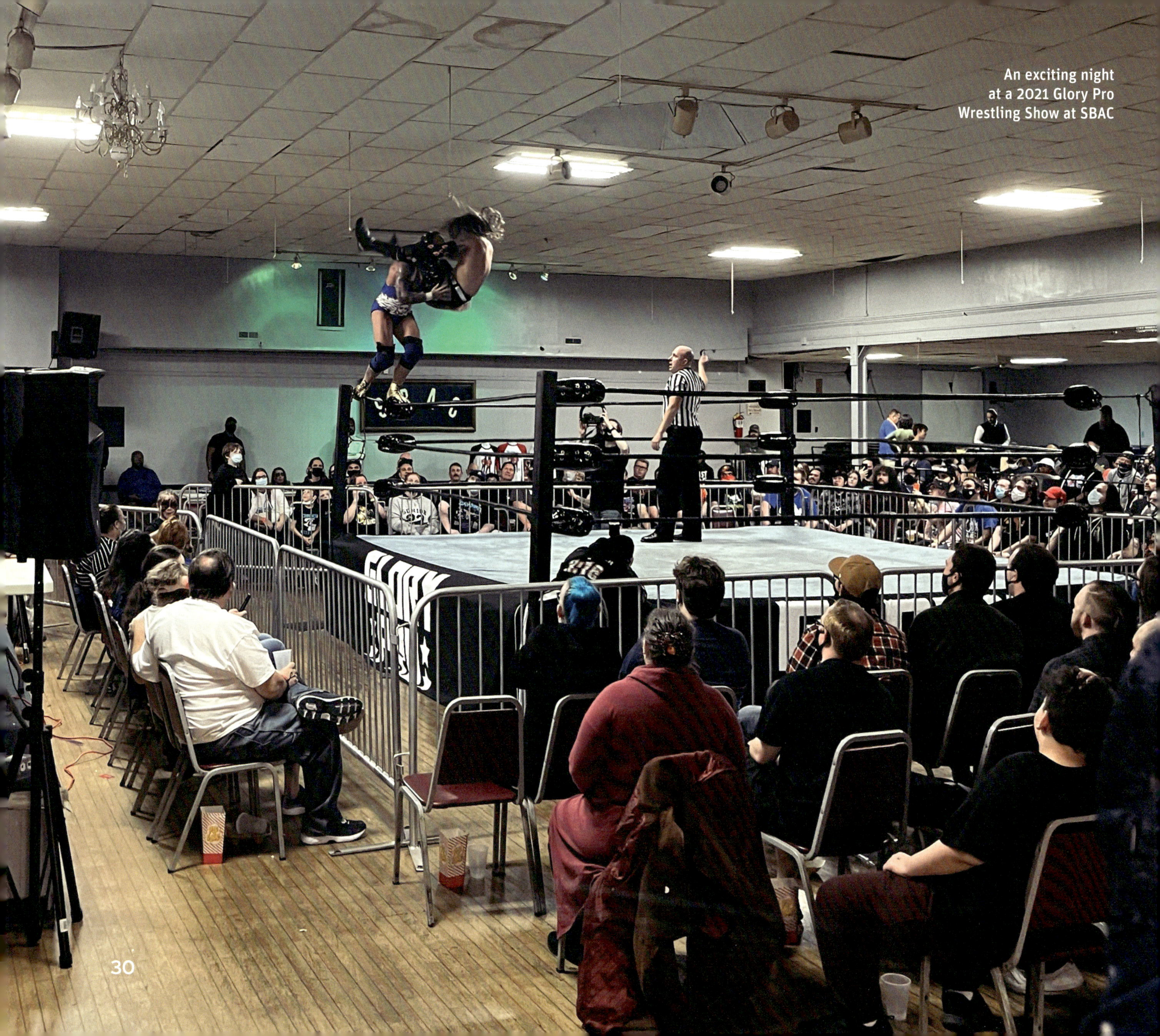

An exciting night at a 2021 Glory Pro Wrestling Show at SBAC

than 40 years now. The club now also hosts Glory Pro Wrestling, which does a few shows a year.

With the SBAC providing a stage for local talent, wrestlers and fans faithfully gather for cheap beers, popcorn, and a raucous performance. Fan participation became a regular part of the show. Working crowds into a frenzy were names such as the Giant Assassin, Big Daddy, Gary "Night Train" Jackson, "Rockin" Al Bauman, Shaft, and Moondog Rover. Local wrestlers made the SBAC a landmark destination for wrestling fans.

"Boxing was a loss leader for us," said SBAC President Kevin Wilkins. "We were putting on boxing shows and losing money. Wrestling—outside of Mardi Gras—was the bread and butter of the club."

When the club was struggling financially in the 2000s and 2010s, wrestling was always there. "We could count on wrestling every month to generate bar revenue," Wilkins said. "That's what we could count on, to try and keep the lights on."

The fight in the ring was always the draw, but the boxers, wrestlers, coaches, promoters, fans, and club members developed a loyal community around the "physical culture" the founding members established in 1899.

—Ryan Buckley and Miriam Moynihan

A series of promotional pictures featuring SBAC wrestlers
(left to right) Giant Assassin, "Little Dynamite" Tony Costa, and Big Daddy

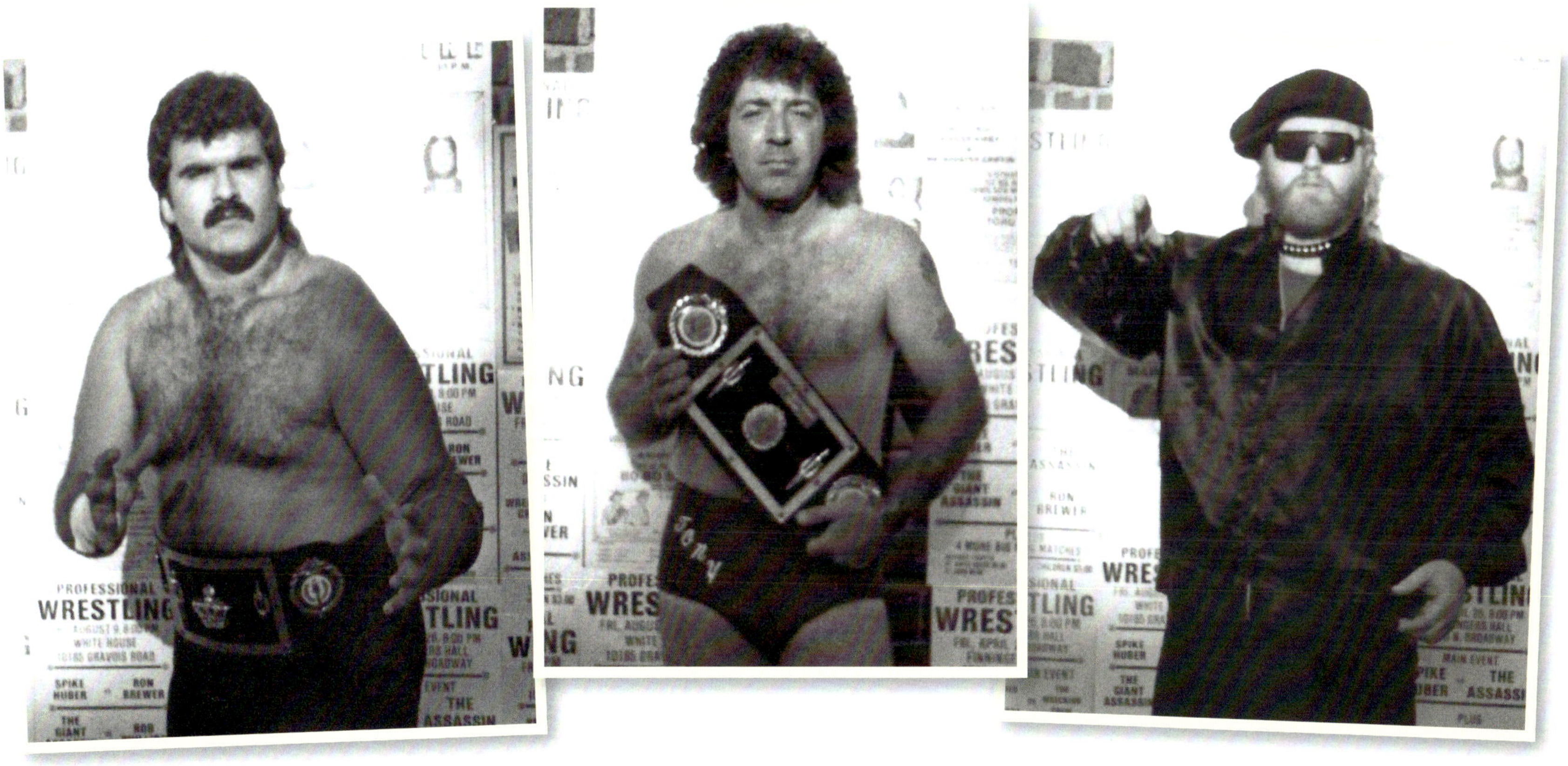

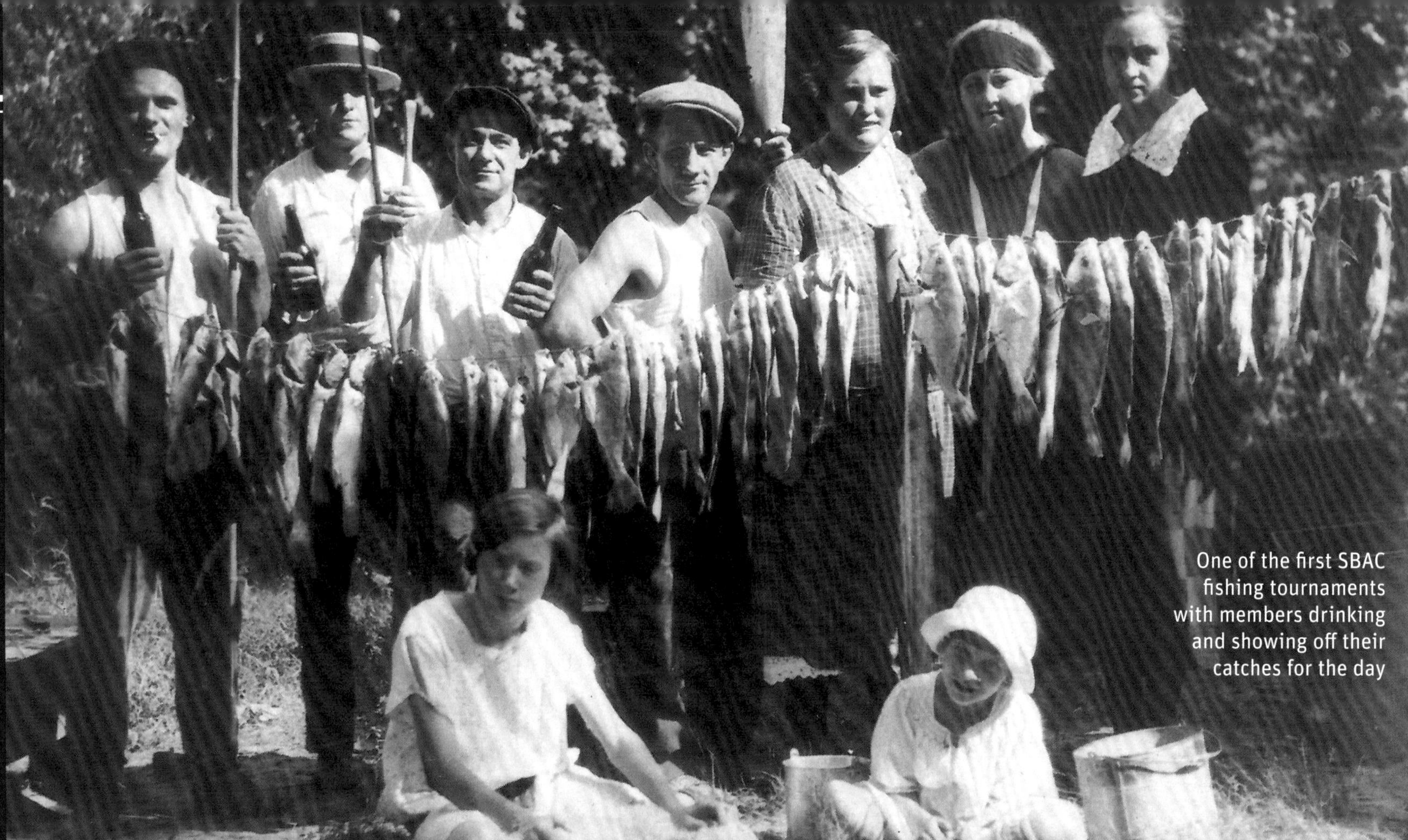

One of the first SBAC fishing tournaments with members drinking and showing off their catches for the day

OTHER SPORTS: BEYOND BOXING AND WRESTLING

KNOWN PRIMARILY for boxing and later for its extravagant wrestling shows, the South Broadway Athletic Club also has hosted and sponsored many sports outside the ring. Between the left hooks and leg drops, a community of camaraderie was cultivated around the physical culture the club embraced.

In the early 1900s, club members gathered to see who could out-pedal each other in bicycle races around the burgeoning city. They also took trips to the countryside to see who could reel in the most fish in their fishing tournaments. The 1910s saw long-distance swimmer Joe Momford and track star Joe Arens as members. There was also a 15-year span starting in 1910 when the club turned out a "crack" baseball team, led by manager George Paul. Bowling also was popular, and in the 1940s the club had eight bowling teams that played at the Downtown Bowl.

When its dance floor was not in use, the club was home to many corkball games. Originating in St. Louis, corkball is a mini-baseball game, played with a smaller ball and narrow bat. With just a batter, pitcher, and catcher—and no base running—corkball can be played inside. As the hits added up, so did the holes in the club's walls; movable nets eventually were added, and multiple games could be played at once. Corkball gave way to fuzzball, similar in play but using a tennis ball with its outer layer burned off instead of a stitched corkball. Recreational leagues became popular in the 1980s, and SBAC was home base to many. As the fuzzball leagues grew, SBAC's Mike Button, Brian Thomason, Rex Bridges, and Nelson Riddle began videotaping, commentating, and interviewing players for a public access television show after getting advice from Pete Parisi of *World Wide Magazine*.

SBAC has been sponsor and namesake to many sports teams, including rugby, baseball, softball, soccer, football, and Gaelic football. The club also provides financial support to youth sports organizations, donating money for jerseys and equipment. Through its 125 years, scores of local athletes have proudly worn SBAC across their chests or competed within its walls.

From its founding to the present, the club's dedication to sports has filled its rosters with members, athletes, and spectators alike.

—Ryan Buckley

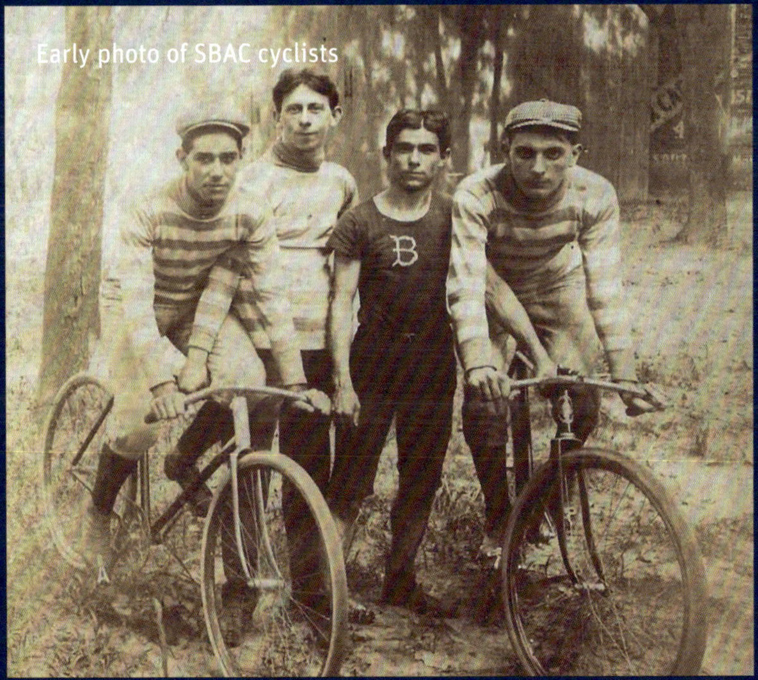

Early photo of SBAC cyclists

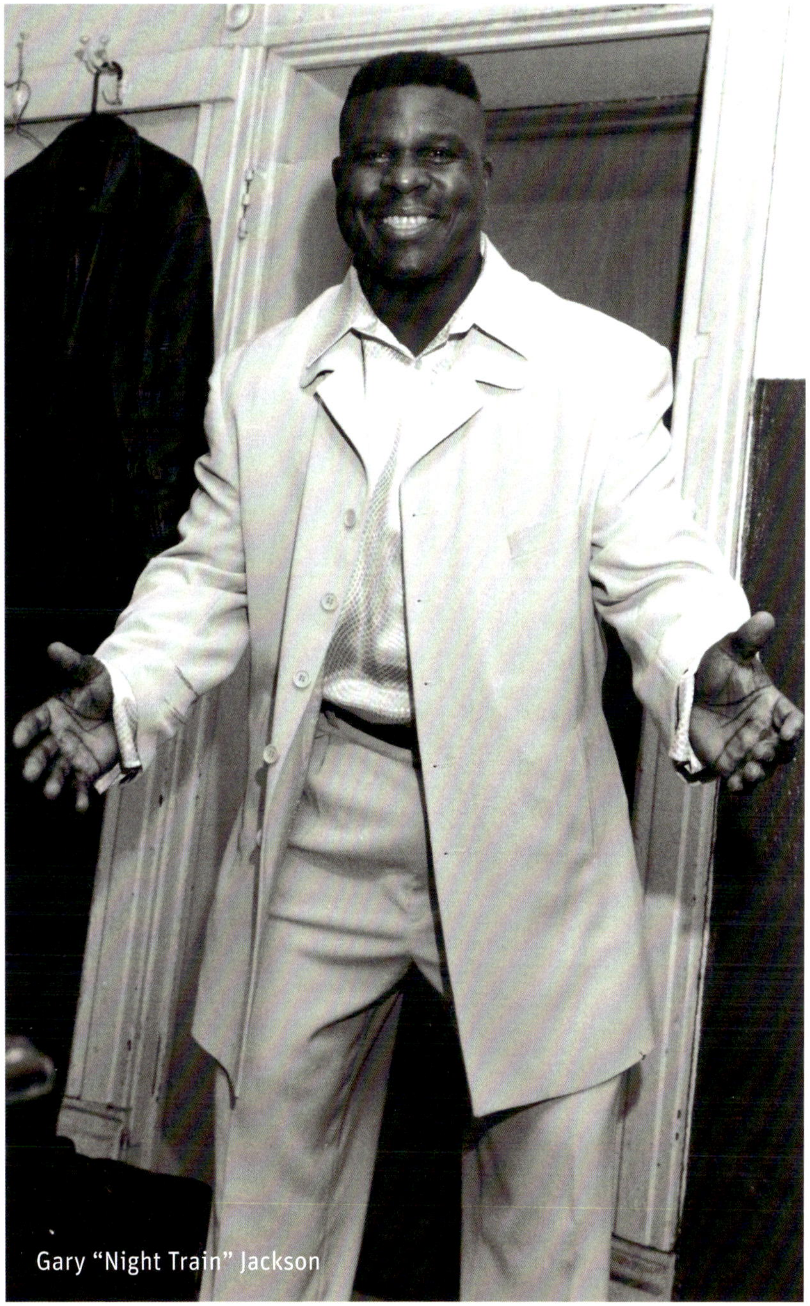

Gary "Night Train" Jackson

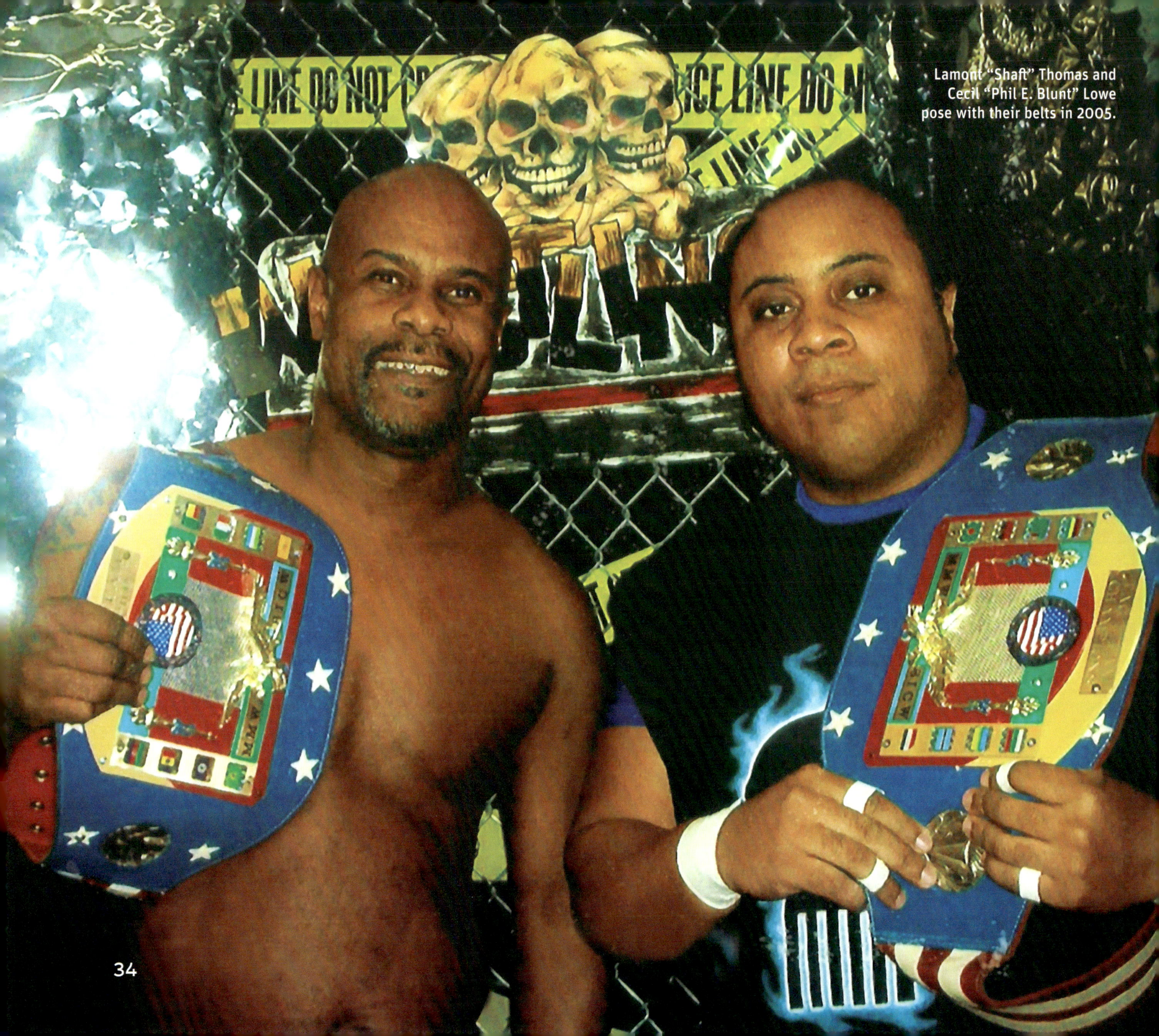

Lamont "Shaft" Thomas and Cecil "Phil E. Blunt" Lowe pose with their belts in 2005.

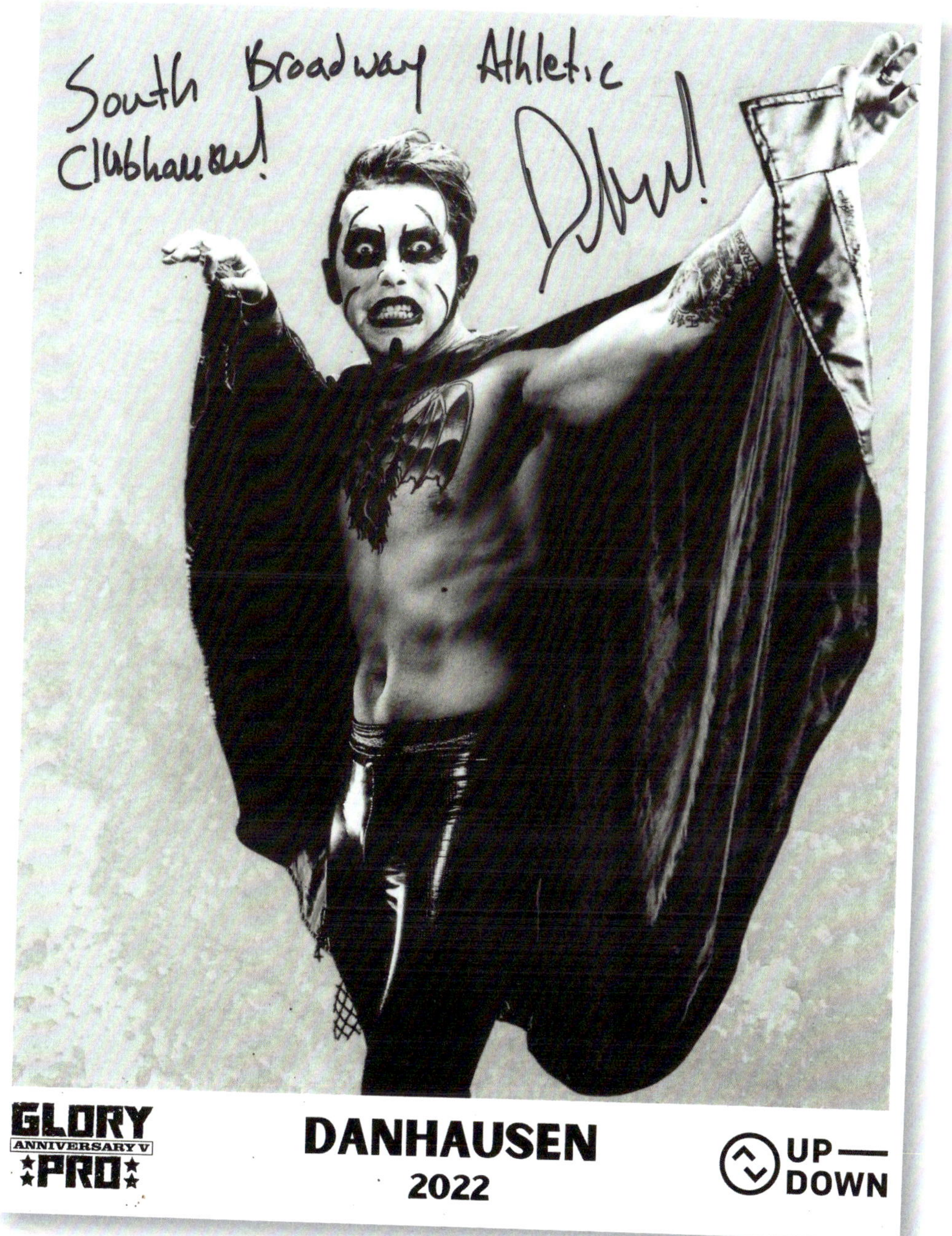

A signed promotional photo of Glory Pro wrestler Danhausen

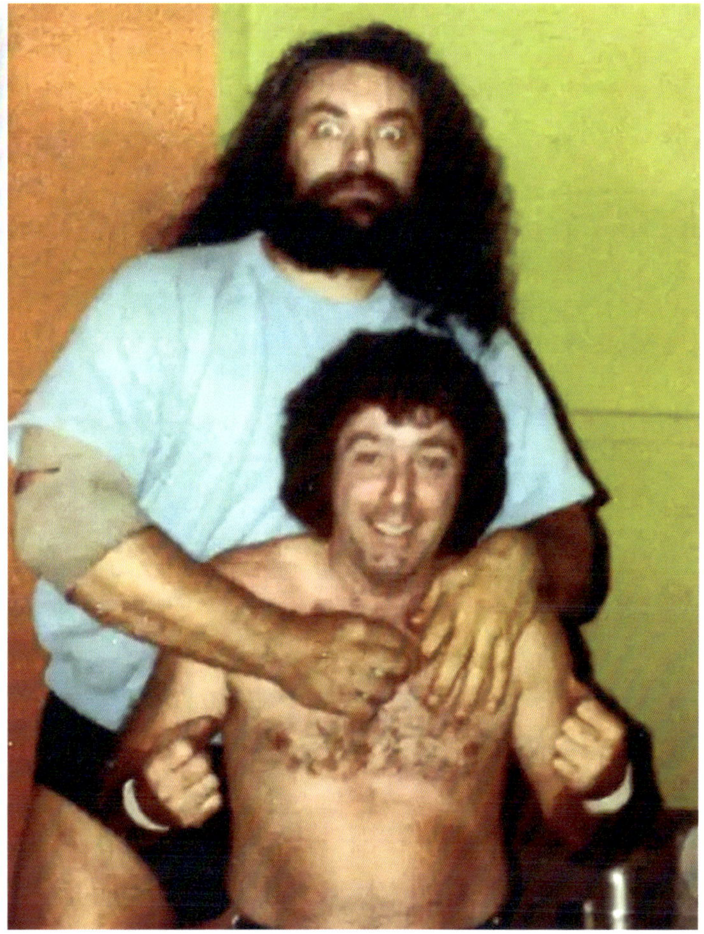

Wrestlers Tony Costa and King Kong Brody pose for a picture.

Children enjoying the entertainment of our 1949 Christmas Party

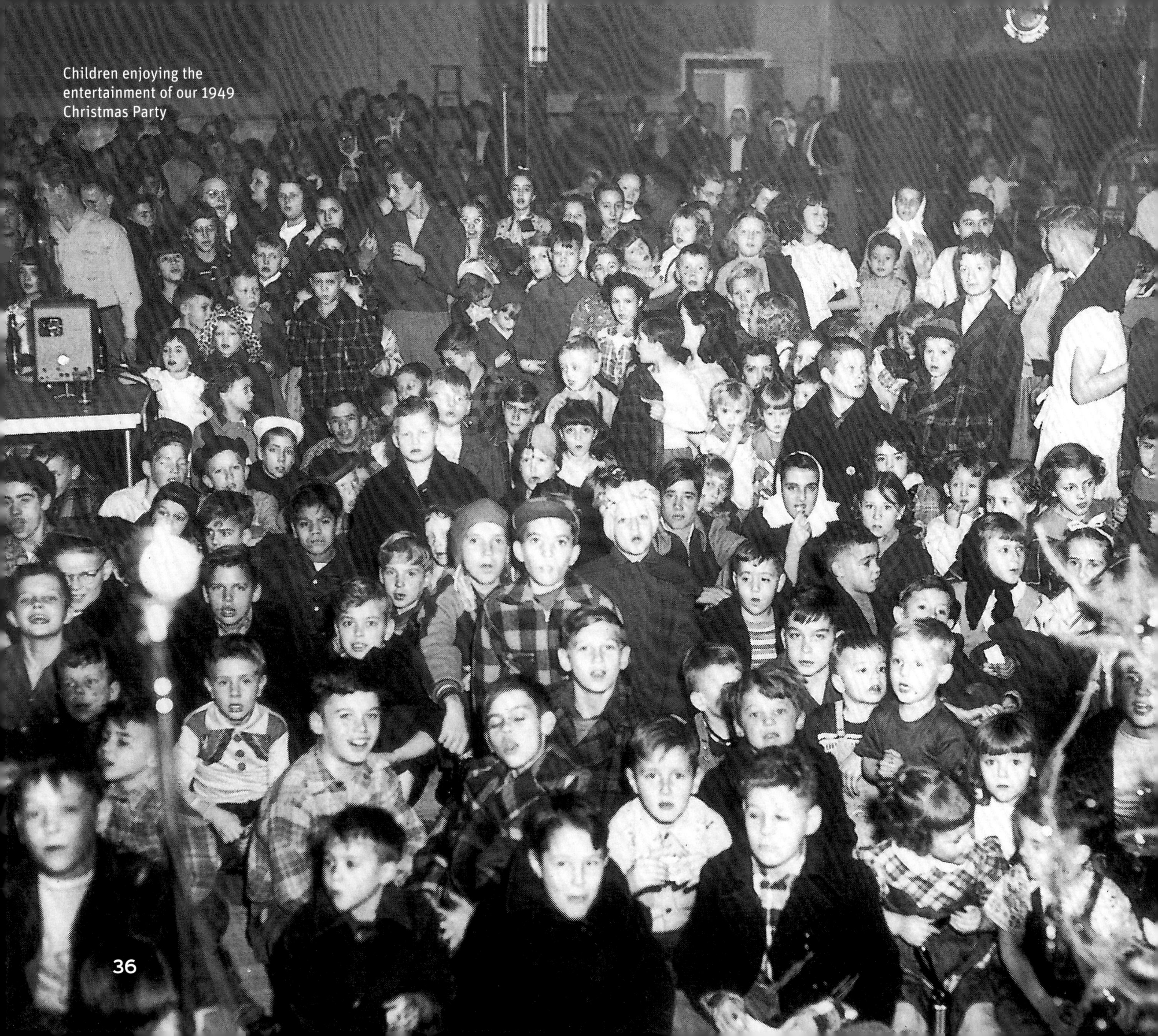

Chapter 3

A Social Place

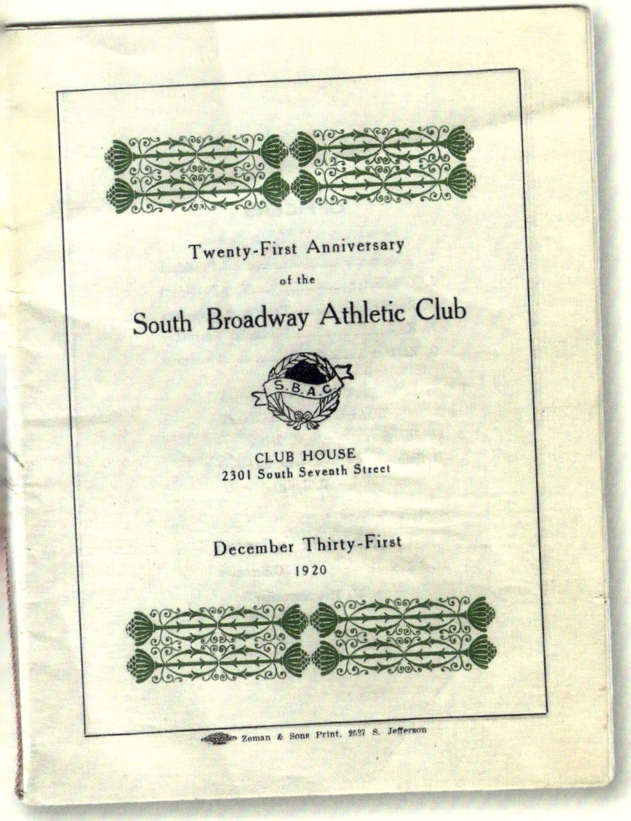

Twenty-First Anniversary booklet from 1920, including menu and order of dances

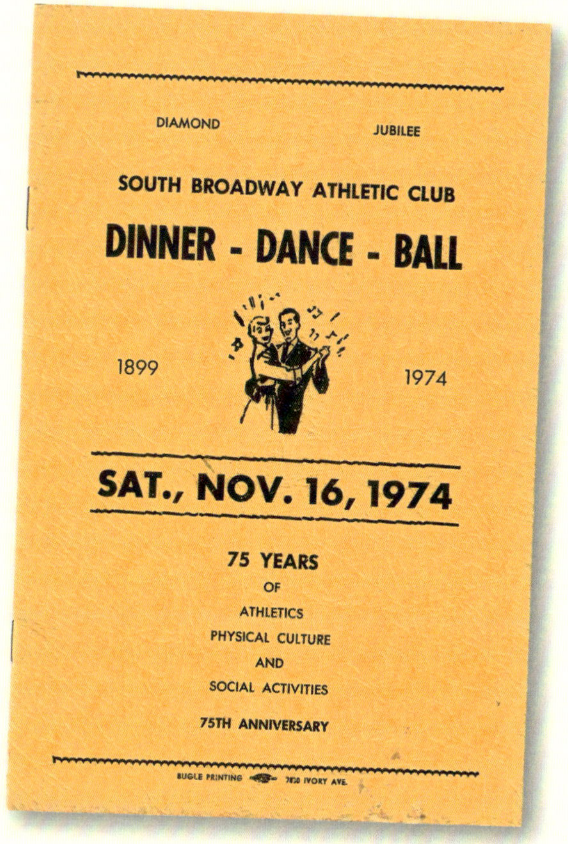

Diamond Jubilee book from 1974, celebrating 75 years of athletics, physical culture, and social activities

AS WRITTEN in our 1899 bylaws, "the promotion of social intercourse among its members" has always—along with sports—ensured the longevity of the SBAC. Social activity continues to drive the 300-plus members of the club. The SBAC is a volunteer-run organization, and keeping the doors open requires the hands of many. With a bar and a large hall well suited for events, the club quickly became a popular place for get-togethers after the SBAC moved to South 7th Street in 1914.

Photos of fishing tournaments, big band concerts, swing dancing, and Christmas parties for underprivileged children fill the club archives. Many St. Louisans recall Rat Pack–style ballroom dances and the annual Homecoming Ball. Wallet-size schedules from the 1960s and 1970s promoted bimonthly social events. Big acts of the

1950s and 1960s, such as the Bob Kuban Brass, graced the stages of the SBAC. In 2018, because of the club's dance hall license, the nationally promoted swing dance event Nevermore Jazz Ball & St. Louis Swing Dance Festival featured all-night dance competitions that attracted hundreds of participants dancing on the hardwood floors of the SBAC from dusk to dawn.

SBAC also has welcomed a large variety of musical events. Senior members of SBAC have fond memories of local Elvis impersonator Steve Davis gracing our stage. The Las Vegas Revue offered the

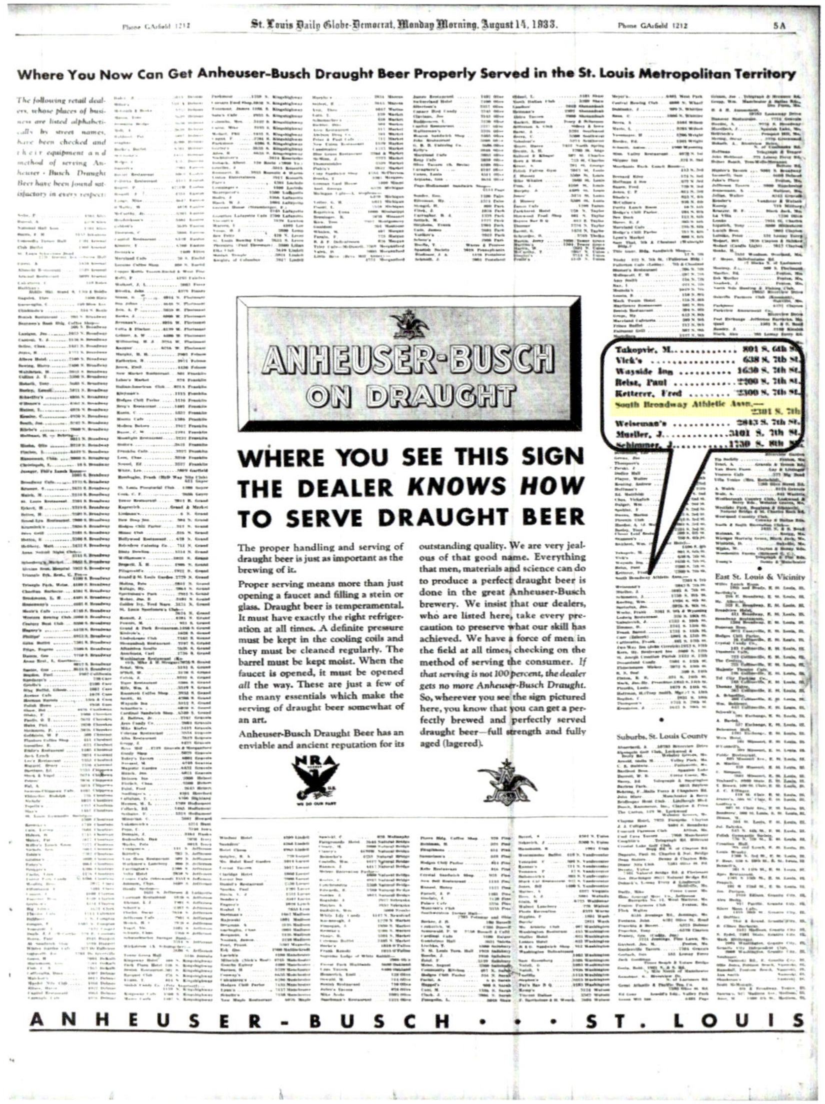

St. Louis Daily Globe-Democrat, Monday Morning, August 14, 1933.

Where You Now Can Get Anheuser-Busch Draught Beer Properly Served in the St. Louis Metropolitan Territory

ANHEUSER-BUSCH ON DRAUGHT

WHERE YOU SEE THIS SIGN THE DEALER *KNOWS HOW* TO SERVE DRAUGHT BEER

The proper handling and serving of draught beer is just as important as the brewing of it.

Proper serving means more than just opening a faucet and filling a stein or glass. Draught beer is temperamental. It must have exactly the right refrigeration at all times. A definite pressure must be kept in the cooling coils and they must be cleaned regularly. The barrel must be kept moist. When the faucet is opened, it must be opened *all* the way. These are just a few of the many essentials which make the serving of draught beer somewhat of an art.

Anheuser-Busch Draught Beer has an enviable and ancient reputation for its outstanding quality. We are very jealous of that good name. Everything that men, materials and science can do to produce a perfect draught beer is done in the great Anheuser-Busch brewery. We insist that our dealers, who are listed here, take every precaution to preserve what our skill has achieved. We have a force of men in the field at all times, checking on the method of serving the consumer. *If that serving is not 100 percent, the dealer gets no more Anheuser-Busch Draught.* So, wherever you see the sign pictured here, you know that you can get a perfectly brewed and perfectly served draught beer—full strength and fully aged (lagered).

Takopvic, M. .... 801 S. 6th St.
Vick's .... 638 S. 7th St.
Wayside Inn .... 1630 S. 7th St.
Reisz, Paul .... 2200 S. 7th St.
Ketterer, Fred .... 2300 S. 7th St.
South Broadway Athletic Assn.—2301 S. 7th
Weiseman's .... 2813 S. 7th St.
Mueller, J. .... 3101 S. 7th St.
Schimmer, J. .... 1730 S. 8th St.

ANHEUSER-BUSCH • • • ST. LOUIS

This 1933 post-Prohibition ad from Anheuser-Busch lists the establishments where you could find "draught beer properly served" including the South Broadway Athletic Club.

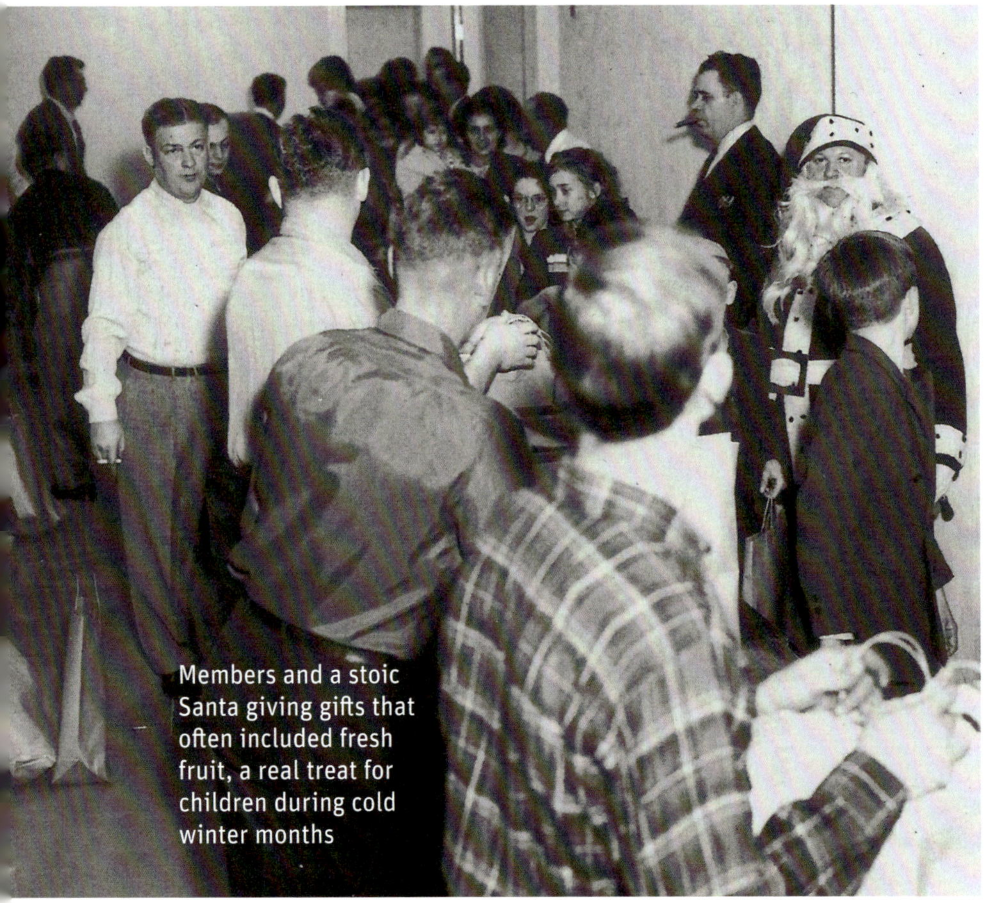

Members and a stoic Santa giving gifts that often included fresh fruit, a real treat for children during cold winter months

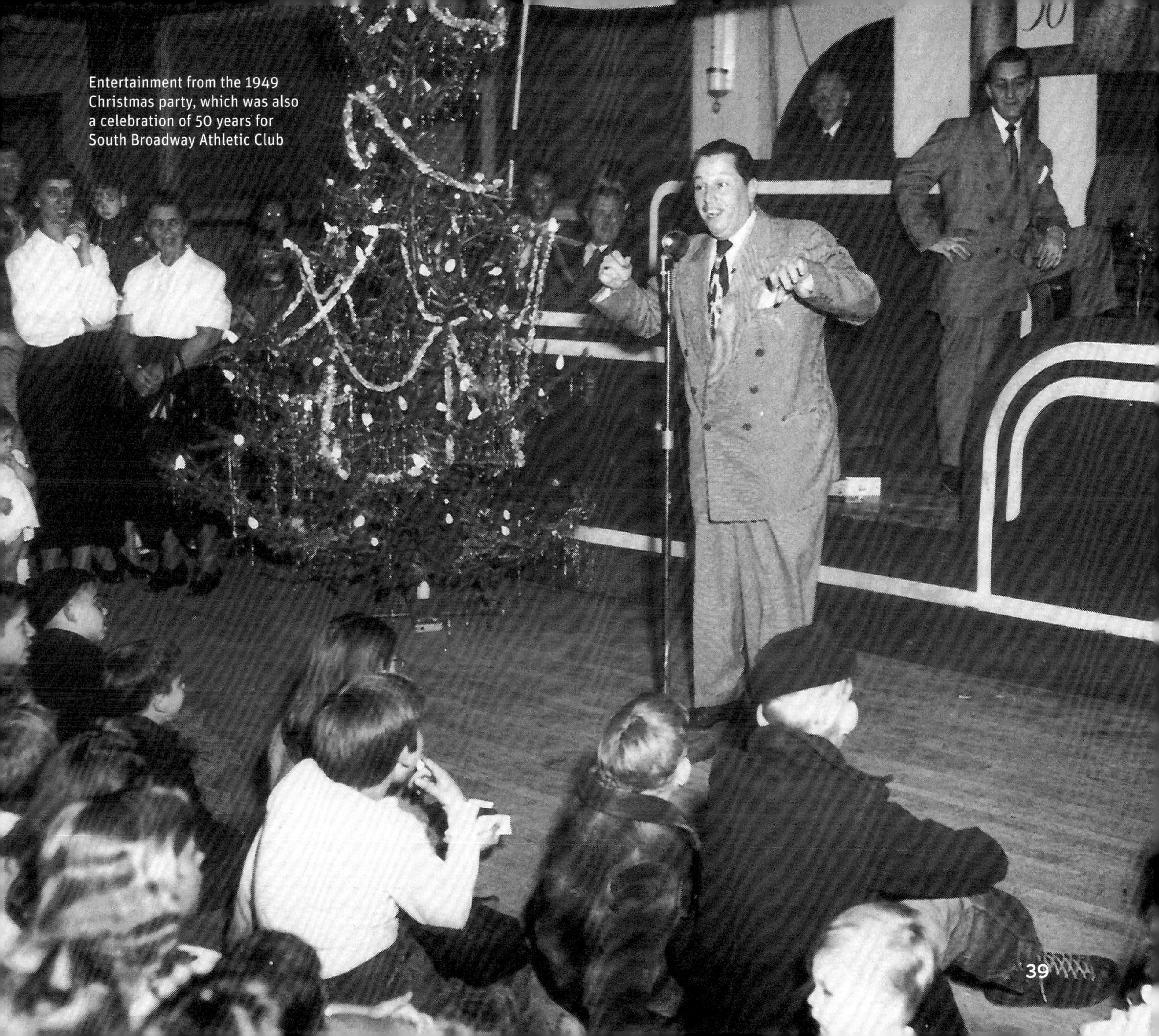

Entertainment from the 1949 Christmas party, which was also a celebration of 50 years for South Broadway Athletic Club

MARDI GRAS

MARDI GRAS MADE its humble beginnings in St. Louis's Soulard neighborhood as a house party. Held at Hillary Clement's home on Russell Boulevard in 1980 and 1981, it was a gathering of friends trying to bring the spirit of the New Orleans celebration to the neighborhood.

The first parade was a short 2.5-block walk up to John D. McGurk's Irish Pub on Russell. In 1982, the first public Mardi Gras was organized by the Soulard Mardi Gras Association. According to Tom Gullickson, owner of 1860 Saloon, "The first Mardi Gras was organized to bring people into Soulard and reacquaint them with the neighborhood that was in the beginning throes of rehabilitation in the early 1980s. It was also a way to bring revenue to the fledgling businesses that were pioneers in the redevelopment of the once-blighted area." The first public Mardi Gras included a poster art contest, a Mardi Gras Ball, a Cajun Cookoff, the first Taste of Soulard, and a Grand Parade.

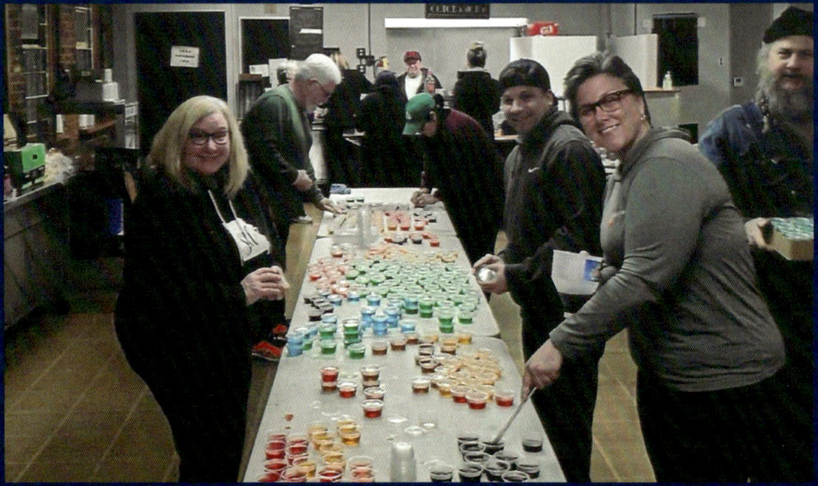

Members Mary Moynihan, Mike Berry, Zach Mertens, Leah Jones, and Brent Jones making more than 2,000 jello shots for Mardi Gras Grand Parade

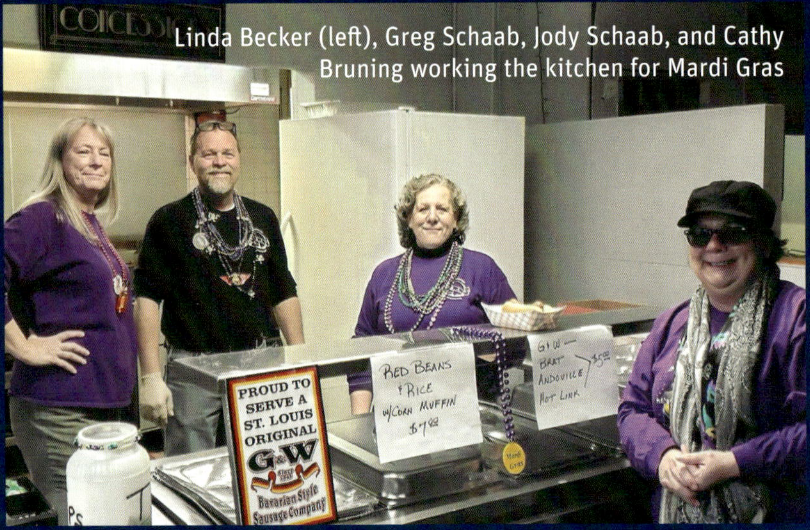

Linda Becker (left), Greg Schaab, Jody Schaab, and Cathy Bruning working the kitchen for Mardi Gras

Through the 1980s, Soulard and its Mardi Gras celebration grew and expanded. A promotion company was hired in 1987 to market the event, and an estimated 50,000 people attended that year. Taste of Soulard was extended and a second Fat Tuesday Parade was added in 1988. Because of growing attendance, the parade was lengthened in 1990, and the route was changed to alleviate congestion in the neighborhood. The Pet Parade was added in 1995, bringing a new family-friendly event that welcomes thousands of St. Louis–area pets marching through the streets. In 1997, the Saturday Parade route was moved to its current route down 7th Street, starting at Busch Stadium, going past the SBAC, and ending at Anheuser-Busch Brewery.

The Fat Tuesday Parade of 1999 ended in turmoil with clashes between partygoers and police. The incident—marked by injuries, arrests, and property damage—was a low point that left the future of Mardi Gras uncertain. The riot led to changes in organization and planning. In 2000, Mardi Gras, Inc., was formed to revitalize and coordinate future Mardi Gras events.

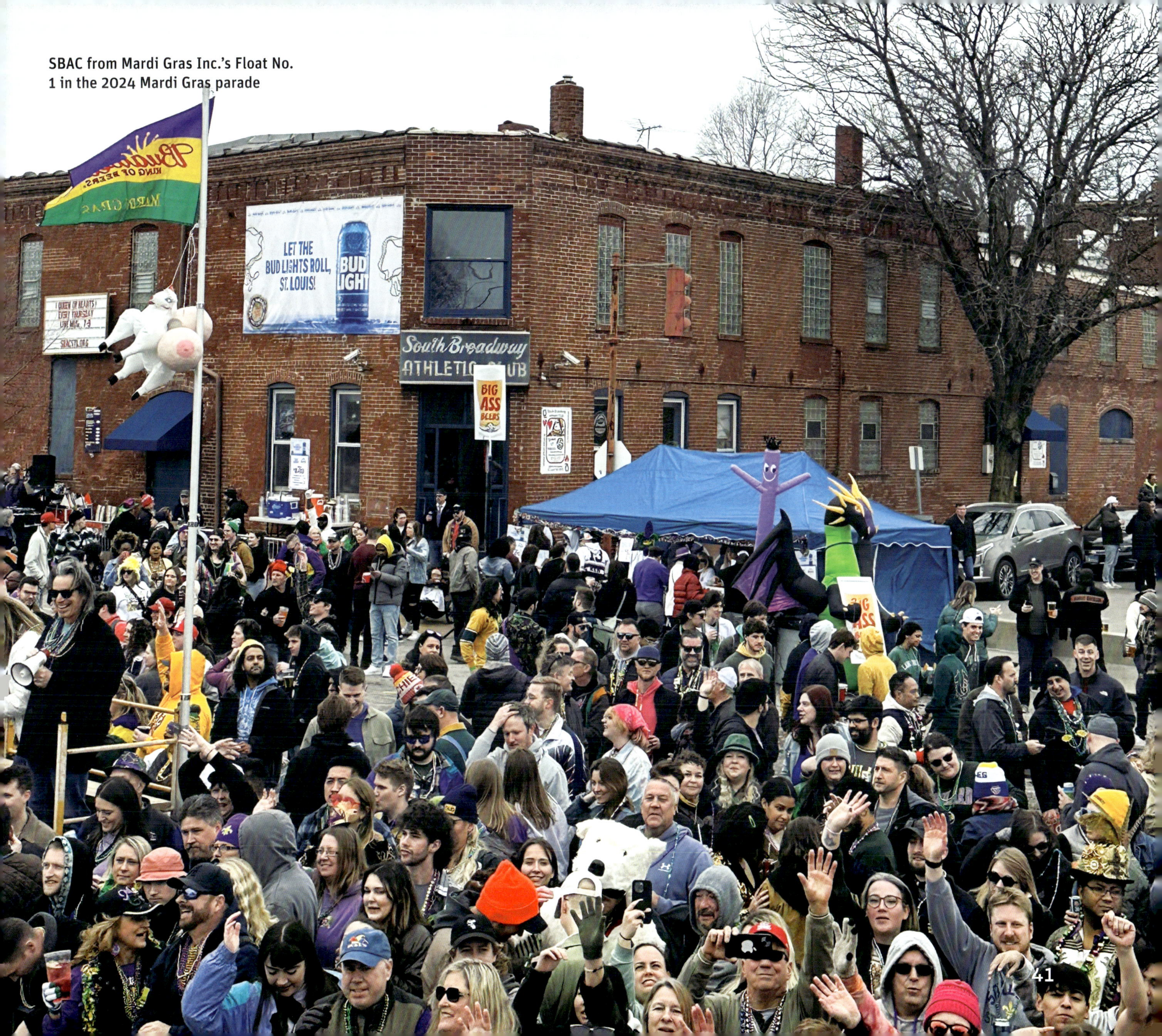

SBAC from Mardi Gras Inc.'s Float No. 1 in the 2024 Mardi Gras parade

Since the 2000s, the celebration has continued to grow, becoming one of the largest annual events in the St. Louis region and second-largest Mardis Gras celebration in the country besides New Orleans. With the event now drawing attendees from all over the world, the planning and organization has become a full-time job, bringing large amounts of revenue to the neighborhood's businesses. Mardi Gras generates about $20 million a year for the local economy.

ARRIVING IN NORTH AMERICA with French colonists in the early 1700s, Mardi Gras (meaning "Fat Tuesday" in French), is a centuries-old celebration of food, drink, music, and dance. Rooted in pagan spring fertility rituals, Mardi Gras was adapted to the Christian Lent tradition. Mardi Gras begins on January 6, known as Twelfth Night, marking the end of the Twelve Days of Christmas and the beginning of Mardi Gras season: a period of extravagant parades, floats, masked balls, and parties with copious amounts of food and alcohol. Culminating on Fat Tuesday, the indulgent celebrations are intended as a purge of sinful behavior prior to the abstinence of the Lent ritual, which beings the following day with Ash Wednesday.

Being in the heart of Soulard, SBAC has been involved with Mardi Gras since its early years. With its large main hall, dance floor, and bar, SBAC has been home to many balls and parties throughout the years. Since 2023, SBAC has hosted the Twelfth Night kickoff celebration, along with a Mardi Gras Ball.

As a stop on the Taste of Soulard tour, the club serves up étouffée in honor of the late member and chef Ray Wiley. The recipe is carried on by his friends and club members every year. On Saturday, when the parade marches down 7th Street, SBAC is lined with bars and food booths serving the scores of parade attendees. Inside, the tables and dance floor are filled with people and music.

Mardi Gras is South Broadway Athletic Club's largest annual event and has helped sustain the club financially for many years.

—Ryan Buckley

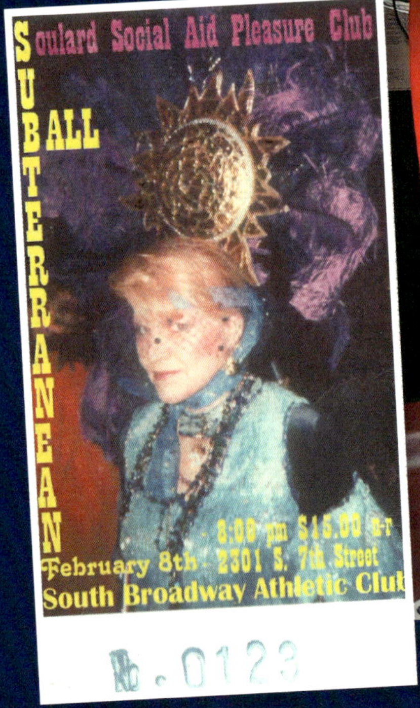

Event ticket for the Soulard Social Aid Pleasure Club "Subterranean Ball"

1860 Saloon, Game Room, and Hardshell Cafe owner Tom Gullickson shows some of his Mardi Gras posters from his many years of involvement in the event.

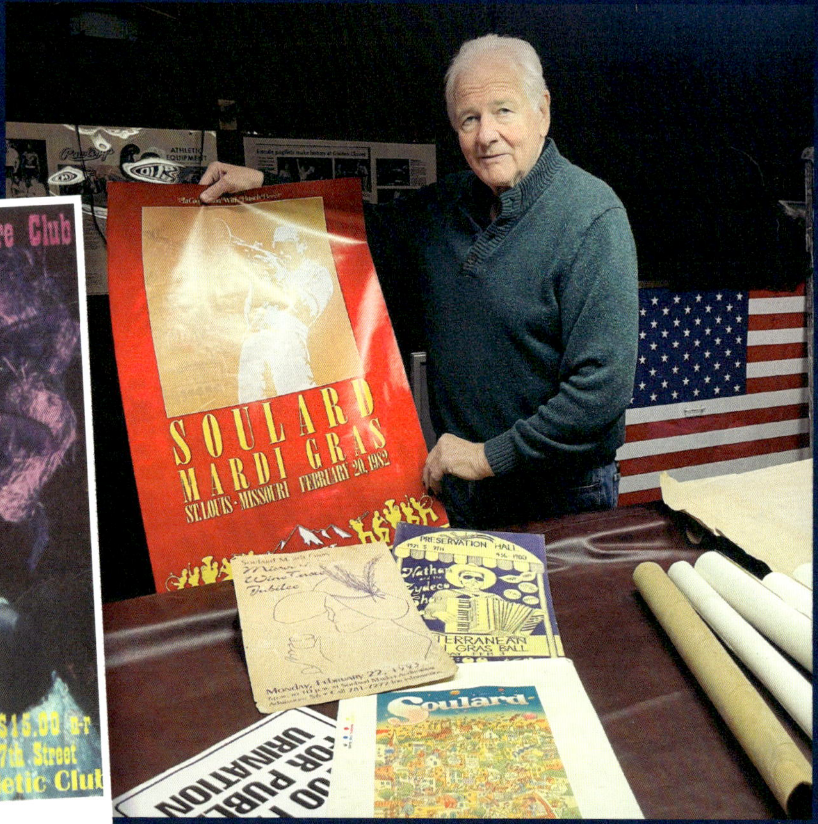

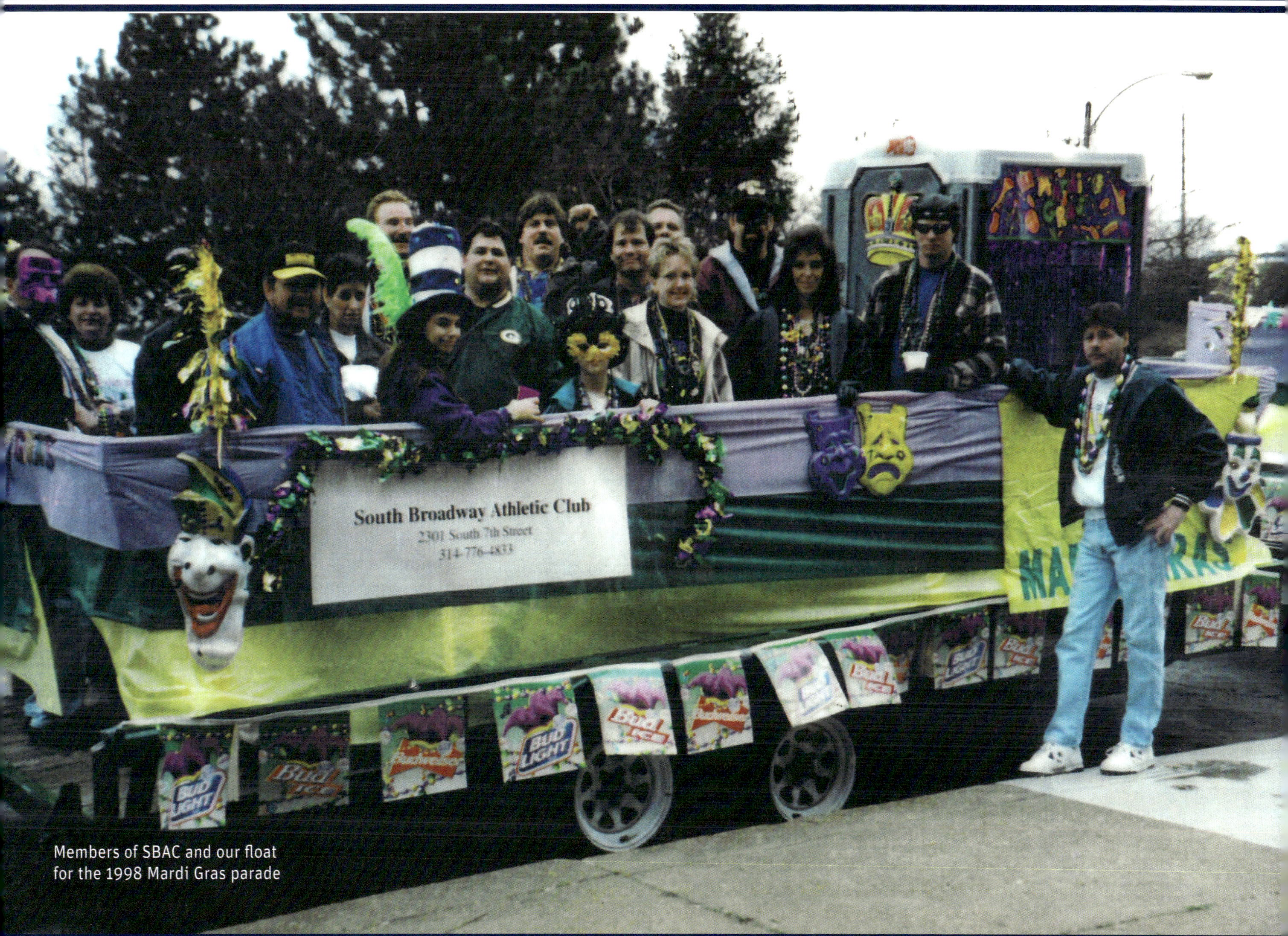

Members of SBAC and our float for the 1998 Mardi Gras parade

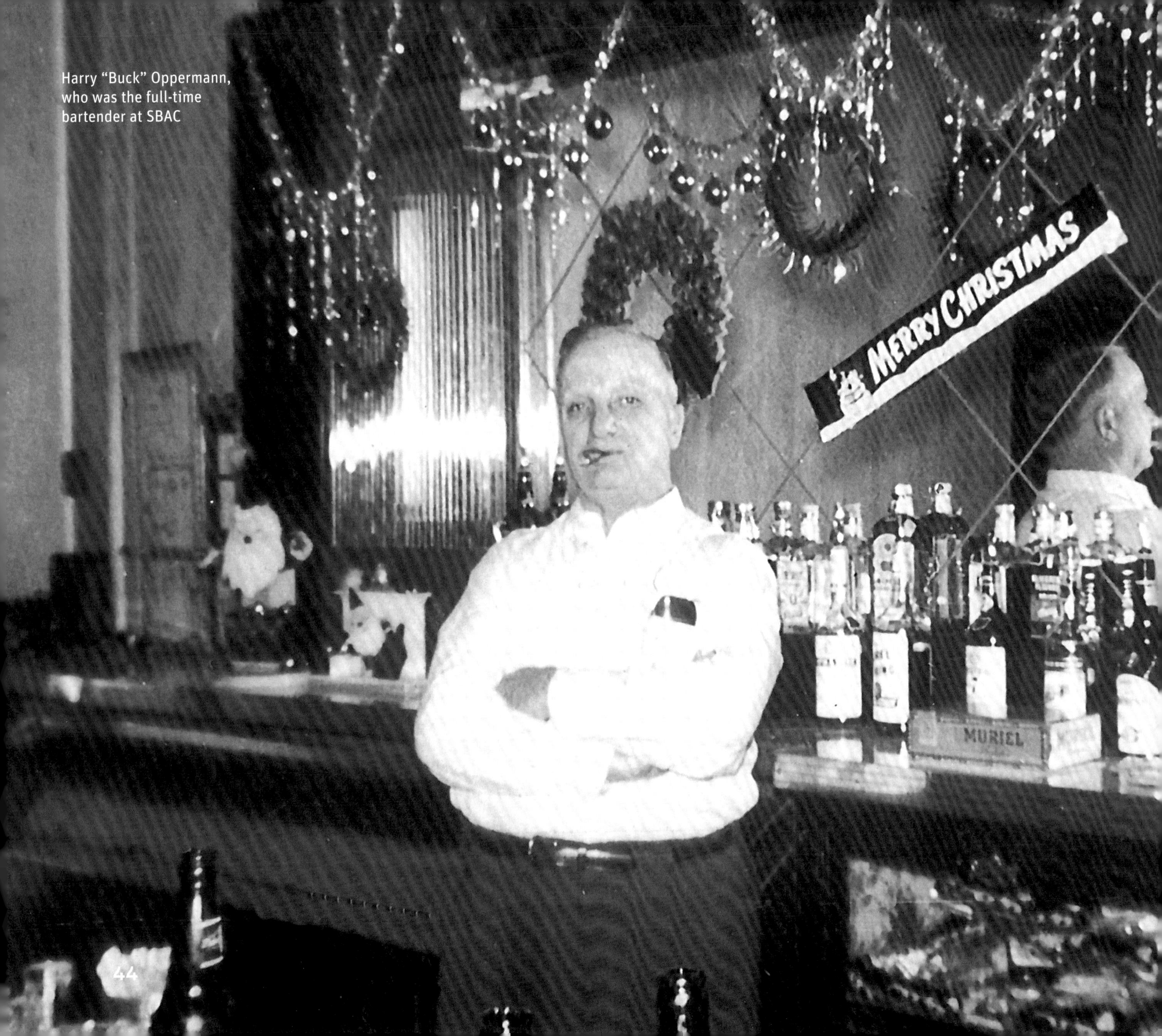

Harry "Buck" Oppermann, who was the full-time bartender at SBAC

I can remember in 1945 when I was 17 years old coming down at S.B.A.C for dances. The price was $3.00 a couple with all the beer. We had live music with Joe Rodree I danced with Ray Dierkes & my sister with Bob Dierkes. We had a ball every Sat. nite.

If you came by yourself it was $1.50. We never had any problems.

Then Hog & I met we married & had our Wedding reception there on Oct. 29, 1949.

Millie & Hog

Handwritten memories from Millie and Hog, who met at a weekly SBAC dance and had their wedding reception at South Broadway on October 29, 1945

Members of the Ladies Auxiliary at the Fall Dance

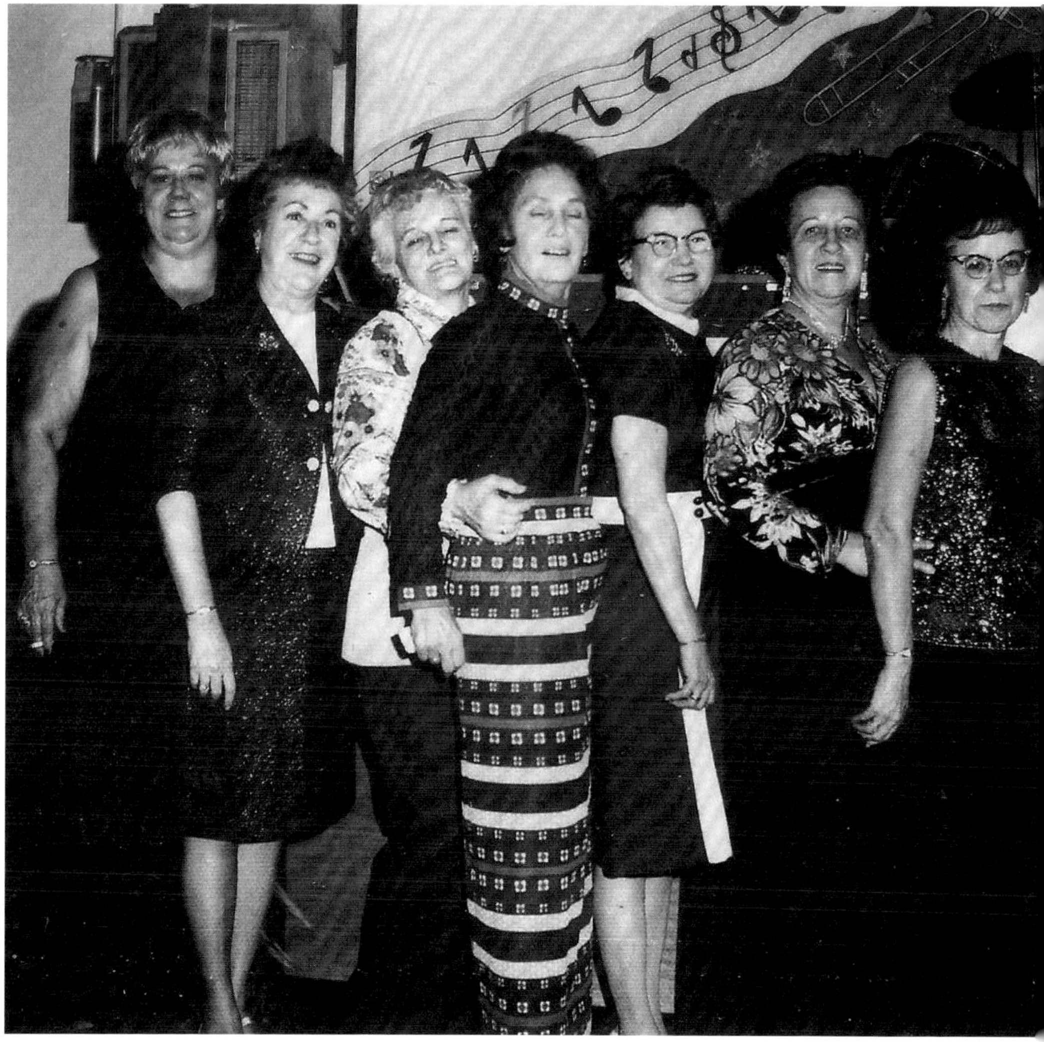

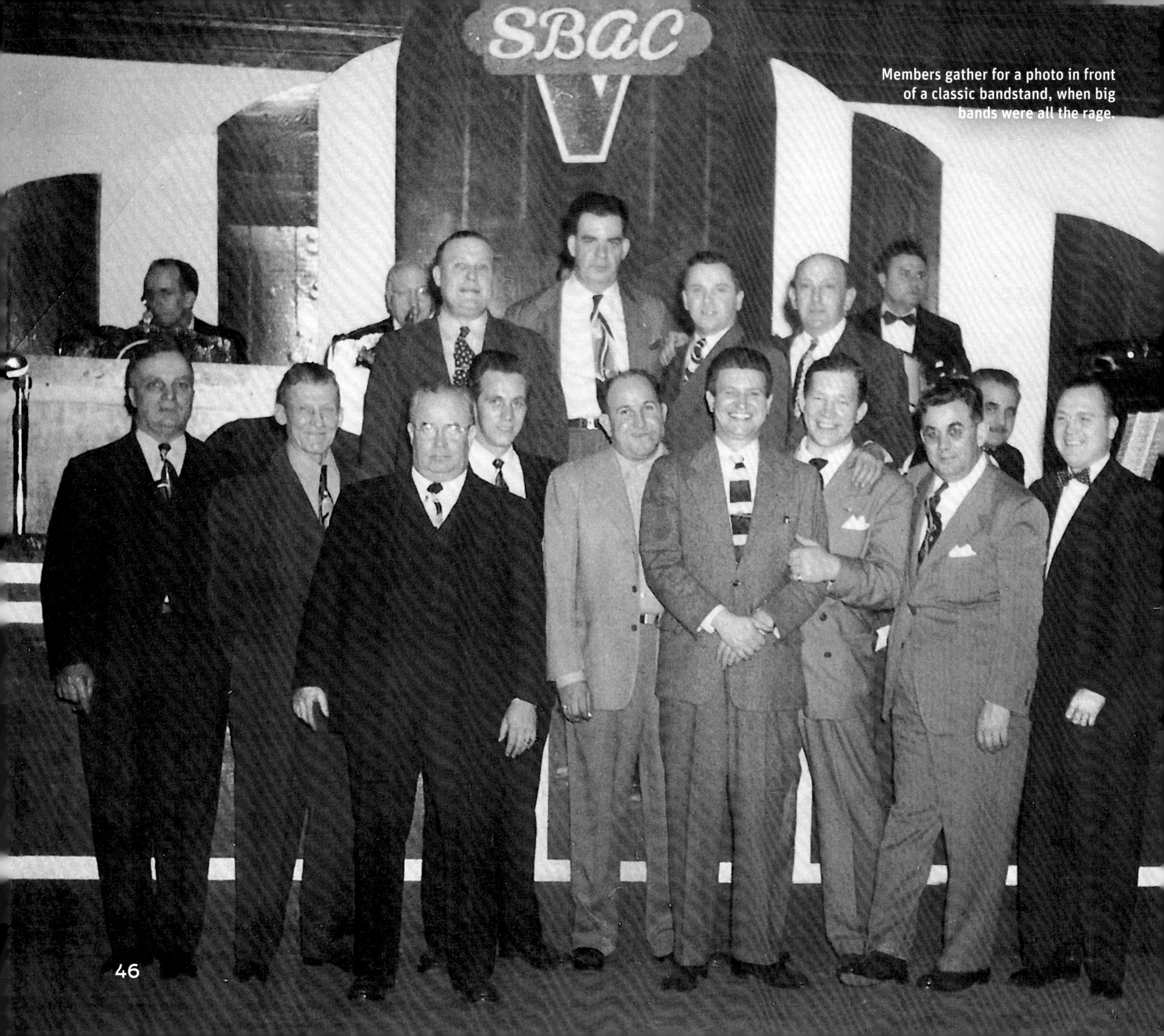

Members gather for a photo in front of a classic bandstand, when big bands were all the rage.

"Memories of Elvis" shows, which were an annual must-see tradition for all of St. Louis. Bluegrass Brunches offered Sunday afternoon bluegrass music paired with the fine cooking skills of the barbecue crew. The SBAC hosted the Punk Rock Pig Roast for the fourth time in 2024.

Local band The Maness Brothers brought the Whiskey War Festival to the Club in 2017. Described as a heavy

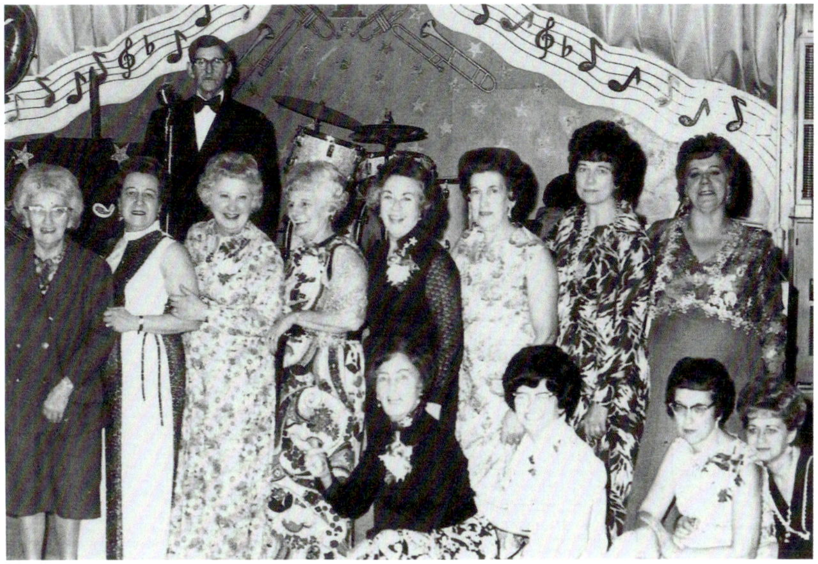

Ladies attending the Diamond Jubilee dance in 1974

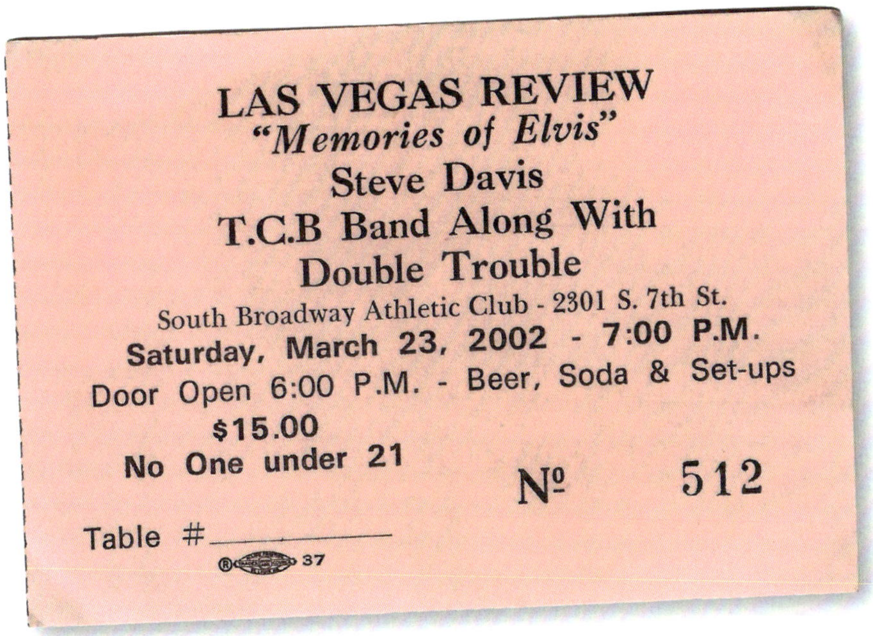

LAS VEGAS REVIEW
"Memories of Elvis"
Steve Davis
T.C.B Band Along With
Double Trouble
South Broadway Athletic Club - 2301 S. 7th St.
Saturday, March 23, 2002 - 7:00 P.M.
Door Open 6:00 P.M. - Beer, Soda & Set-ups
$15.00
No One under 21
№ 512
Table #
37

Ticket for the 2002 Las Vegas Review "Memories of Elvis"

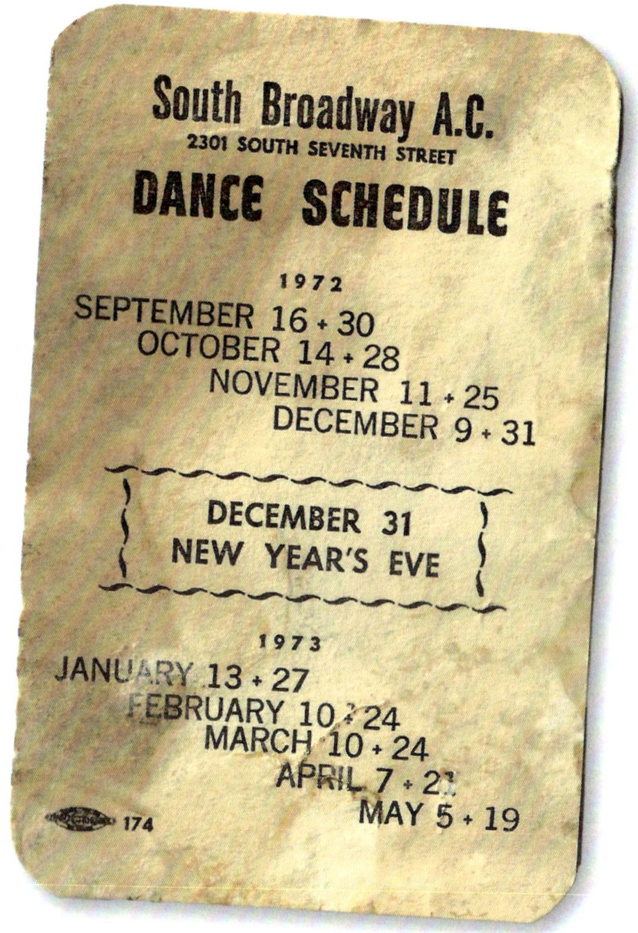

South Broadway A.C.
2301 SOUTH SEVENTH STREET
DANCE SCHEDULE
1972
SEPTEMBER 16 + 30
OCTOBER 14 + 28
NOVEMBER 11 + 25
DECEMBER 9 + 31
DECEMBER 31
NEW YEAR'S EVE
1973
JANUARY 13 + 27
FEBRUARY 10 + 24
MARCH 10 + 24
APRIL 7 + 2
MAY 5 + 19
174

Event ticket for the 1972 Dance Schedule

LADIES AUXILIARY

FOR 50 YEARS, whenever an SBAC event needed a touch of hospitality—whether it was boxing, wrestling, bingo, or a funeral luncheon—the Ladies Auxiliary was there to provide it.

South Broadway was founded in 1899 as a men's club, and in 1966 the general membership voted to form the Ladies Auxiliary. Those meeting notes recorded: "Cards are to be mailed to members' wives, informing them of said proposition and get their reactions!" Little did they know at the time that the Ladies Auxiliary would prove vital in keeping the SBAC afloat in the years to come.

Having an official women's arm helped foster a sense of family and community in the club. It also provided for some much-needed organization and help at events. The Ladies Auxiliary was involved in almost every major event hosted by the SBAC.

The women's organization developed into a robust and organized group, with its own officers, bank accounts, meetings, and newsletter. The women ran the kitchen for all major events, and their food sales helped pay certain bills and fund key upgrades such as bathroom fixtures, outdoor furniture, and repair of the floor in the Shenandoah entrance. At its height, there were 30 to 40 women involved in the group, most of whom were wives of club members. The last Lady President, as the head officer was called, was Cheryl Bauman. She recalled how the women were divided into four teams, with each team taking responsibility for staffing the kitchen (or whatever was needed) one weekend a month.

In the early 2000s and 2010s, when the club was struggling financially, the Ladies Auxiliary was there to help. The SBAC was strapped for cash, so the women would often loan the club money to pay for necessary expenditures for the annual Soulard Mardi Gras—the biggest revenue generator of the year and vital to the club's existence.

Eventually, in 2016 when new leadership took over, the Ladies Auxiliary was approached about disbanding the anachronistic auxiliary group and joining the club as fully fledged members. They agreed it was time, and their remaining funds were used to buy a new freezer for the kitchen.

Since then the club has operated as one organization. Yet, from 1966 to 2016, the Ladies Auxiliary played a vital role in keeping the club together. There is little dispute that if not for the Ladies Auxiliary, the SBAC would not be here today.

—Miriam Moynihan

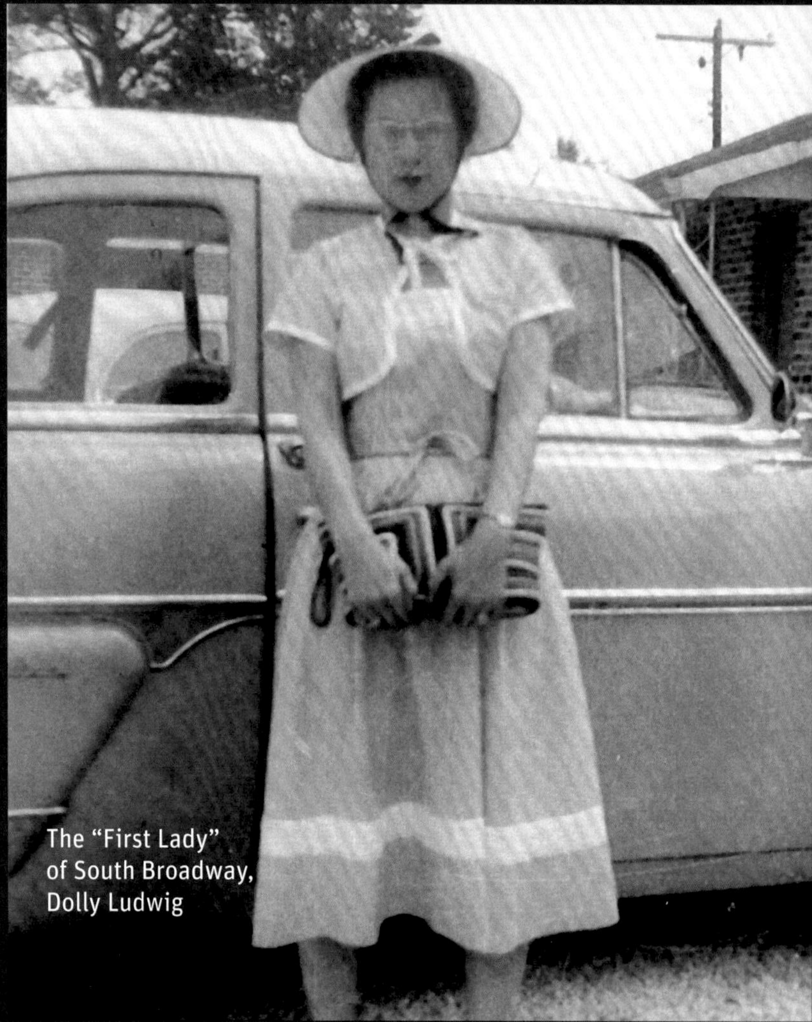

The "First Lady" of South Broadway, Dolly Ludwig

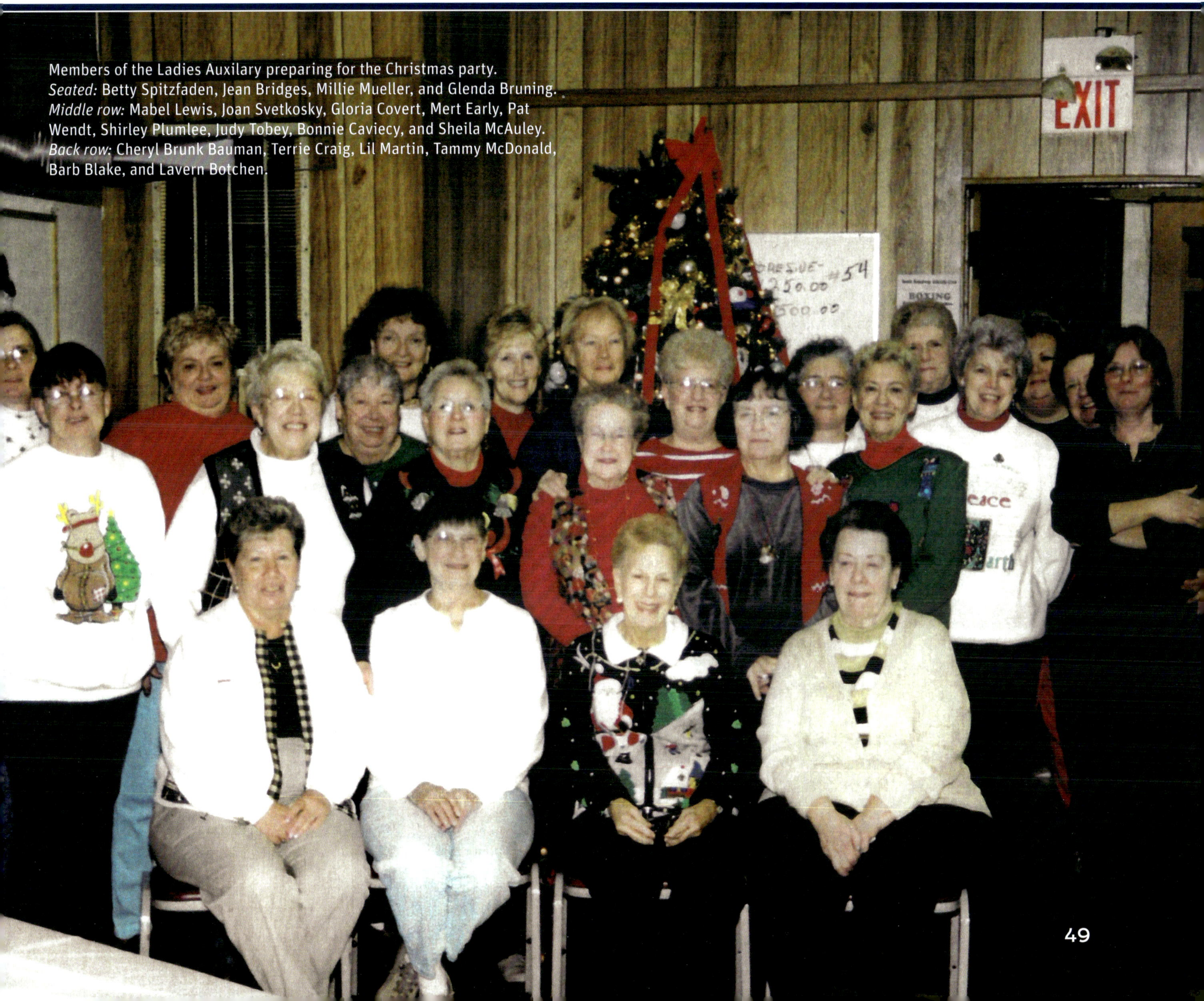

Members of the Ladies Auxilary preparing for the Christmas party. *Seated:* Betty Spitzfaden, Jean Bridges, Millie Mueller, and Glenda Bruning. *Middle row:* Mabel Lewis, Joan Svetkosky, Gloria Covert, Mert Early, Pat Wendt, Shirley Plumlee, Judy Tobey, Bonnie Caviecy, and Sheila McAuley. *Back row:* Cheryl Brunk Bauman, Terrie Craig, Lil Martin, Tammy McDonald, Barb Blake, and Lavern Botchen.

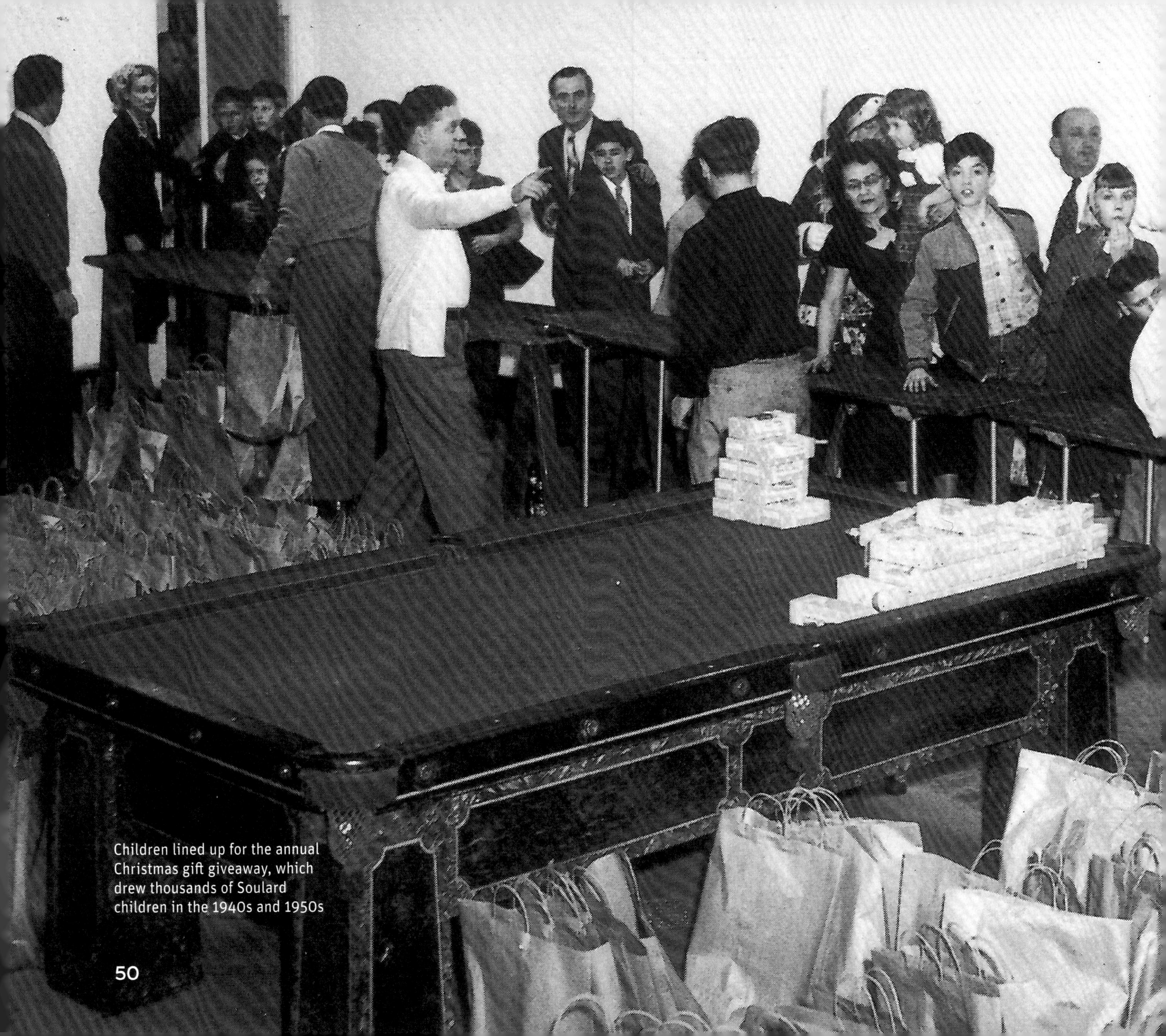

Children lined up for the annual Christmas gift giveaway, which drew thousands of Soulard children in the 1940s and 1950s

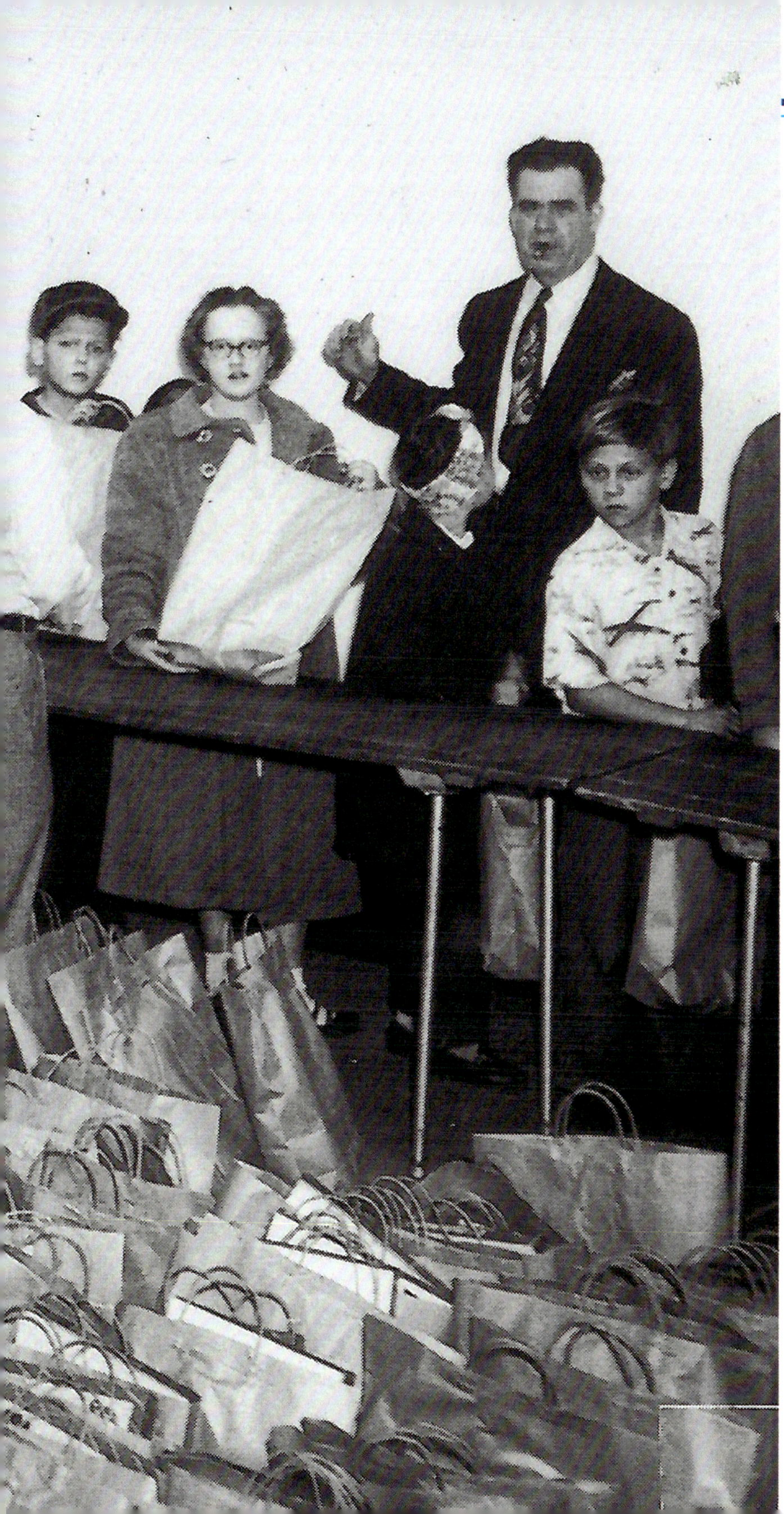

blues-rock showcase, Whiskey War attracted bands from across the Midwest and as far away as Alaska. For the past seven years, South Broadway has presented The *Last Waltz* show on the night before Thanksgiving. This event, growing out of the Stag Nite All-Stars collaboration (which began at the old Magee's Bar), brings an ever-rotating collection of the finest musicians in St. Louis performing the songs from the iconic Martin Scorsese film *The Last Waltz*, which documented The Band's 1976 farewell concert.

1978-79 Fish Fry, Dance, and *Amateur Sport Show Schedule*

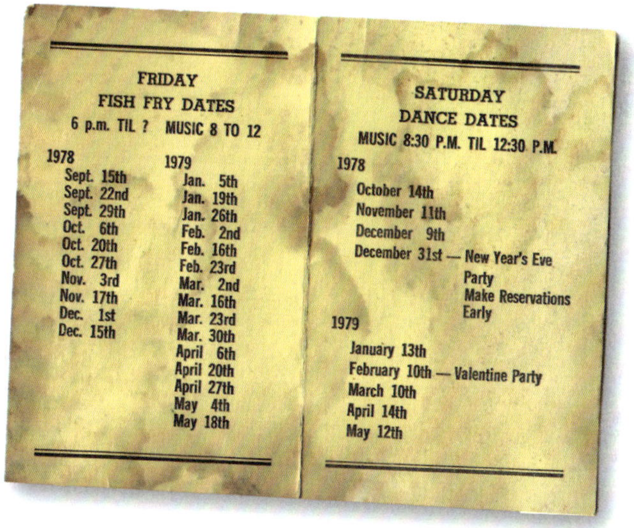

FRIDAY
FISH FRY DATES
6 p.m. TIL ? MUSIC 8 TO 12

1978
Sept. 15th
Sept. 22nd
Sept. 29th
Oct. 6th
Oct. 20th
Oct. 27th
Nov. 3rd
Nov. 17th
Dec. 1st
Dec. 15th

1979
Jan. 5th
Jan. 19th
Jan. 26th
Feb. 2nd
Feb. 16th
Feb. 23rd
Mar. 2nd
Mar. 16th
Mar. 23rd
Mar. 30th
April 6th
April 20th
April 27th
May 4th
May 18th

SATURDAY
DANCE DATES
MUSIC 8:30 P.M. TIL 12:30 P.M.

1978
October 14th
November 11th
December 9th
December 31st — New Year's Eve Party
Make Reservations Early

1979
January 13th
February 10th — Valentine Party
March 10th
April 14th
May 12th

1989 Cinema Races

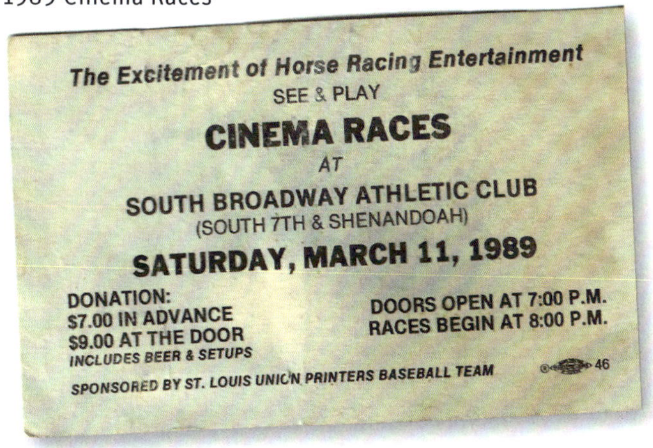

The Excitement of Horse Racing Entertainment
SEE & PLAY
CINEMA RACES
AT
SOUTH BROADWAY ATHLETIC CLUB
(SOUTH 7TH & SHENANDOAH)
SATURDAY, MARCH 11, 1989

DONATION:
$7.00 IN ADVANCE
$9.00 AT THE DOOR
INCLUDES BEER & SETUPS

DOORS OPEN AT 7:00 P.M.
RACES BEGIN AT 8:00 P.M.

SPONSORED BY ST. LOUIS UNION PRINTERS BASEBALL TEAM

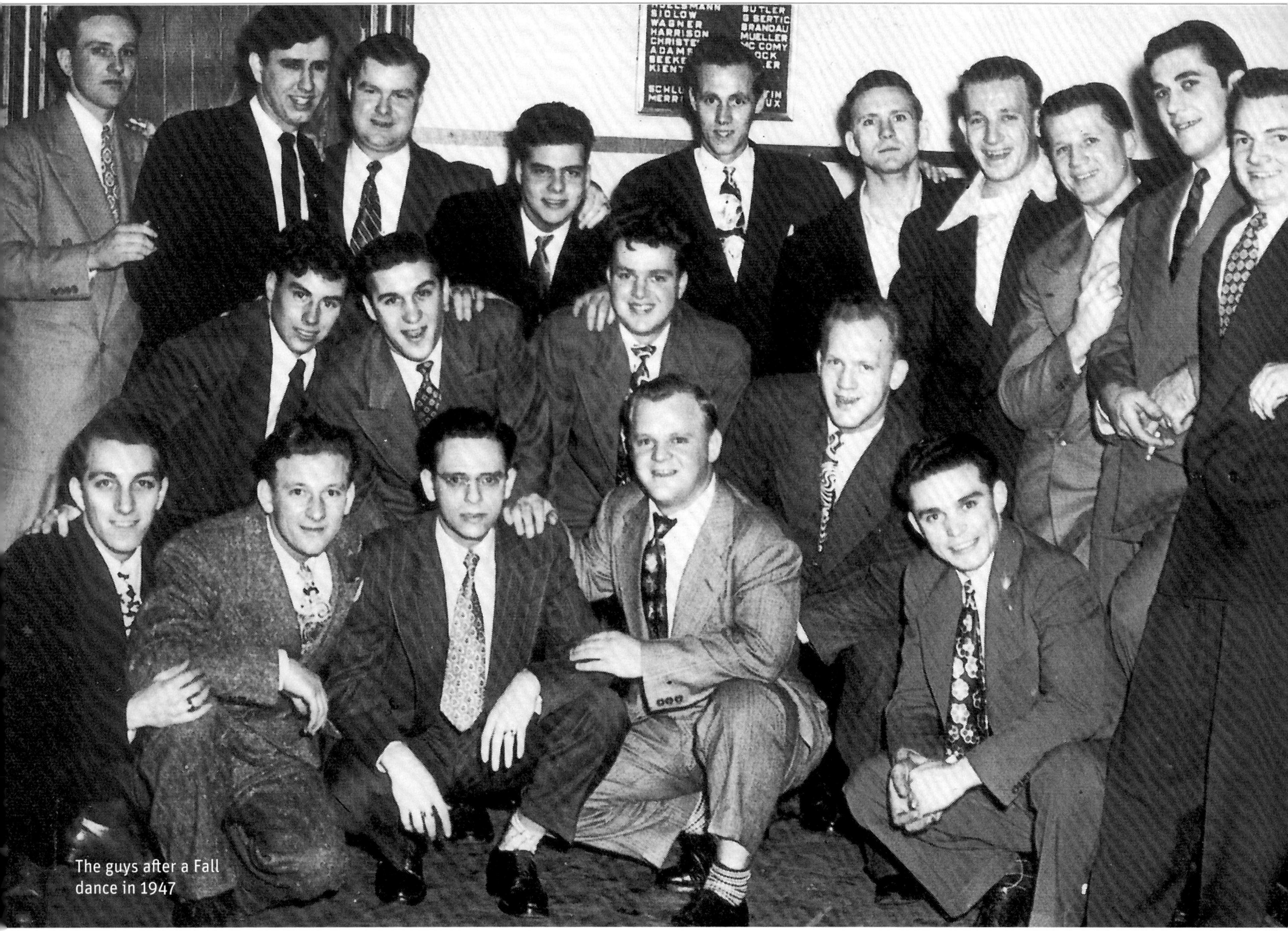

The guys after a Fall dance in 1947

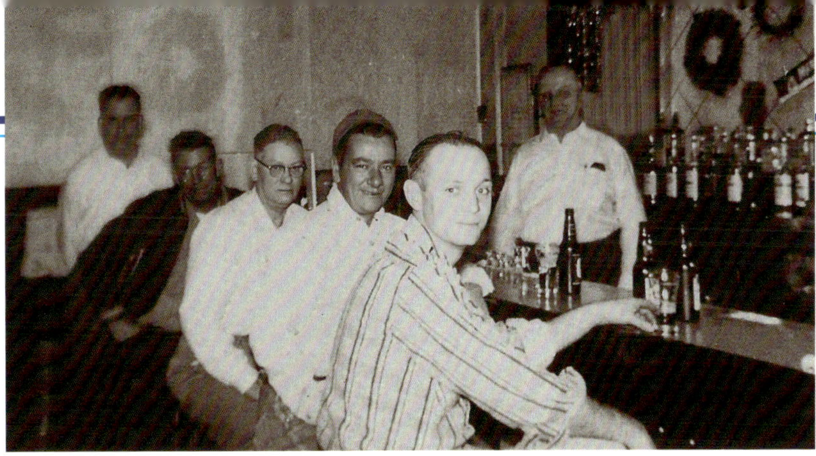

Members bellied up to the bar: George Ludwig (left), Carl Godbey, Monty Simpson, Bill Schlueter, and Ralph Riess, with Harry "Buck" Oppermann behind the bar

From the mid-1990s through early 2010s, the largest social event and fundraiser for SBAC was the weekly bingo events. These game nights became so popular that they were expanded to three nights per week, and seating in the back Members Only room had to be opened to handle the crowds. Still filling the back room for many years are the traditional South City Meat Shoots.

Another popular event in the mid-2000s was Spaghetti Wrestling. Promoted as a fundraiser, spaghetti wrestling brought neighborhood icons together to battle it out in a pool of spaghetti,

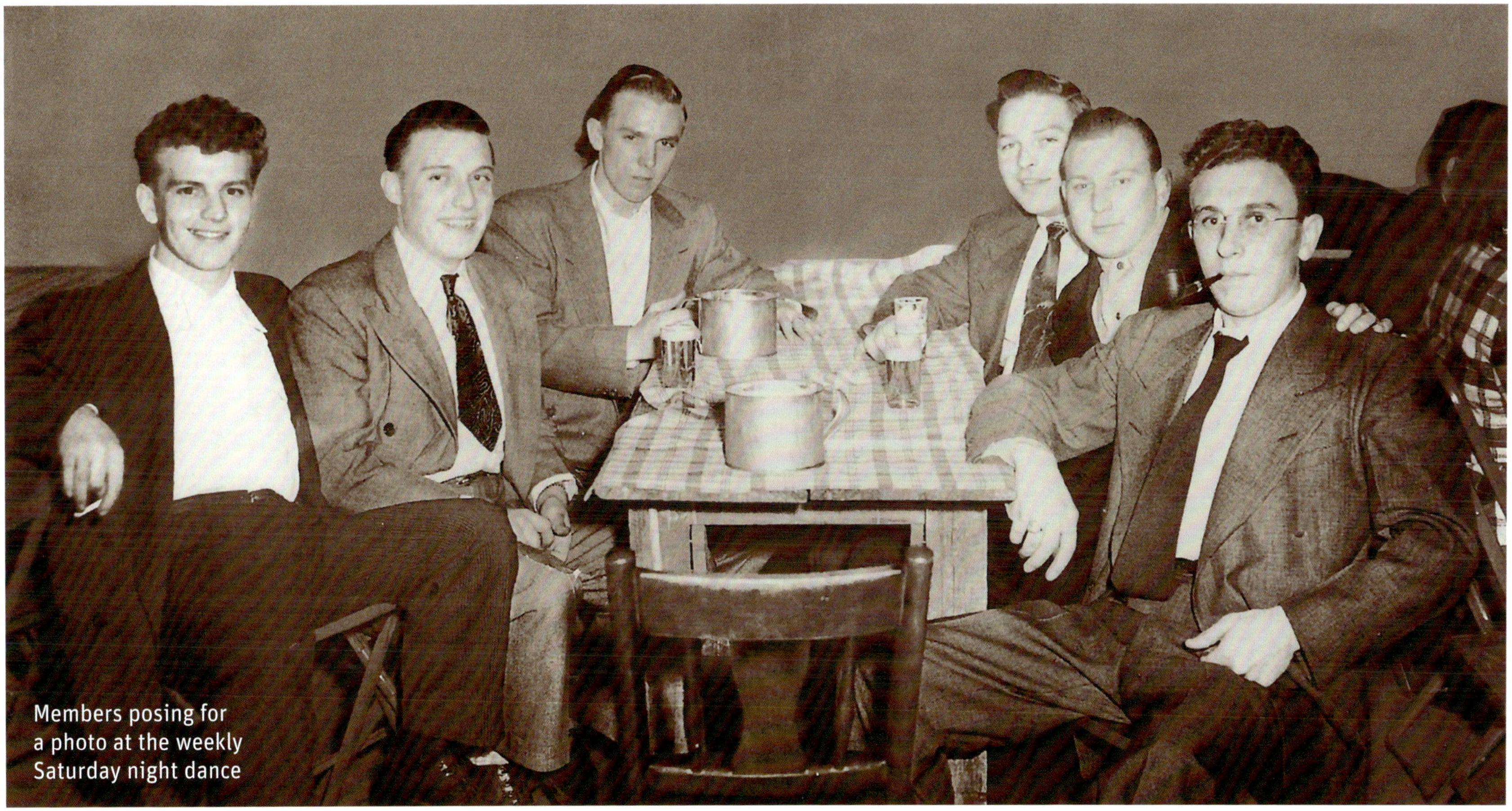

Members posing for a photo at the weekly Saturday night dance

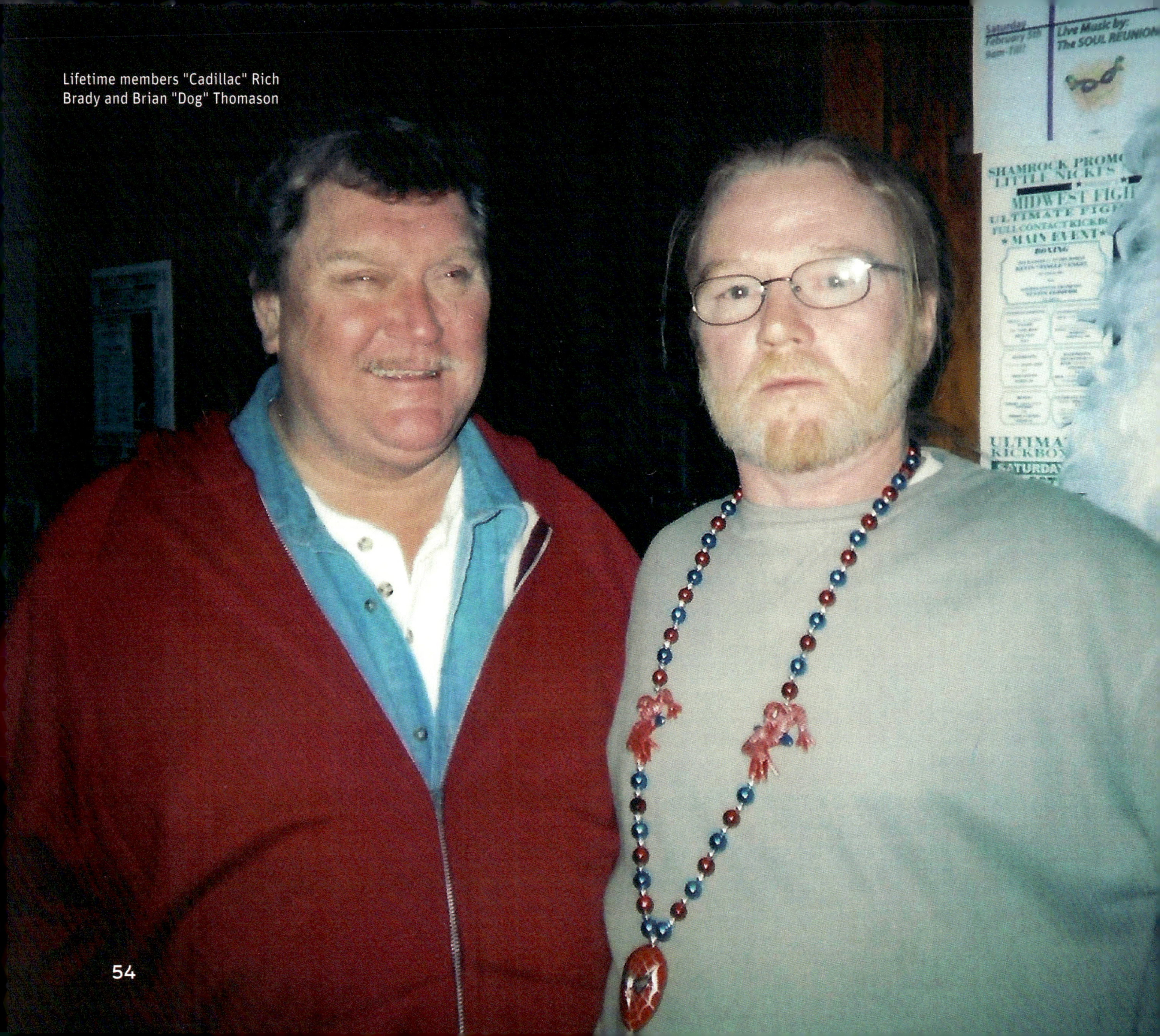

Lifetime members "Cadillac" Rich Brady and Brian "Dog" Thomason

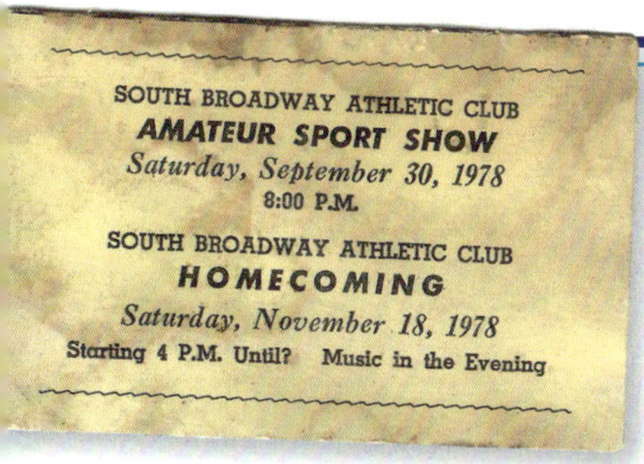

SOUTH BROADWAY ATHLETIC CLUB
AMATEUR SPORT SHOW
Saturday, September 30, 1978
8:00 P.M.

SOUTH BROADWAY ATHLETIC CLUB
HOMECOMING
Saturday, November 18, 1978
Starting 4 P.M. Until? Music in the Evening

A ticket for an amateur sports show and homecoming event

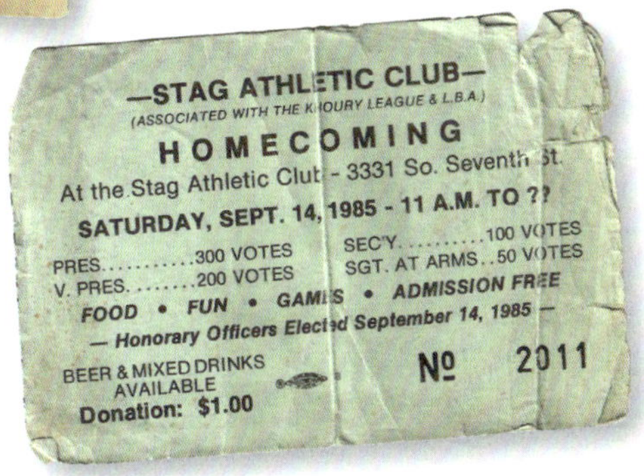

—STAG ATHLETIC CLUB—
(ASSOCIATED WITH THE KHOURY LEAGUE & L.B.A.)
HOMECOMING
At the Stag Athletic Club - 3331 So. Seventh St.
SATURDAY, SEPT. 14, 1985 - 11 A.M. TO ??
PRES............300 VOTES SEC'Y..........100 VOTES
V. PRES.........200 VOTES SGT. AT ARMS..50 VOTES
FOOD • FUN • GAMES • ADMISSION FREE
— Honorary Officers Elected September 14, 1985 —
BEER & MIXED DRINKS AVAILABLE
Donation: $1.00
№ 2011

A ticket for the 1985 Stag Athletic Club Homecoming

supplied by local restaurateur Joanie Spurgeon of Joanie's Pizza fame. Attendees would feast on an all-you-can-eat spaghetti dinner while cheering on those wrestling in a pool of sloppy pasta.

The Friday Fish Fry was a staple of the club in the early days. A flier from the 1978–79 season shows three weeks per month when the SBAC doors were open on Friday nights for fried fish and beer socials. In recent years, members have reintroduced the Fish Fry as a Good Friday event to bring members and neighbors together.

Social events keep our members involved and excited about continuing the legacy of the South Broadway Athletic Club. As new generations of members take on the traditions of the past 125 years and work to ensure the next century and more of our organization, we always welcome new ideas for events. Many recent events, such as Queen of Hearts raffles, trivia nights, washer tournaments, and Ladies Night Bunko, have provided a boost needed to attract new members. The past few years have proven the future is bright for SBAC. As lifetime member and SBAC Hall of Famer Rick Lanius always said, "It's a grand old club!"

— Dan Guenther

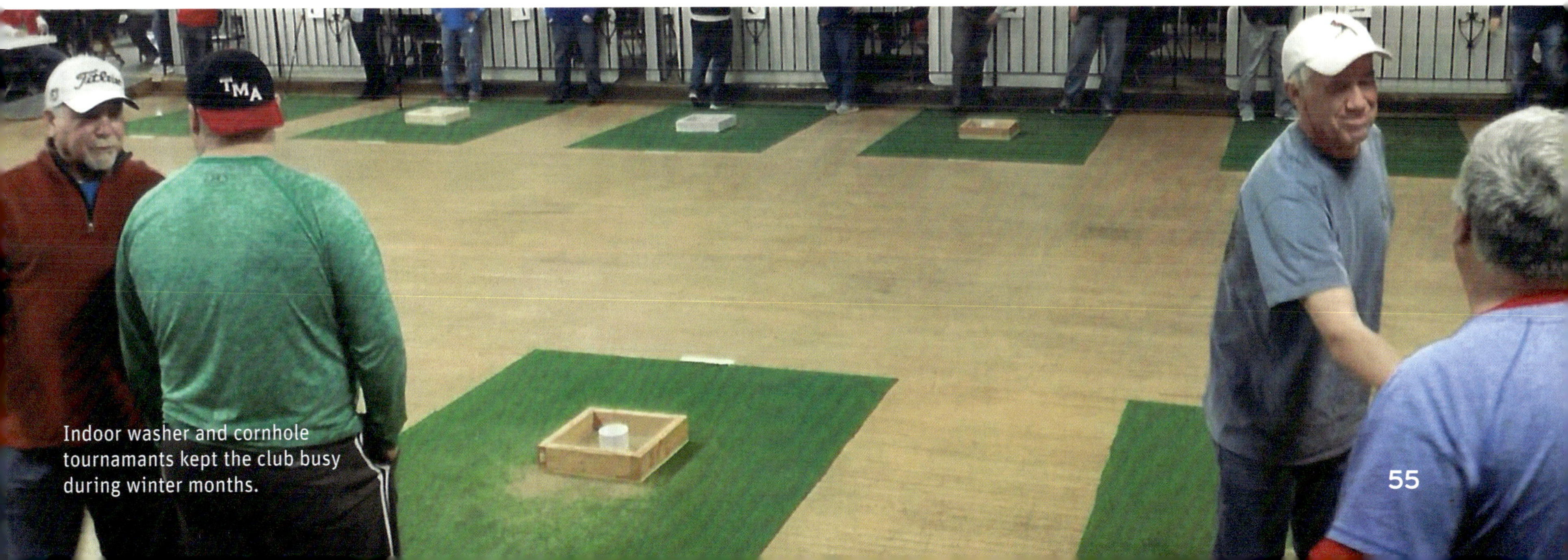

Indoor washer and cornhole tournamants kept the club busy during winter months.

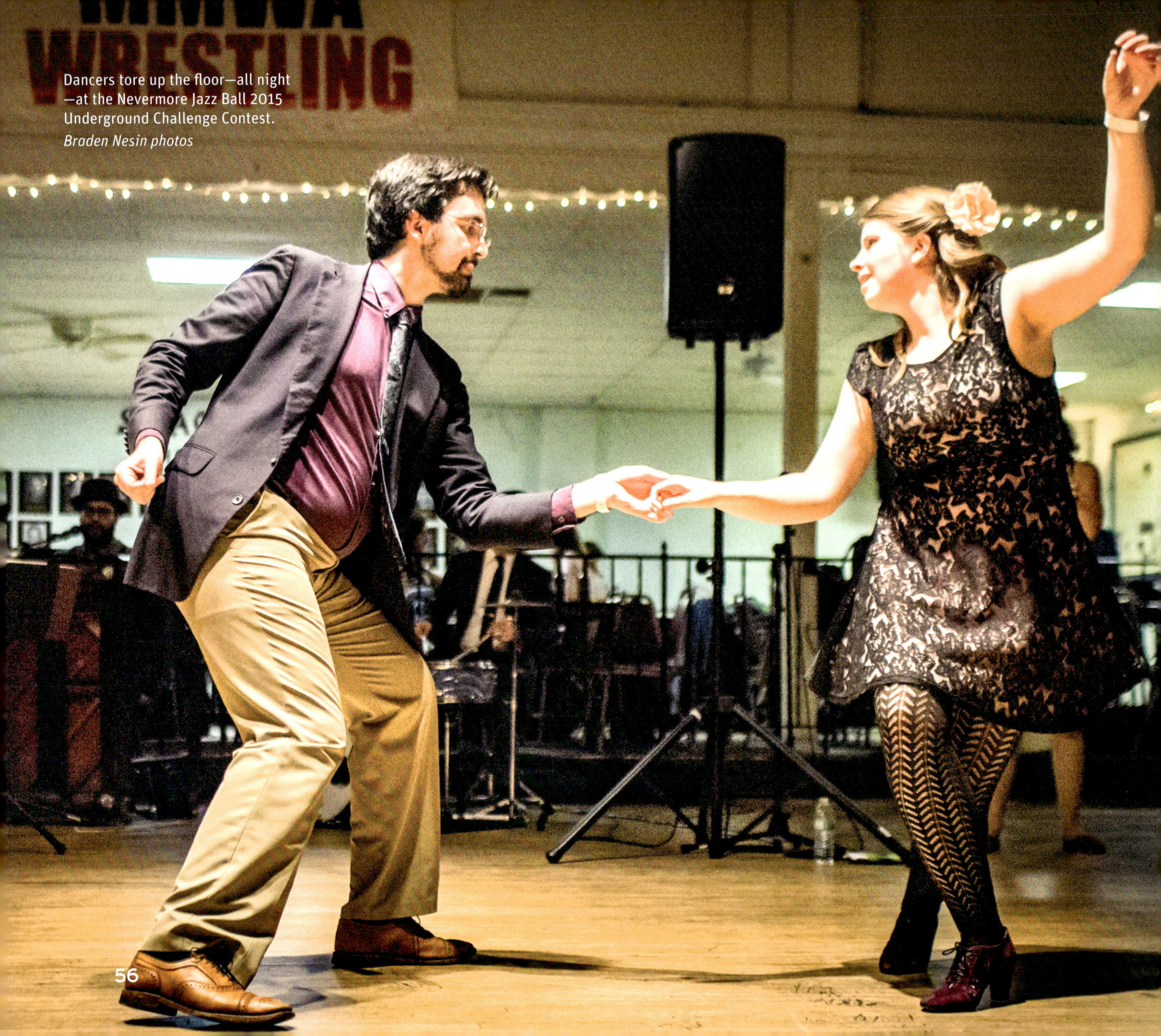

Dancers tore up the floor—all night—at the Nevermore Jazz Ball 2015 Underground Challenge Contest.
Braden Nesin photos

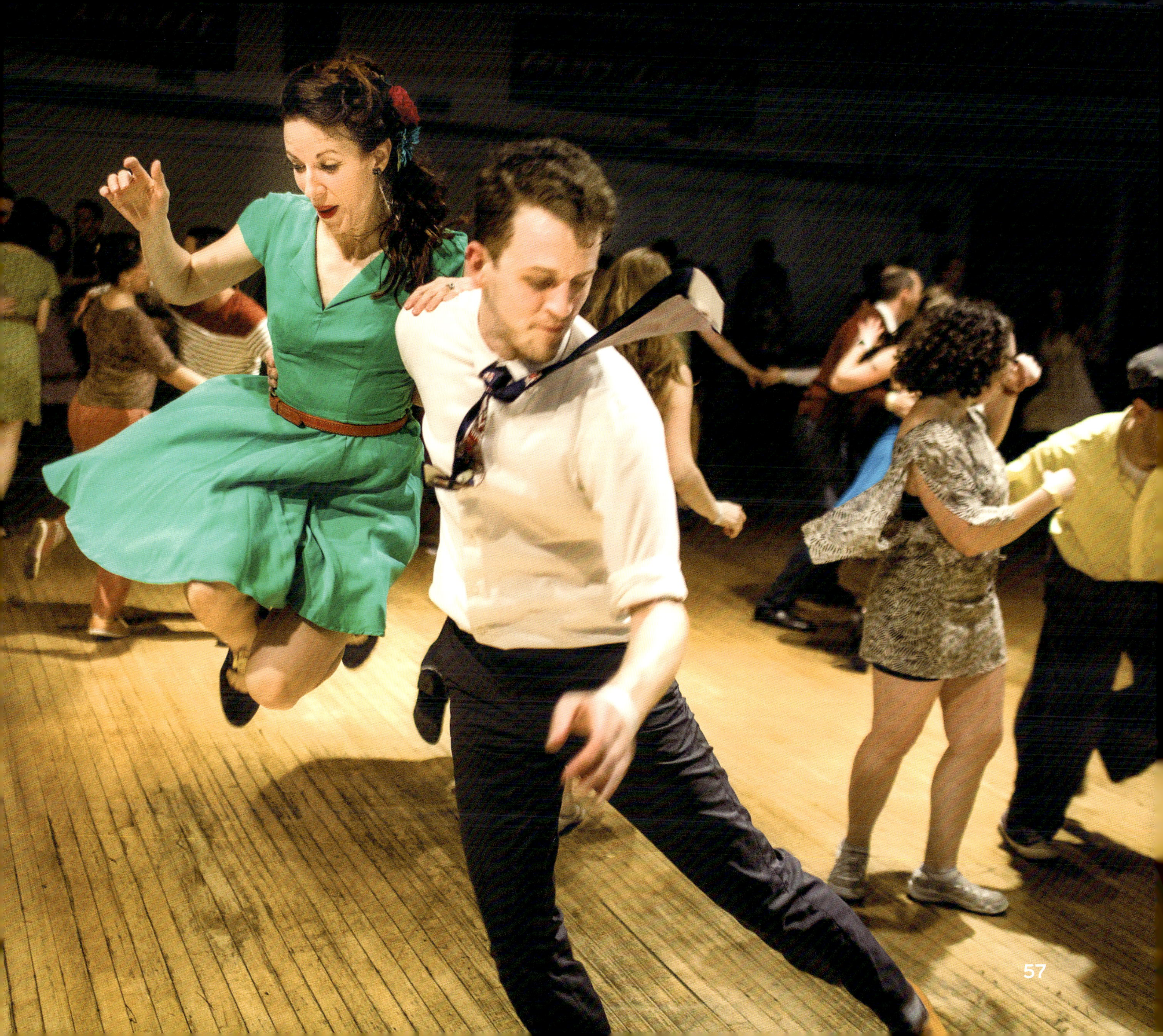

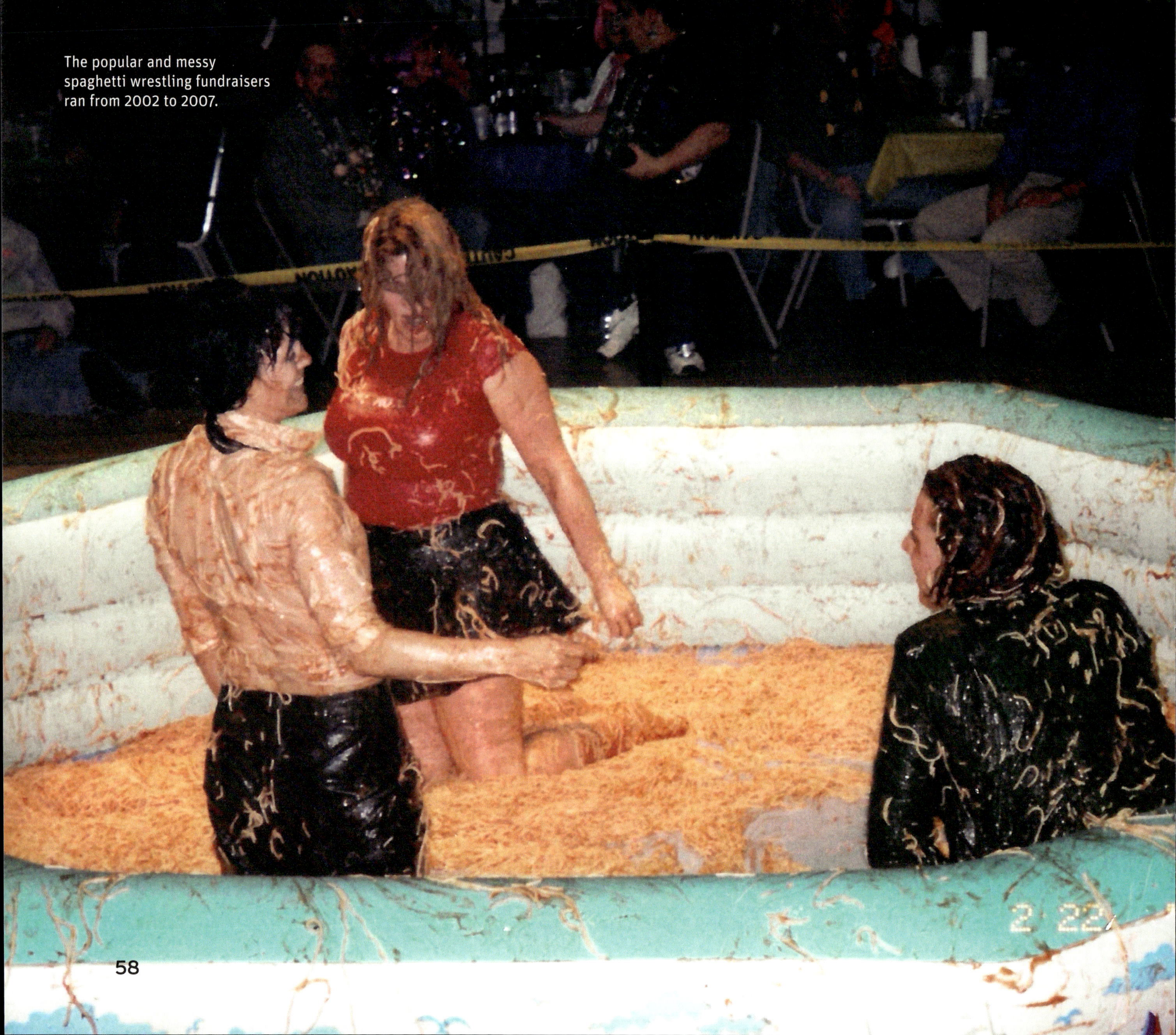

The popular and messy spaghetti wrestling fundraisers ran from 2002 to 2007.

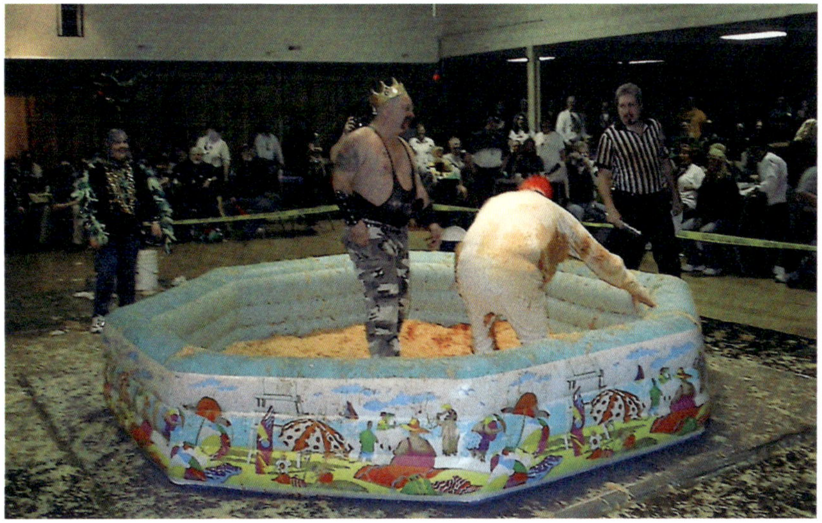

Costumes and characters made spaghetti wrestling the place to be in St. Louis.

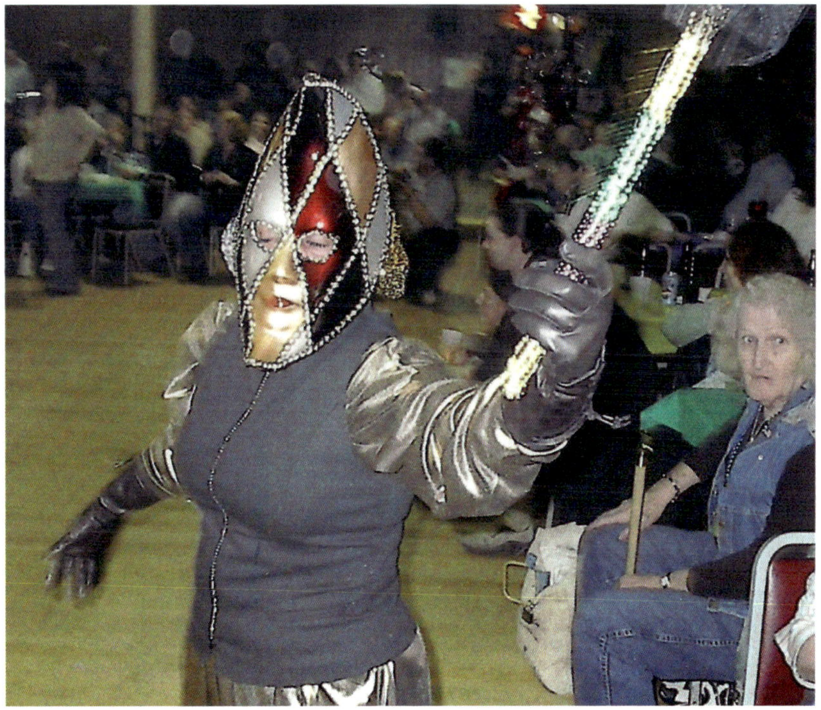

Historical Note

Soulard Evolution

Beginning with French settlement in the 18th century, Soulard was the port of entry for people emigrating from across Europe. Waves of Germans, Bohemians, and Eastern and Southern Europeans had built the Soulard neighborhood and given it a distinctive charm and sense of home.

Even after the United States virtually shut the door to immigration in 1924, Soulard continued to be the city's port of entry. The new residents, however, were not from foreign countries. They were White rural Americans. Like the Great Migration of Blacks from the deep South, this migration of Whites had left behind sharecropping and depressed small-town economies to find opportunities in industrializing cities. In St. Louis, they found rooms or apartments alongside the Eastern European families in the Soulard neighborhood. Their children filled the classrooms at St. Louis Public Schools, then one of the leading systems in the United States. Some of these new residents found a home at the SBAC.

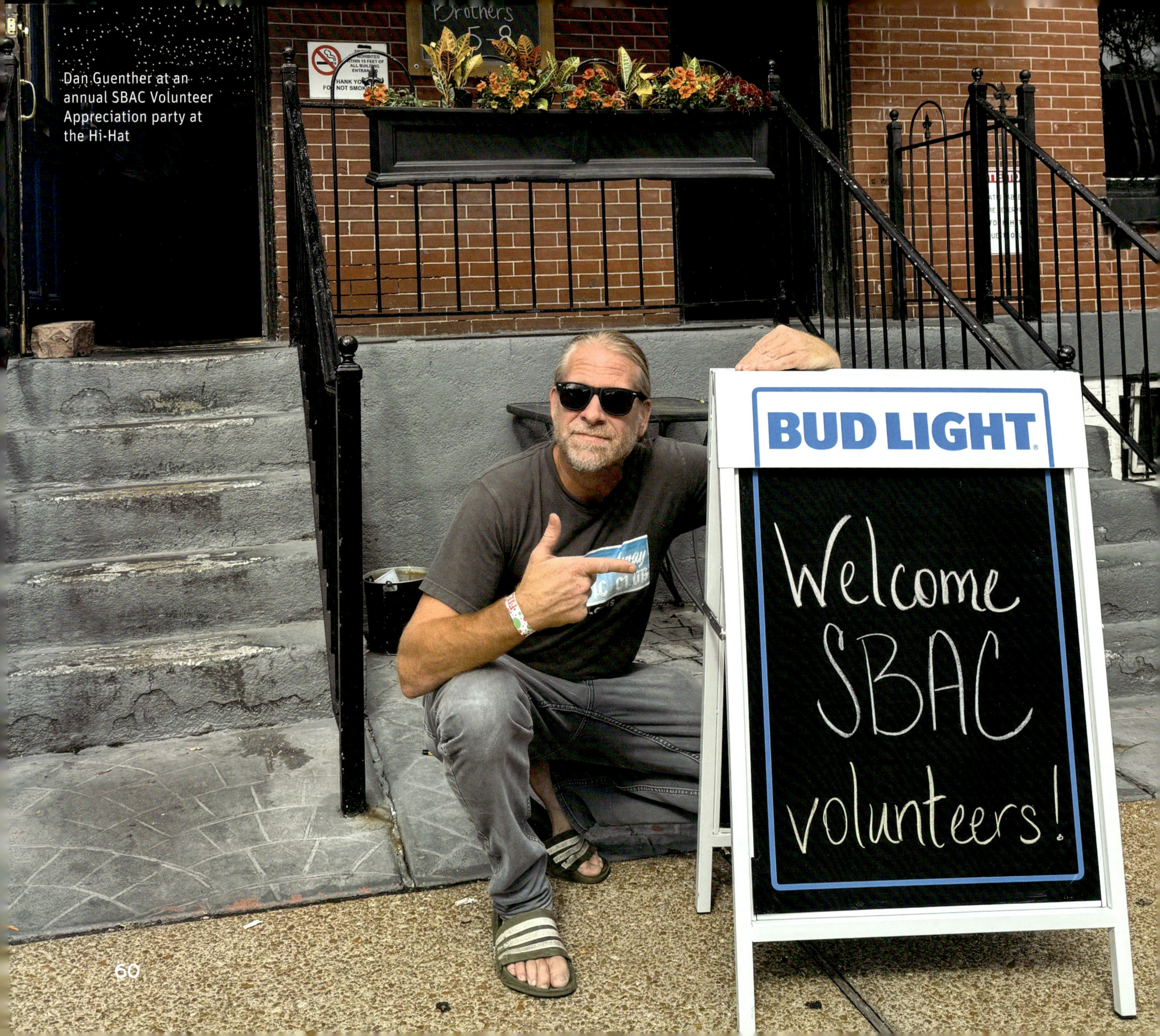

Dan Guenther at an annual SBAC Volunteer Appreciation party at the Hi-Hat

Chapter 4

Club as Community

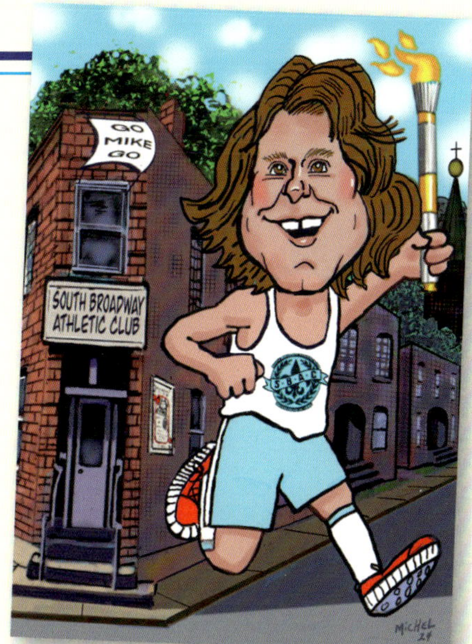

Lifetime member Mike Button carrying the 1996 Olympic torch for the SBAC

Bill Michel illustration

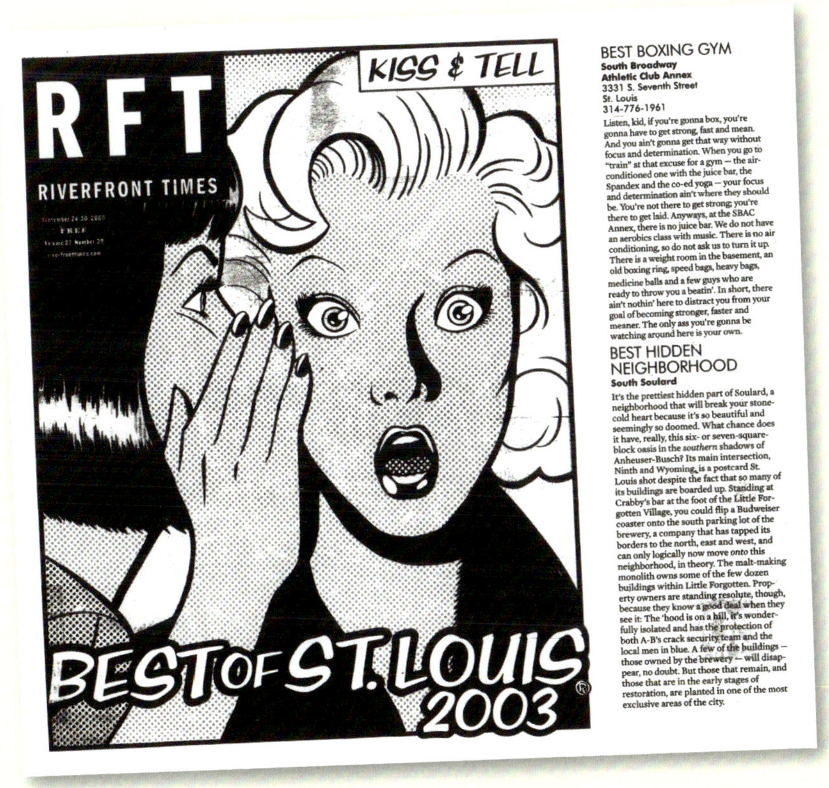

KISS & TELL

RFT

RIVERFRONT TIMES

BEST OF ST. LOUIS 2003

BEST BOXING GYM

South Broadway Athletic Club Annex
3331 S. Seventh Street
St. Louis
314-776-1961

Listen, kid, if you're gonna box, you're gonna have to get strong, fast and mean. And you ain't gonna get that way without focus and determination. When you go to "train" at that excuse for a gym — the air-conditioned one with the juice bar, the Spandex and the co-ed yoga — your focus and determination ain't where they should be. You're not there to get strong; you're there to get laid. Anyways, at the SBAC Annex, there is no juice bar. We do not have an aerobics class with music. There is no air conditioning, so do not ask us to turn it up. There is a weight room in the basement, an old boxing ring, speed bags, heavy bags, medicine balls and a few guys who are ready to throw you a beatin'. In short, there ain't nothin' here to distract you from your goal of becoming stronger, faster and meaner. The only ass you're gonna be watching around here is your own.

BEST HIDDEN NEIGHBORHOOD

South Soulard

It's the prettiest hidden part of Soulard, a neighborhood that will break your stone-cold heart because it's so beautiful and seemingly so doomed. What chance does it have, really, this six- or seven-square-block oasis in the *southern* shadows of Anheuser-Busch? Its main intersection, Ninth and Wyoming, is a postcard St. Louis shot despite the fact that so many of its buildings are boarded up. Standing at Crabby's bar at the foot of the Little Forgotten Village, you could flip a Budweiser coaster onto the south parking lot of the brewery, a company that has tapped its borders to the north, east and west, and can only logically now move *onto* this neighborhood, in theory. The malt-making monolith owns some of the few dozen buildings within Little Forgotten. Property owners are standing resolute, though, because they know a good deal when they see it: The 'hood is on a hill, it's wonderfully isolated and has the protection of both A-B's crack security team and the local men in blue. A few of the buildings — those owned by the brewery — will disappear, no doubt. But those that remain, and those that are in the early stages of restoration, are planted in one of the most exclusive areas of the city.

Riverfront Times article with SBAC winning best boxing gym (Best of St. Louis 2003)

THERE IS A LONG history of athletic clubs in St. Louis representing diverse communities, and the SBAC is no exception. While the founders in 1899 may have been looking to bring like-minded individuals together for sport, recreation, and fellowship, the history of the SBAC is that of a club that represents our community and gives back to our neighbors.

The founders were predominantly young German immigrants in the Soulard neighborhood. As the club evolved, many athletic and social organizations merged with South Broadway, as memberships waned or groups were looking for a more permanent location for their organizations. The Stag AC, the Monkeys AC, the Pirates AC, and the Millard Fillmore AC were all athletic clubs that brought all their members to the SBAC.

Of all the athletic organizations to merge with the SBAC, the most influential was Millard Fillmore AC, located at 11th Street and Barton in the Soulard neighborhood. In the 1970s and '80s,

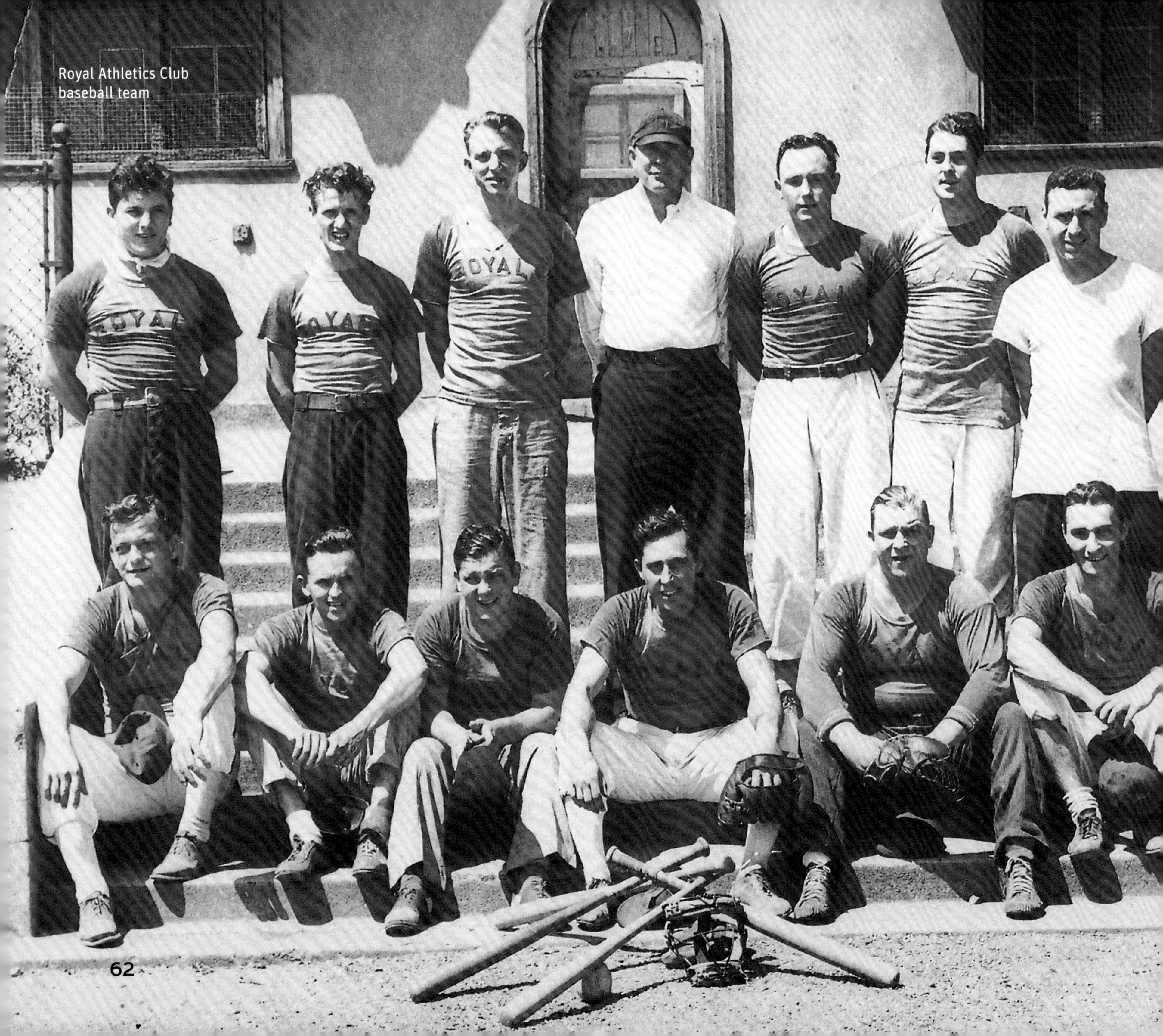

Royal Athletics Club
baseball team

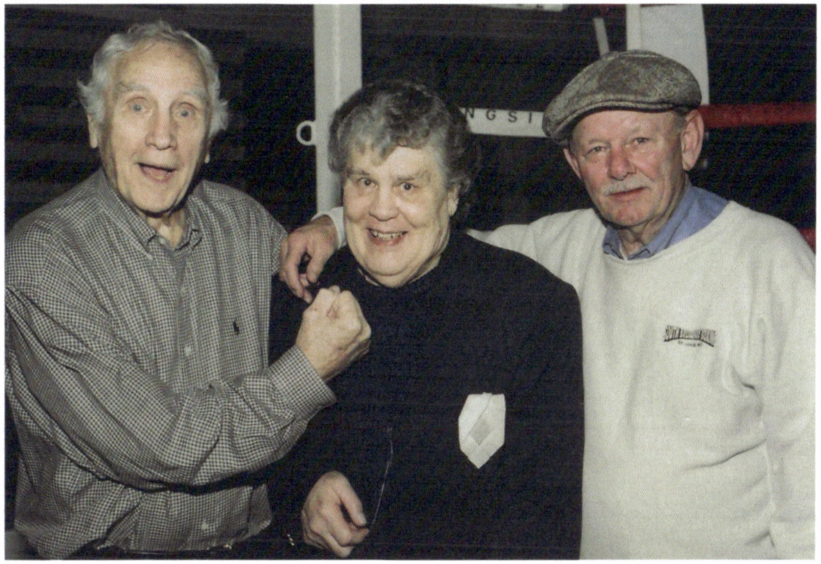

Boxing legends Mike Buha, Billy Stephan, and Coach Jim Hathman

Historical Note

Prizes

Titles and medals were great recognition for a victorious sportsman. The proud South Broadway merchants and businessmen, however, made sure that when the SBAC club members won a contest in the ring or a tournament that they were presented something of worth. The South Broadway merchants and businessmen contributed liberally for prizes—an overcoat or suit of clothes valued at $25, a watch worth $25, or a diamond stud costing $30. A supporter and local businessman, Bill Westhus, described the prizes for the fighters as "something that is some good to them."

Millard Fillmore was a group of young men in their mid 20s who would get together to compete against other athletic clubs in soccer, touch football, corkball, softball, and baseball. Former SBAC President George Bruning Jr., whose son Dale played softball for Millard Fillmore, attended one of their meetings and invited the members to come down and join the SBAC. This merging of clubs brought more than 80 new members to the SBAC in 1984. A few of those former Millard Fillmore AC members, including Dale Bruning, Mike Button, Craig Neumeister, and Brian Thomason, are still active at SBAC and celebrating 40 years as members.

Gateway Motors sponsored corkball team members
Martin Tyberend (left), Harry Oppermann, and Charlie Bolfing.

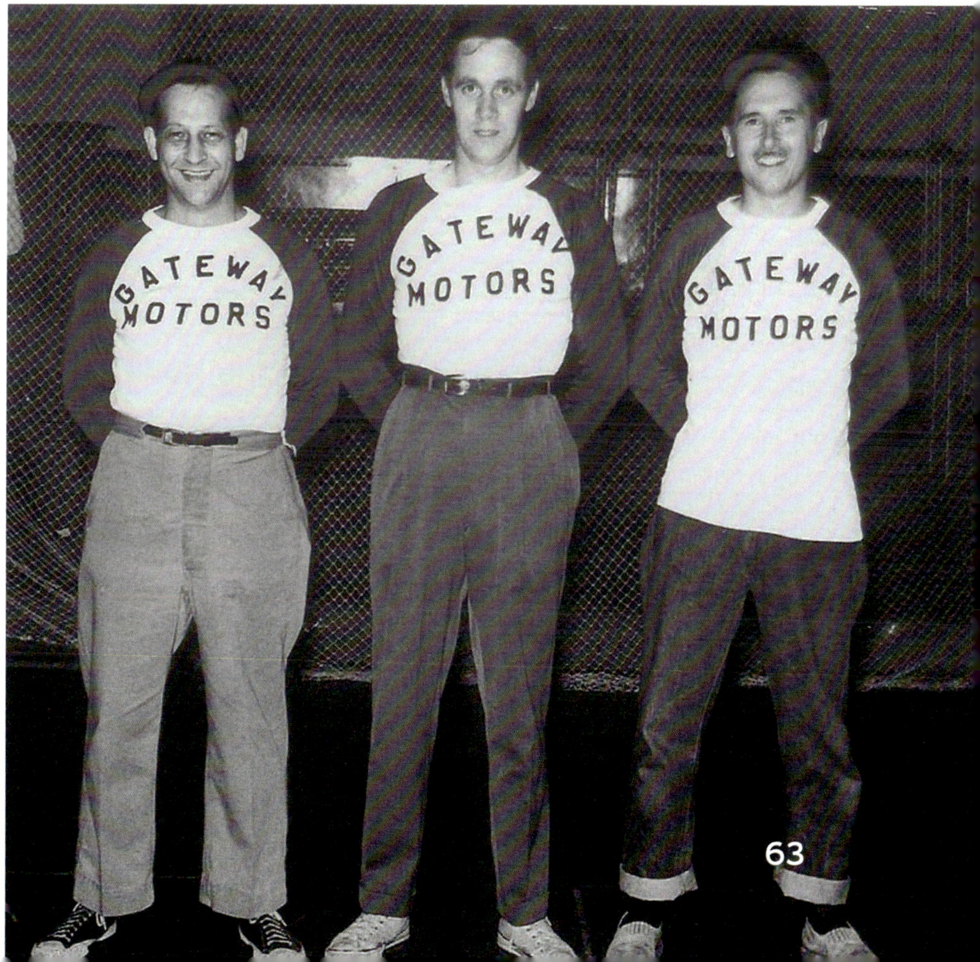

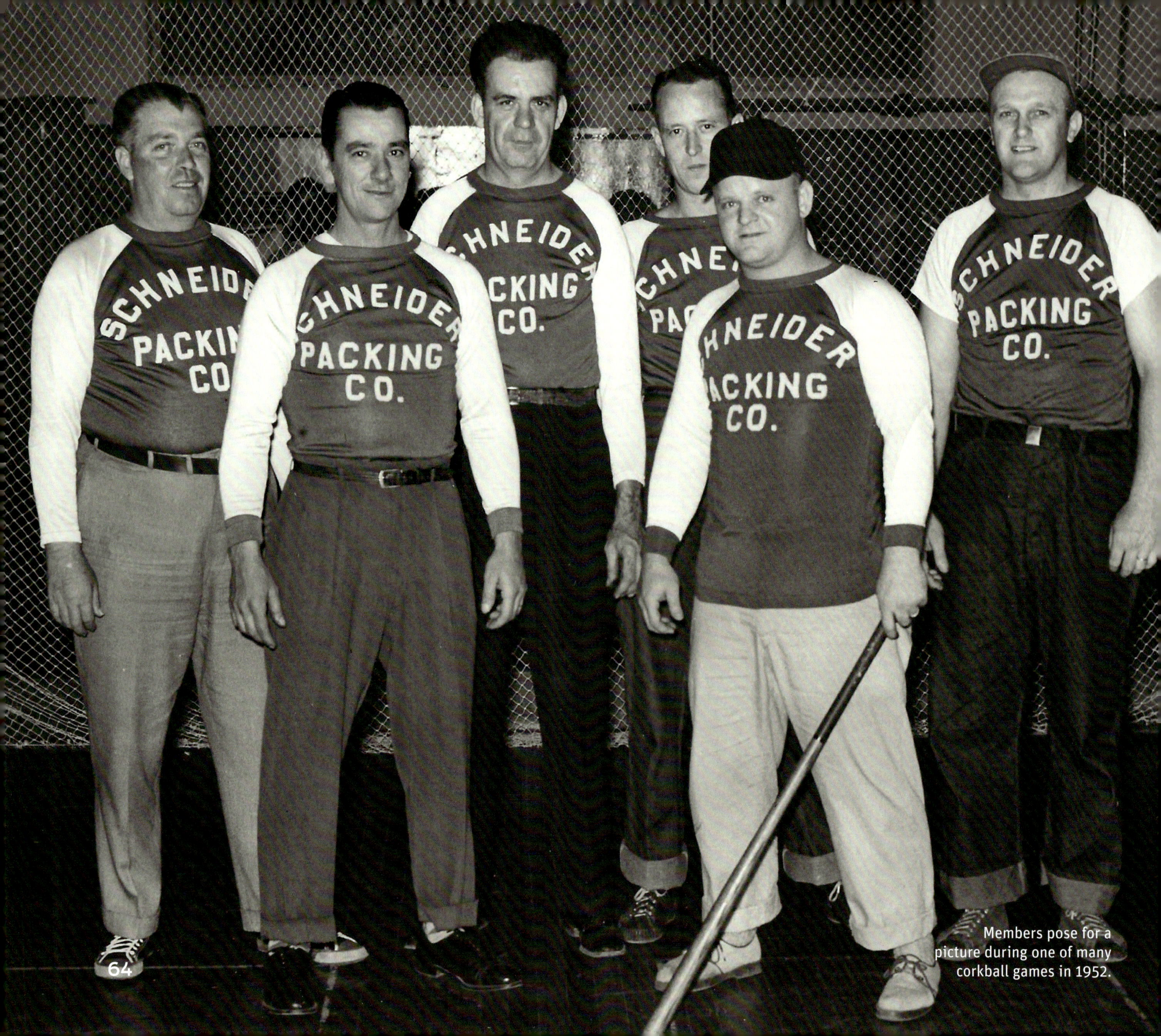

Members pose for a picture during one of many corkball games in 1952.

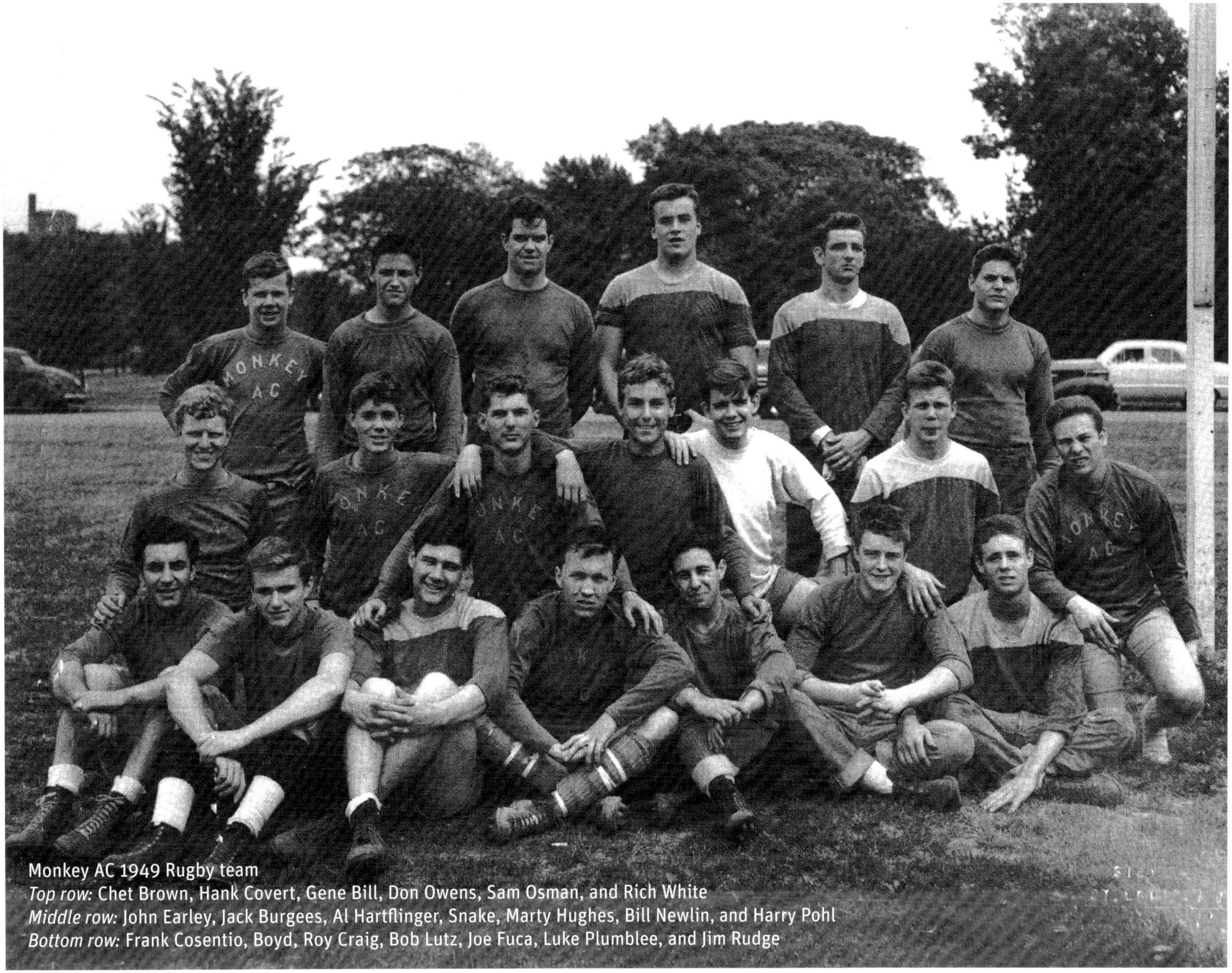

Monkey AC 1949 Rugby team
Top row: Chet Brown, Hank Covert, Gene Bill, Don Owens, Sam Osman, and Rich White
Middle row: John Earley, Jack Burgees, Al Hartflinger, Snake, Marty Hughes, Bill Newlin, and Harry Pohl
Bottom row: Frank Cosentio, Boyd, Roy Craig, Bob Lutz, Joe Fuca, Luke Plumblee, and Jim Rudge

Keeping with our long tradition of supporting youth sports in St. Louis, each year members vote to make financial contributions to local athletic groups. The South City Composite Otters mountain biking club, youth soccer teams, boxing programs, and baseball teams have all been sponsored by South Broadway. The SBAC sponsored the regional Gaelic Football Club over the past two years and enjoys supporting the team on the field for competition against other Soulard-sponsored establishments.

In years past, the SBAC was known for its annual Christmas

Historical Note
Rivalry

Using drama and hyperbole, the sports writers at the *St. Louis Post-Dispatch* seemed to fan rivalries between local athletic clubs—especially between the South Broadway Athletic Club and the Missouri Athletic Club. The MAC, which had only opened its doors in 1903, was located on the sophisticated end of Washington Avenue near department stores and towers of commerce. The SBAC, surrounded by factories, breweries, and tenements, was the established club. The sports coverage in the *Post-Dispatch* used the term *hoi polloi* (an ancient Greek term for "the masses" or "the many" commonly used for the working class) in reference to the SBAC. References were made to the MAC's bloated bar bills, gilded café, and richly upholstered furniture. By comparison at the SBAC, the beer that was brewed in the neighborhood flowed liberally. The conversation around SBAC was described as "a din of Teutonic chatter."

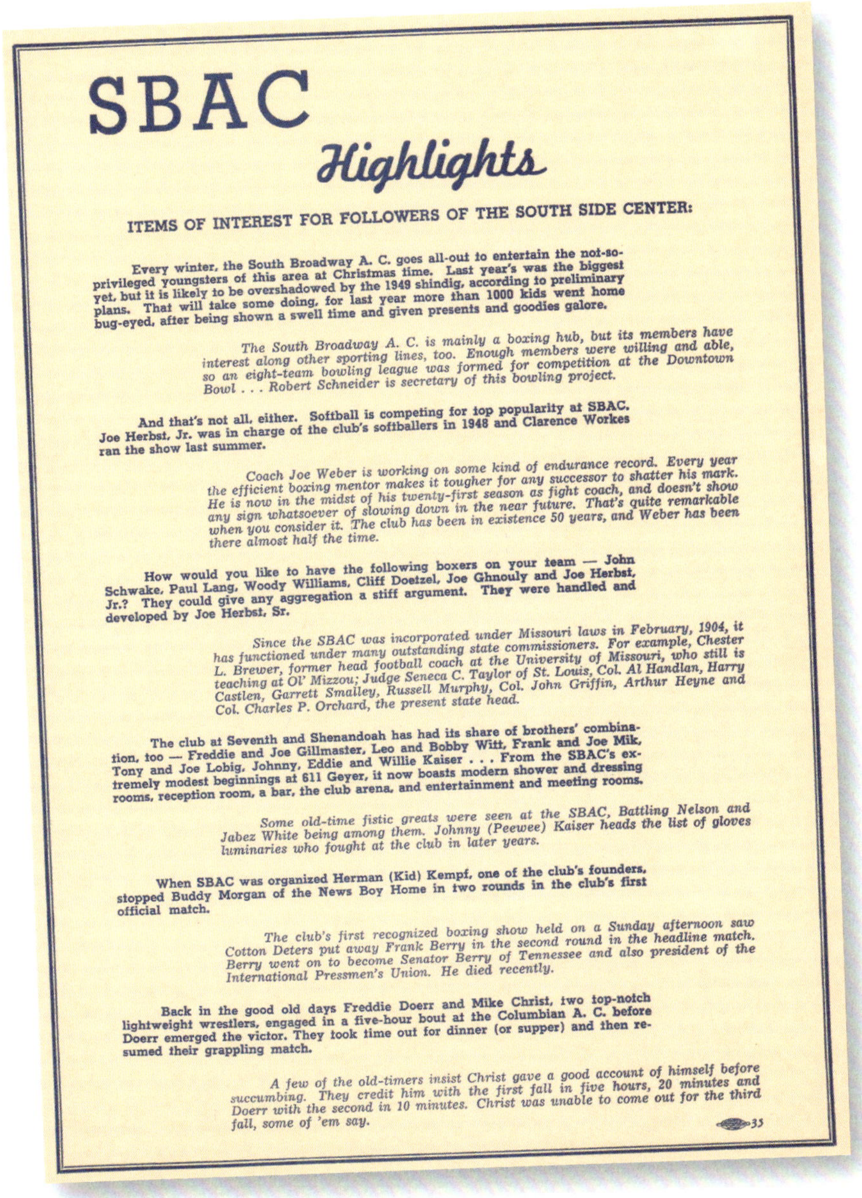

SBAC *Highlights*

ITEMS OF INTEREST FOR FOLLOWERS OF THE SOUTH SIDE CENTER:

Every winter, the South Broadway A. C. goes all-out to entertain the not-so- privileged youngsters of this area at Christmas time. Last year's was the biggest yet, but it is likely to be overshadowed by the 1949 shindig, according to preliminary plans. That will take some doing, for last year more than 1000 kids went home bug-eyed, after being shown a swell time and given presents and goodies galore.

The South Broadway A. C. is mainly a boxing hub, but its members have interest along other sporting lines, too. Enough members were willing and able, so an eight-team bowling league was formed for competition at the Downtown Bowl . . . Robert Schneider is secretary of this bowling project.

And that's not all, either. Softball is competing for top popularity at SBAC. Joe Herbst, Jr. was in charge of the club's softballers in 1948 and Clarence Workes ran the show last summer.

Coach Joe Weber is working on some kind of endurance record. Every year the efficient boxing mentor makes it tougher for any successor to shatter his mark. He is now in the midst of his twenty-first season as fight coach, and doesn't show any sign whatsoever of slowing down in the near future. That's quite remarkable when you consider it. The club has been in existence 50 years, and Weber has been there almost half the time.

How would you like to have the following boxers on your team — John Schwake, Paul Lang, Woody Williams, Cliff Doetzel, Joe Ghnouly and Joe Herbst, Jr.? They could give any aggregation a stiff argument. They were handled and developed by Joe Herbst, Sr.

Since the SBAC was incorporated under Missouri laws in February, 1904, it has functioned under many outstanding state commissioners. For example, Chester L. Brewer, former head football coach at the University of Missouri, who still is teaching at Ol' Mizzou; Judge Seneca C. Taylor of St. Louis, Col. Al Handlan, Harry Castlen, Garrett Smalley, Russell Murphy, Col. John Griffin, Arthur Heyne and Col. Charles P. Orchard, the present state head.

The club at Seventh and Shenandoah has had its share of brothers' combina- tion, too — Freddie and Joe Gillmaster, Leo and Bobby Witt, Frank and Joe Mik, Tony and Joe Lobig, Johnny, Eddie and Willie Kaiser . . . From the SBAC's ex- tremely modest beginnings at 611 Geyer, it now boasts modern shower and dressing rooms, reception room, a bar, the club arena, and entertainment and meeting rooms.

Some old-time fistic greats were seen at the SBAC, Battling Nelson and Jabez White being among them. Johnny (Peewee) Kaiser heads the list of gloves luminaries who fought at the club in later years.

When SBAC was organized Herman (Kid) Kempf, one of the club's founders, stopped Buddy Morgan of the News Boy Home in two rounds in the club's first official match.

The club's first recognized boxing show held on a Sunday afternoon saw Cotton Deters put away Frank Berry in the second round in the headline match. Berry went on to become Senator Berry of Tennessee and also president of the International Pressmen's Union. He died recently.

Back in the good old days Freddie Doerr and Mike Christ, two top-notch lightweight wrestlers, engaged in a five-hour bout at the Columbian A. C. before Doerr emerged the victor. They took time out for dinner (or supper) and then re- sumed their grappling match.

A few of the old-timers insist Christ gave a good account of himself before succumbing. They credit him with the first fall in five hours, 20 minutes and Doerr with the second in 10 minutes. Christ was unable to come out for the third fall, some of 'em say.

35

SBAC Highlights stories for the 50th anniversary book (1949)

SBAC sponsored the Mathews-Dickey Boys Club Football team in 1993.

Thank you
SOUTH BROADWAY ATHLETIC CLUB
for being our
SPONSOR
Your dedication and support are greatly appreciated

Mathews-Dickey Football
13 Thirteen Light

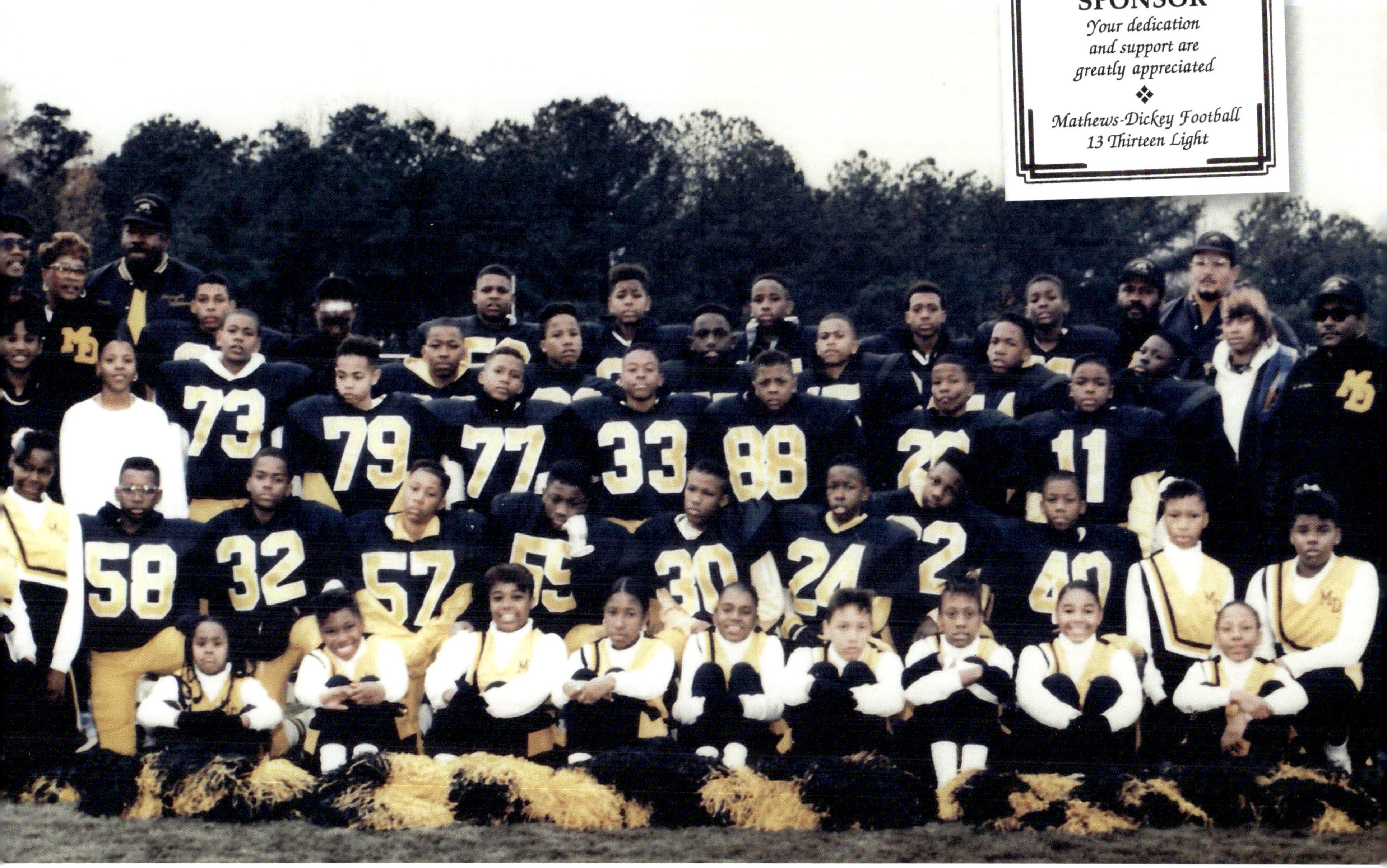

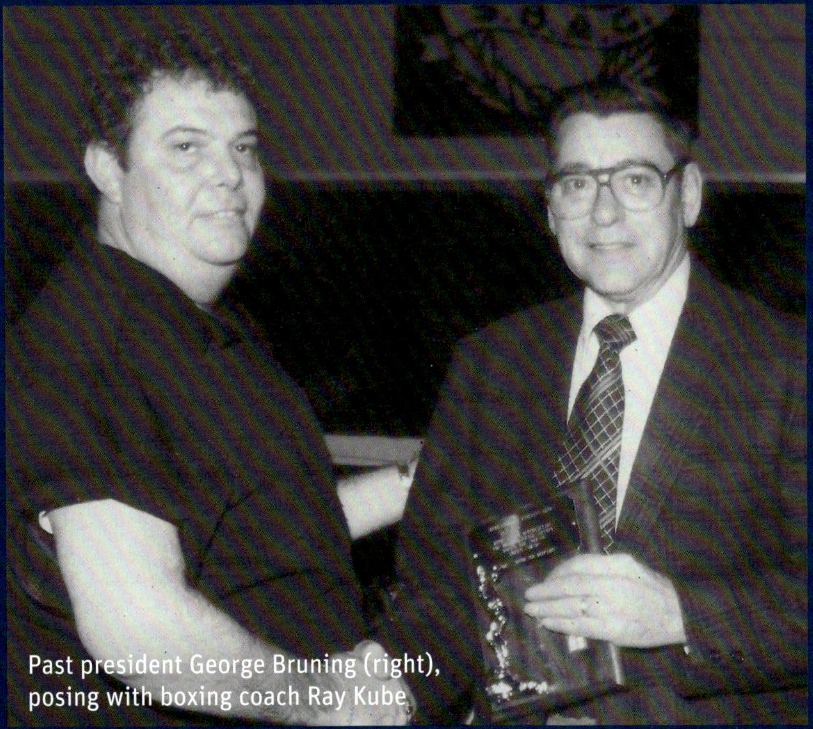

Past president George Bruning (right), posing with boxing coach Ray Kube

THE BRUNING FAMILY

ONLY ONE FAMILY can claim the title as longest-running members of the SBAC, and that's the four generations of Brunings. George Sr., George Jr. and Glenda, Dale Sr. and Cathy, Craig, and Dale Bruning Jr. have all been integral to South Broadway. Dale recalls his grandfather, George Sr., being an active member of the club throughout the 1940s. George Sr. is remembered as running the kitchen back in the days when the SBAC was still a men-only club. George Sr. was also the organizer of our annual children's Christmas parties and key to the Golden Jubilee celebration.

George Bruning Jr. joined the SBAC in 1949. George Jr. was a three-term president and one-term vice president, and he spent eight years as treasurer for the SBAC. George Jr. has been credited for revitalizing membership during the 1980s and '90s while also working to bring amateur boxing back to the SBAC during that time. George Jr.'s son, Dale, recalls the Diamond Jubilee 75th Anniversary in 1974 and being impressed with how formally members dressed for SBAC events, always wearing suits and ties when producing shows. The Diamond Jubilee celebration was a tuxedo-and-gown event.

Dale Bruning joined in August 1984 and is currently celebrating 40 years of membership in SBAC. Originally, Dale was a member of the Millard Fillmore Athletic Club of Soulard, one of the many clubs in St. Louis that focused on sports. During those days of the early 1980s, Dale's father, George Jr., was the president of SBAC. President Bruning, looking to bring new members into the SBAC, went to a Millard Filmore meeting and talked more than 40 young men into joining, creating a new class of SBAC members to carry on the club traditions.

—Dan Guenther

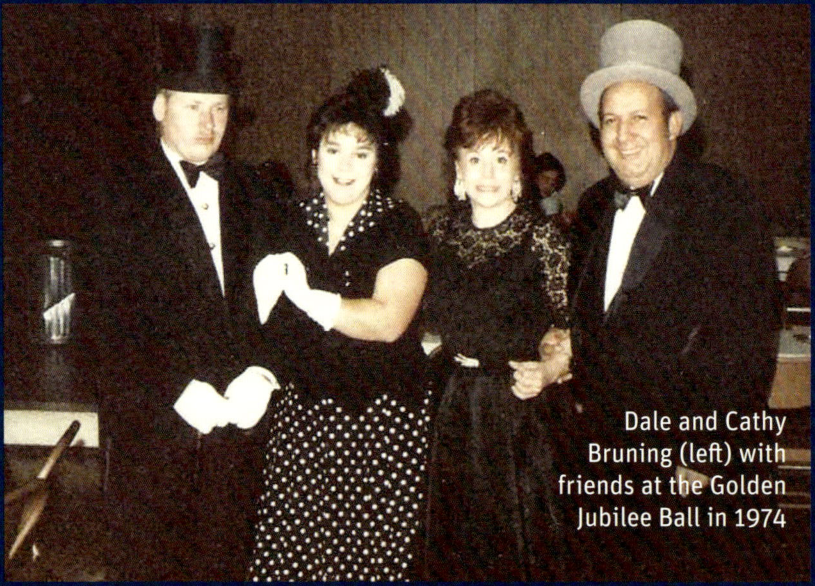

Dale and Cathy Bruning (left) with friends at the Golden Jubilee Ball in 1974

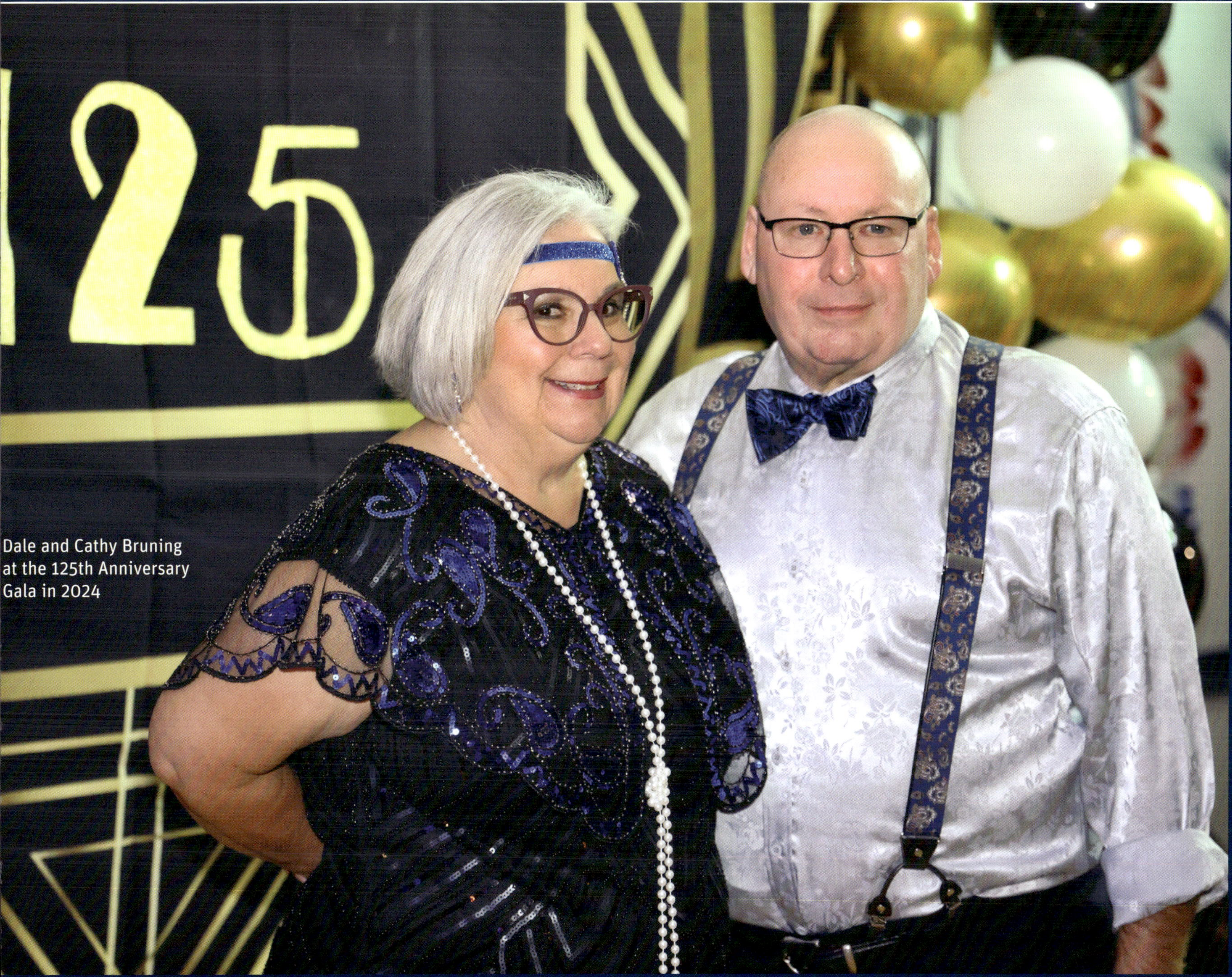

Dale and Cathy Bruning
at the 125th Anniversary
Gala in 2024

events, where children would line up to receive a holiday gift. In the 1940s through the 1960s, children were thrilled to receive a paper bag with an apple or orange as a holiday gift. One longtime member recalls the thrill of receiving fresh fruit in the middle of winter. A document from 1949 stated, "Every winter, the club went all out to provide for our underprivileged children, and at the 1949 Christmas party, more than 1,000 kids went home bug-eyed, after being shown a swell time and given presents and goodies galore."

Another memorable charitable event was during 1990, when our nation entered Operation Desert Storm. The members of our Ladies Auxiliary organized a Care Package Drive and sent hundreds of packages to service members operating overseas.

More recently, the social and barbecue club SOL (Sooner or

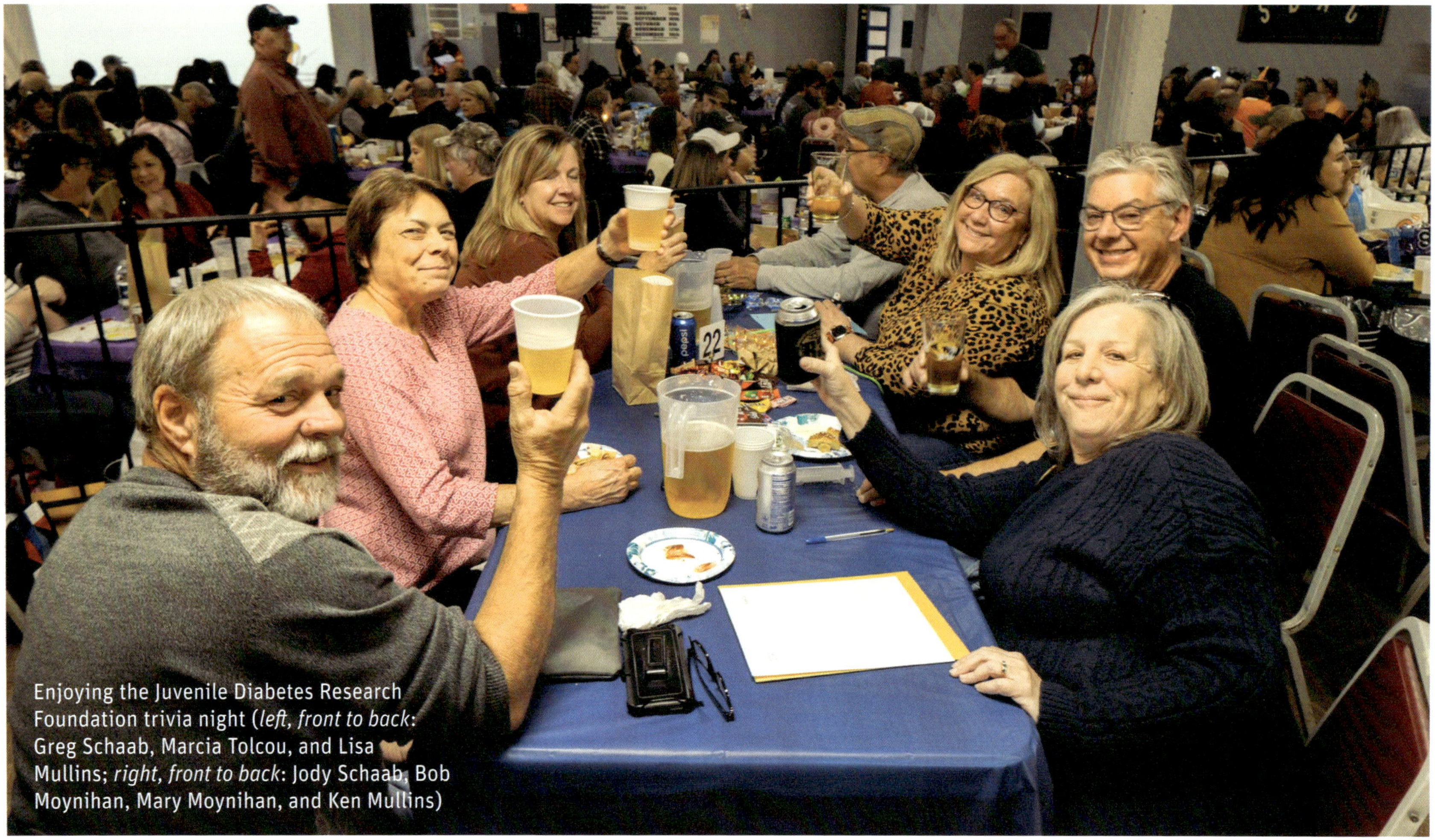

Enjoying the Juvenile Diabetes Research Foundation trivia night (*left, front to back*: Greg Schaab, Marcia Tolcou, and Lisa Mullins; *right, front to back*: Jody Schaab, Bob Moynihan, Mary Moynihan, and Ken Mullins)

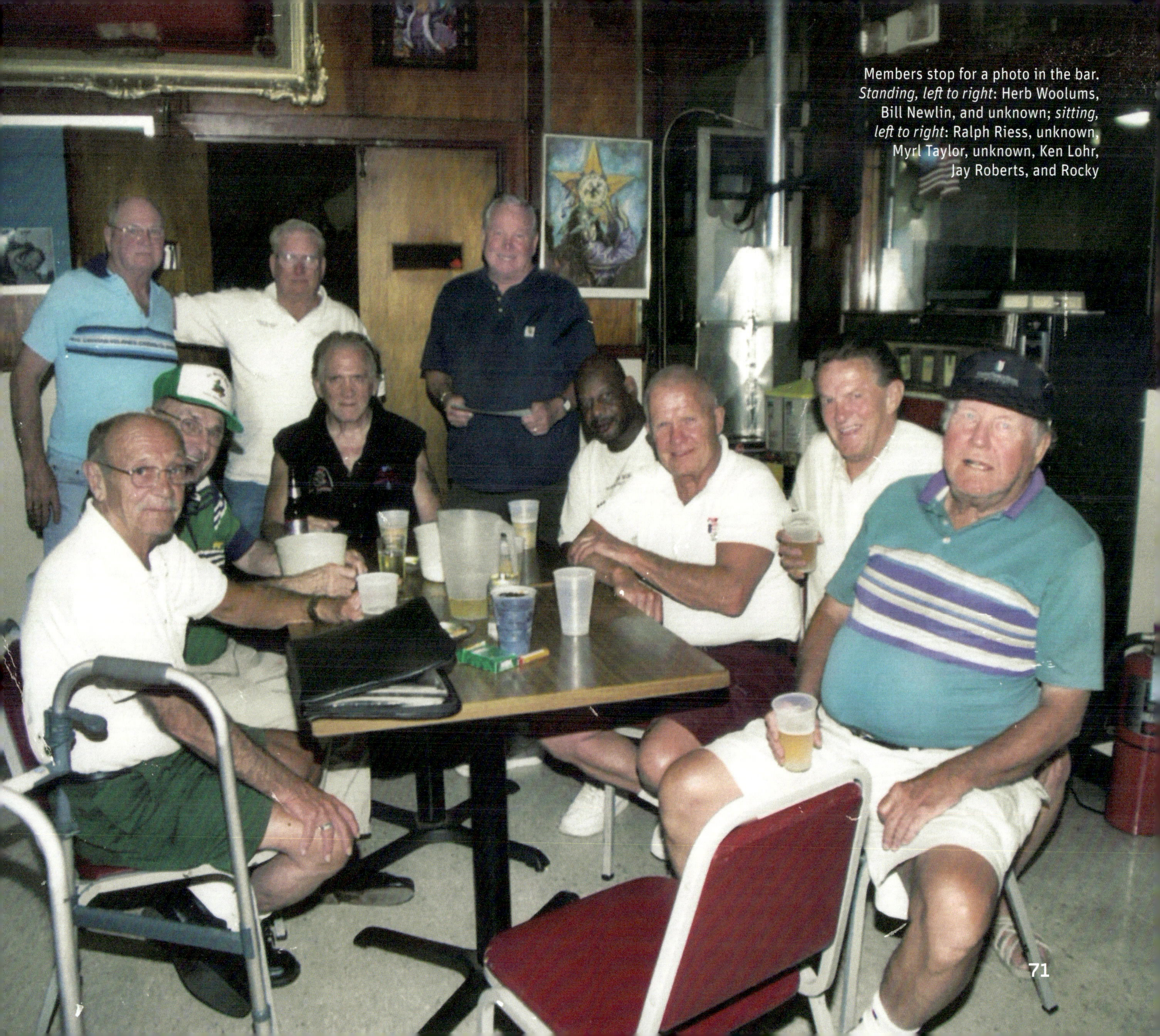

Members stop for a photo in the bar. *Standing, left to right*: Herb Woolums, Bill Newlin, and unknown; *sitting, left to right*: Ralph Riess, unknown, Myrl Taylor, unknown, Ken Lohr, Jay Roberts, and Rocky

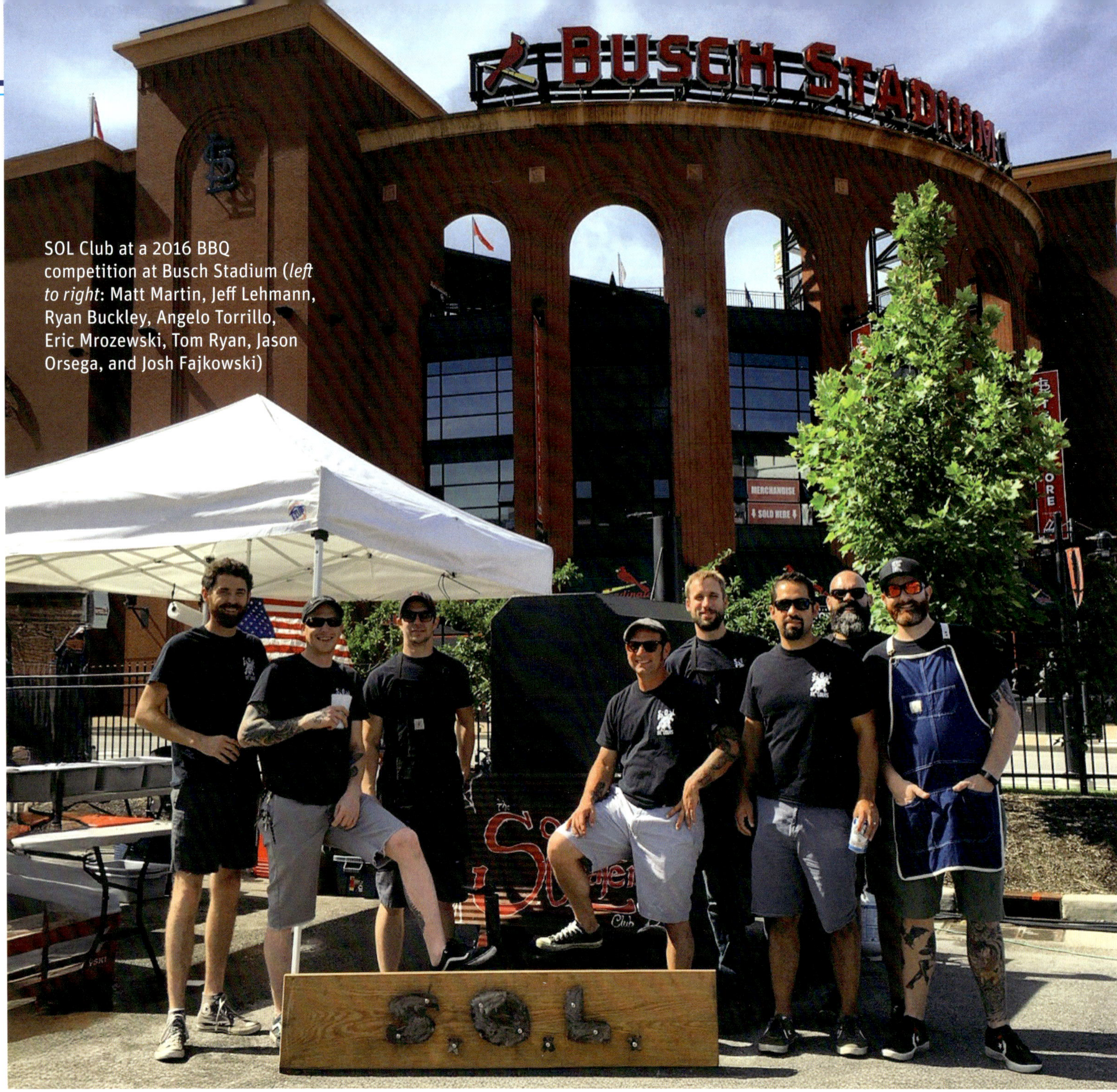

SOL Club at a 2016 BBQ competition at Busch Stadium (*left to right*: Matt Martin, Jeff Lehmann, Ryan Buckley, Angelo Torrillo, Eric Mrozewski, Tom Ryan, Jason Orsega, and Josh Fajkowski)

Later) would bring their award-winning barbecue to SBAC and add a new dimension to fundraising for the club. The 17 members who joined in 2016 quickly found a home at South Broadway and have been instrumental in its revival. SOL has shared their talents with the SBAC by organizing our fundraiser Bluegrass Brunch, participating in the annual Punk Rock Pig Roast, providing corned beef for the Pogues Tribute Shows, and grilling hundreds of brats for the Soulard Oktober Festival. Some of the SOL crew have even donated their time as board members over the years.

The SBAC offers time and resources in giving to charitable

Members volunteering for the ARJ Back to School drive: Marcia Tolcou (left), Connie Bafaro, Jody Schaab, and Sarah Folkemer. Chris Sanchez is behind them.

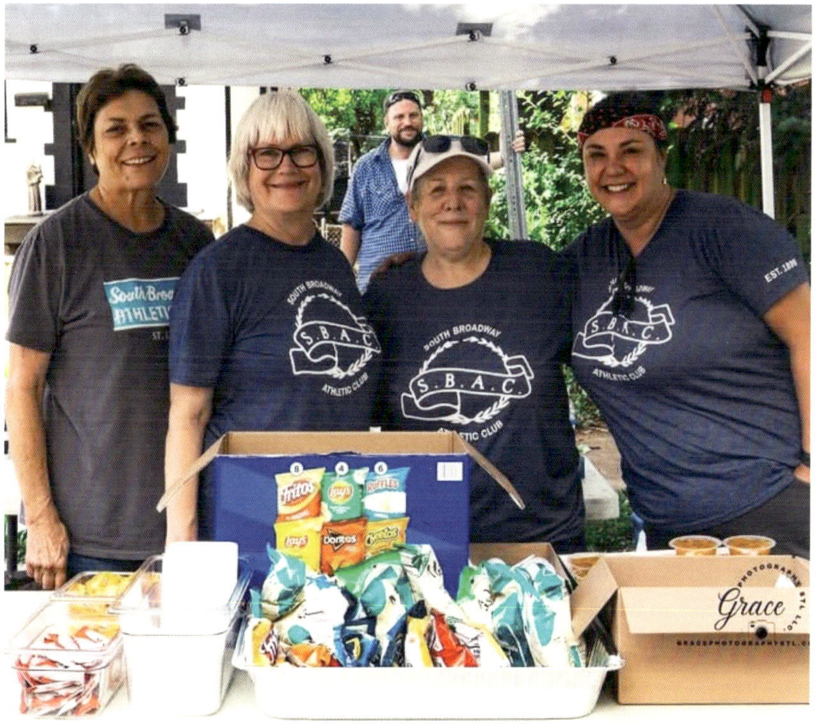

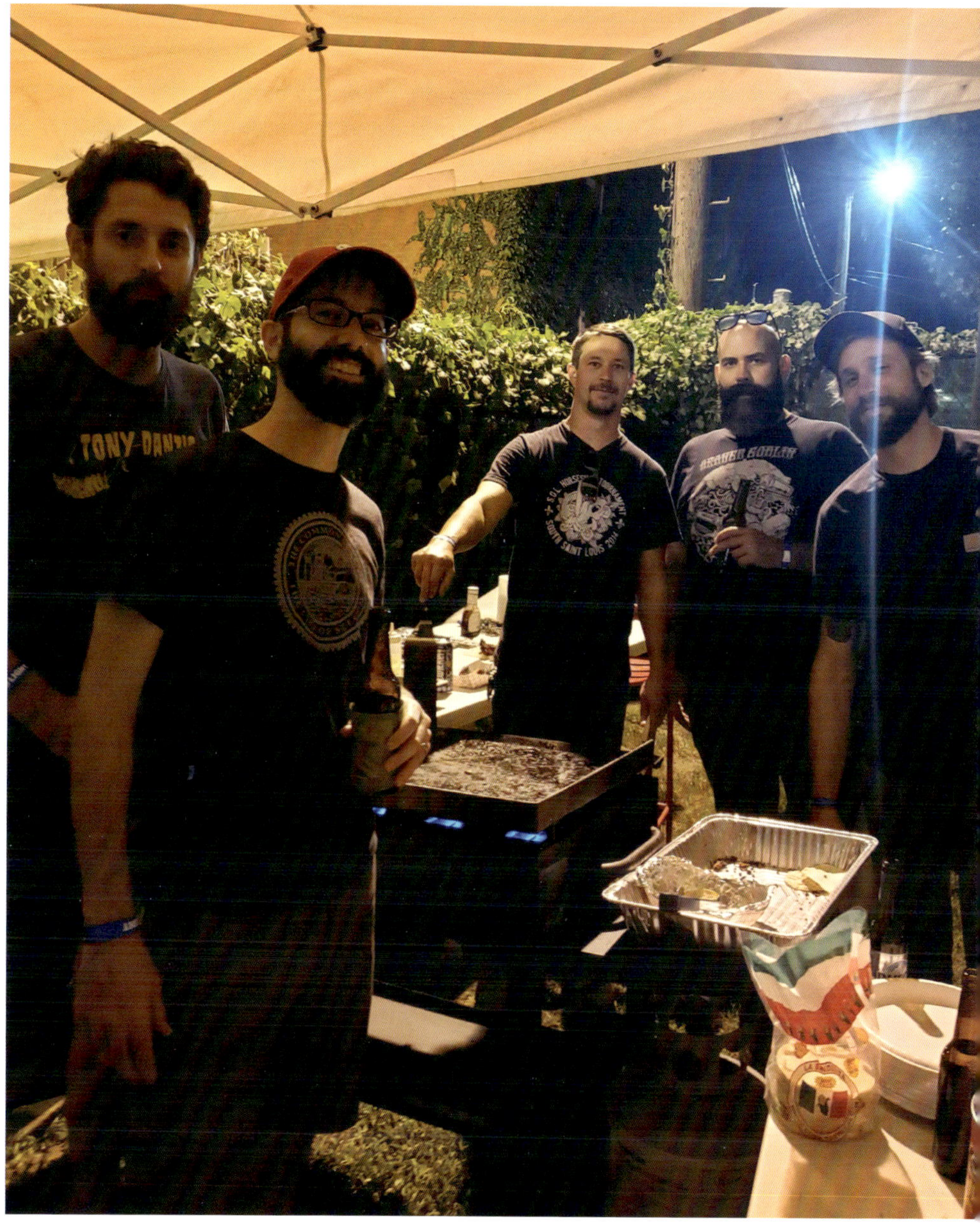

SOL Club members cooking for the Whiskey War Fest: Matt Martin (left), Matt Berra, Ryan Buckley, Jason Orsega, and Eric Mrozewski

A NEIGHBORHOOD OF CLUBS

SOULARD HAS ALWAYS been a neighborhood of clubs, committees, associations, and social groups of all types. The neighborhood was originally settled by Austrians and Germans fleeing the failed revolutions of 1848 and the repressive governments of King Frederick and Emperor Ferdinand. In their new home in the New World, they settled in South St. Louis, in areas such as Frenchtown and Bohemian Hill, in what was at the time one of the fastest-growing cities in the country.

As is often the case throughout human history, alcohol was the bedrock of their social foundations. Most of the bars and beer gardens in the neighborhood were company bars, owned by the numerous independent breweries that cropped up around Soulard's extensive natural cave system. But the center of Soulard's drinking culture was the Union Park Pleasure Resort, six square blocks on Russell Avenue filled with athletic competitions, dancing, music—and, of course, lots and lots of local beer. Singing was another fixture of German life, usually organized in small groups called Saengerbund or Saengerchor, in family homes or local businesses. The most important singing society was the Liederkranz, located near Soulard at 13th and Chouteau, where the upper crust of St. Louis German society would sing and drink the nights away.

Given their love for alcohol, it's a little paradoxical that the other great focus of social life in Soulard was physical fitness and athletic clubs. These stem from the Turner movement, founded in Germany by the inventor of gymnastics, who developed a doctrine of physical education and public health. Turnvereins, the gyms formed by the group, started popping up all over St. Louis, with Soulard's own South St. Louis Turnverein founded in 1864. Instilling in their members a love of physical fitness, the Turnvereins heralded many of the other athletic clubs that would pop up on in Soulard, such as the Monkeys AC, the Millard Fillmore AC, the Pirates AC, and the Stag AC, all of which would later be incorporated into SBAC.

In a way, SBAC is carrying on the long tradition of the old German clubs and social groups in Soulard, where athletic competition is a useful pretense for drinking with your friends.

—Mitchell Goist

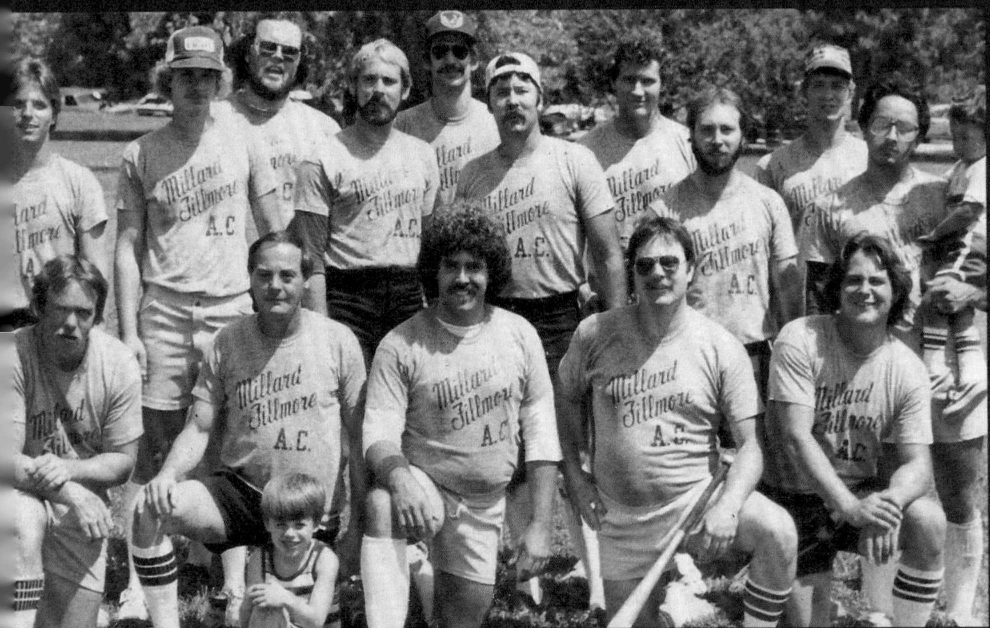

Millard Fillmore AC's 1982 champions
(*top row, left to right*: Rick Zacker, Craig Neumeister, Steve Boyer, John Ward, Jerry Boyer, Harold Zata, Rex Bridges, Paul Renner, and Eddy Sanchez; *kneeling, left to right*: Ernie Gore, Jerry Dempsey, Bob Benson, Andy Dicus, and Mike Button)

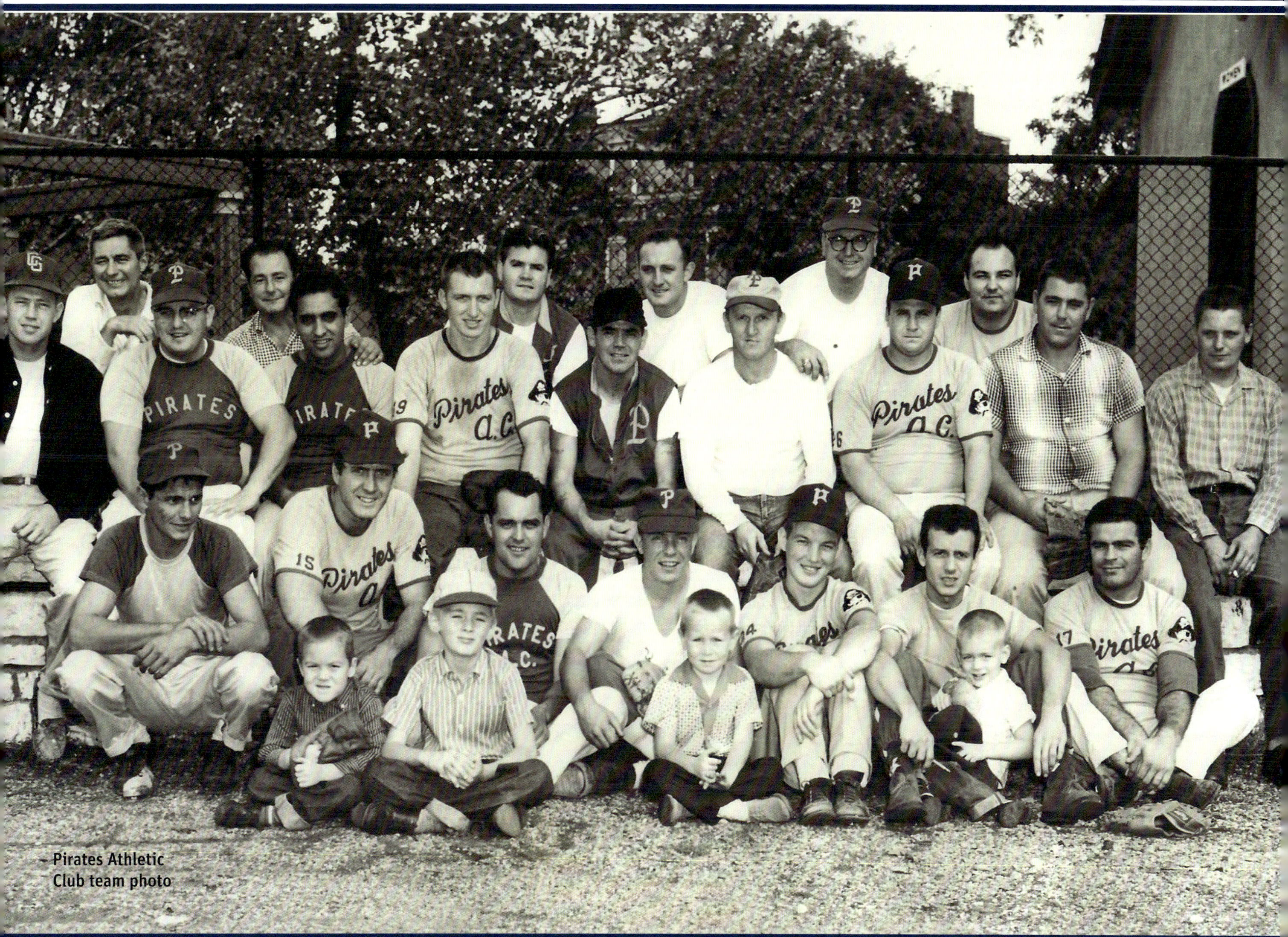

Pirates Athletic Club team photo

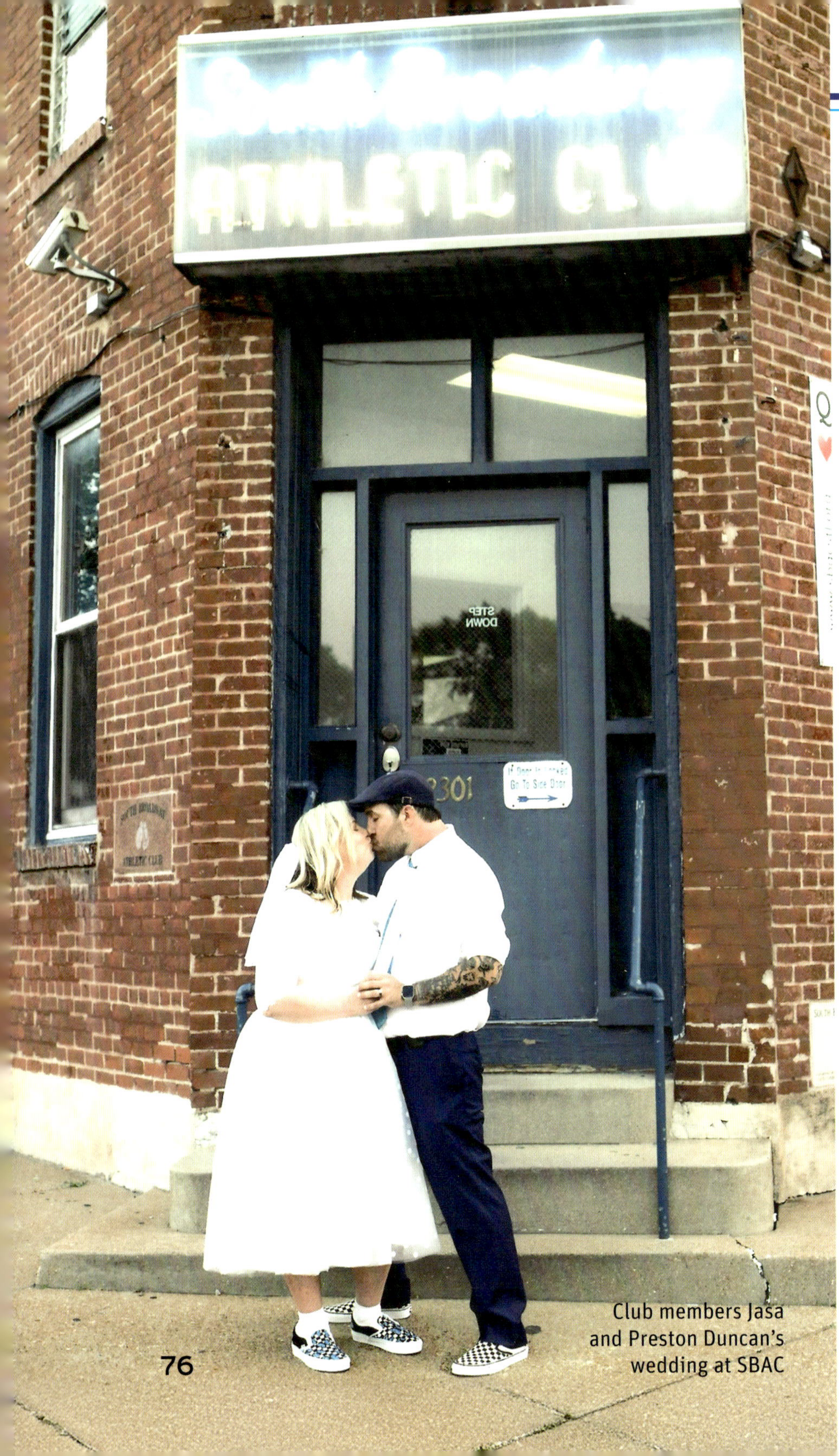

Club members Jasa and Preston Duncan's wedding at SBAC

organizations throughout the City of St. Louis. Each month, the community outreach committee picks a local organization to support with donations. A few notable charitable organizations include the Society of St. Vincent de Paul and St. Agatha Parish, where food items are donated to stock their pantry shelves; the ARJ Community Foundation, where members have sponsored back-to-school supply donations, Toys for Tots Christmas toy drives and the annual April Showers Women's Care Package drive;

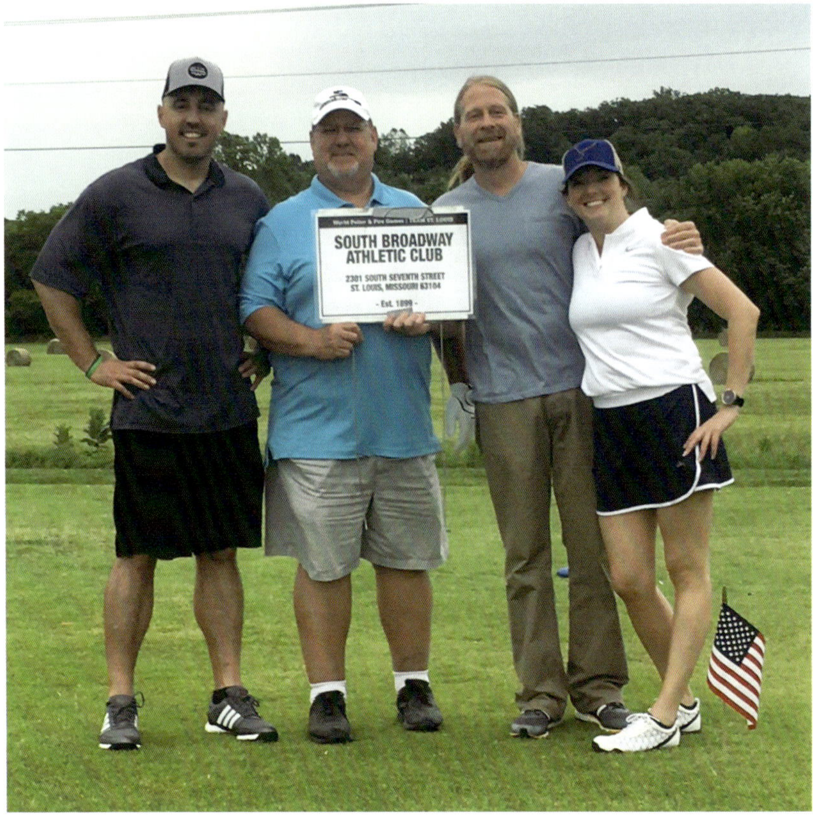

Members participating in the Theresa J. Winkler Memorial Golf Tournament: Kevin Wilkins (left), Glen Hearold, Dan Guenther, and Samantha Winkler

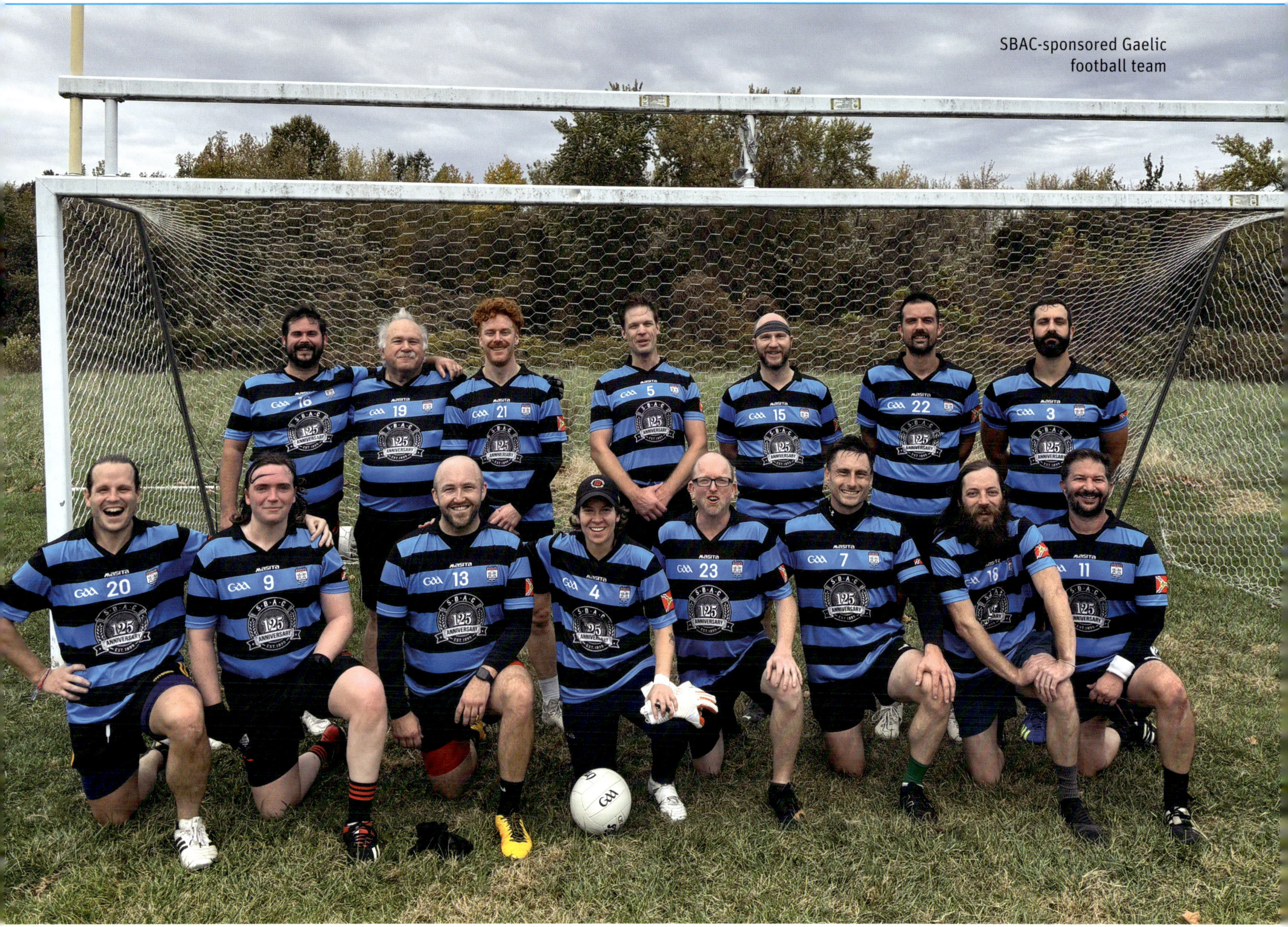

SBAC-sponsored Gaelic football team

SOULARD ORGANIZATIONS

THE SOUTH BROADWAY Athletic Club has always had a tight bond with the Soulard neighborhood, from neighborhood improvement to celebrating Mardi Gras and hosting parties.

The club donates space to several organizations for meetings and parties, including Mardi Gras, Inc., which holds its 12th Night and Scavenger Hunt parties at the SBAC. Their nonprofit arm, the Mardi Gras Foundation, is an important booster to the neighborhood. The Mardi Gras Foundation raises funds through producing Mardi Gras and the Mayor's Ball to provide community improvement grants to the Soulard neighborhood, along with some downtown projects at the mayor's discretion.

"It's important for them to keep the money generated in the neighborhood working for the neighborhood," SBAC president Kevin Wilkins said.

To date the group has issued more than $350,000 through grants. Some of their projects include:

- Park benches and permanent electric power for events at Soulard Market Park
- Ornamental iron fencing in that park and in Pontiac Park
- Playground equipment, lighting and landscaping, and several local parks and schools
- Funding for Frenchtown Dog Park

The Soulard Restoration Group, which has brought an influx of new members to the SBAC, holds its annual membership drive at the club, as well as its afterparty for the annual Parlour Tour. It's the largest neighborhood group in Soulard and has an immense amount of information on ordinances, code, and rehabbing, along with great events all year.

The SBAC also offers space for the Community Improvement District (CID) joint meeting with Soulard Special Business District for their review, and their safety and general meetings. The CID replaces and waters new trees, puts Soulard banners on streetlights, installs trash cans, maintains trash pickup, and has an alley-cleaning initiative.

—Miriam Moynihan

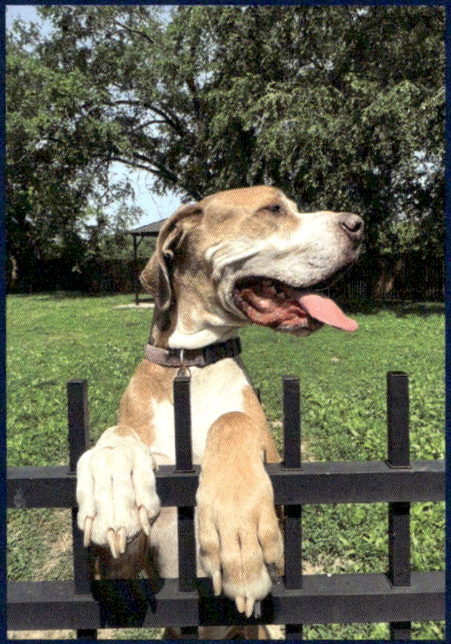

The Mardi Gras Foundation helped fund the Frenchtown Dog Park.

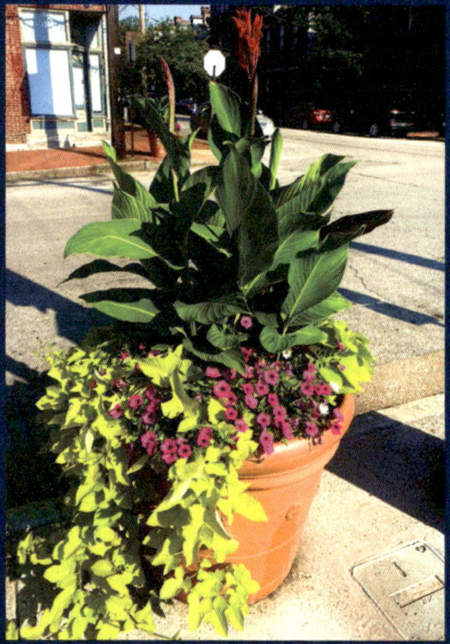

The Soulard Restoration Group has contributed beautification funding to the plant containers located in the area and the restoration of Soulard Station.

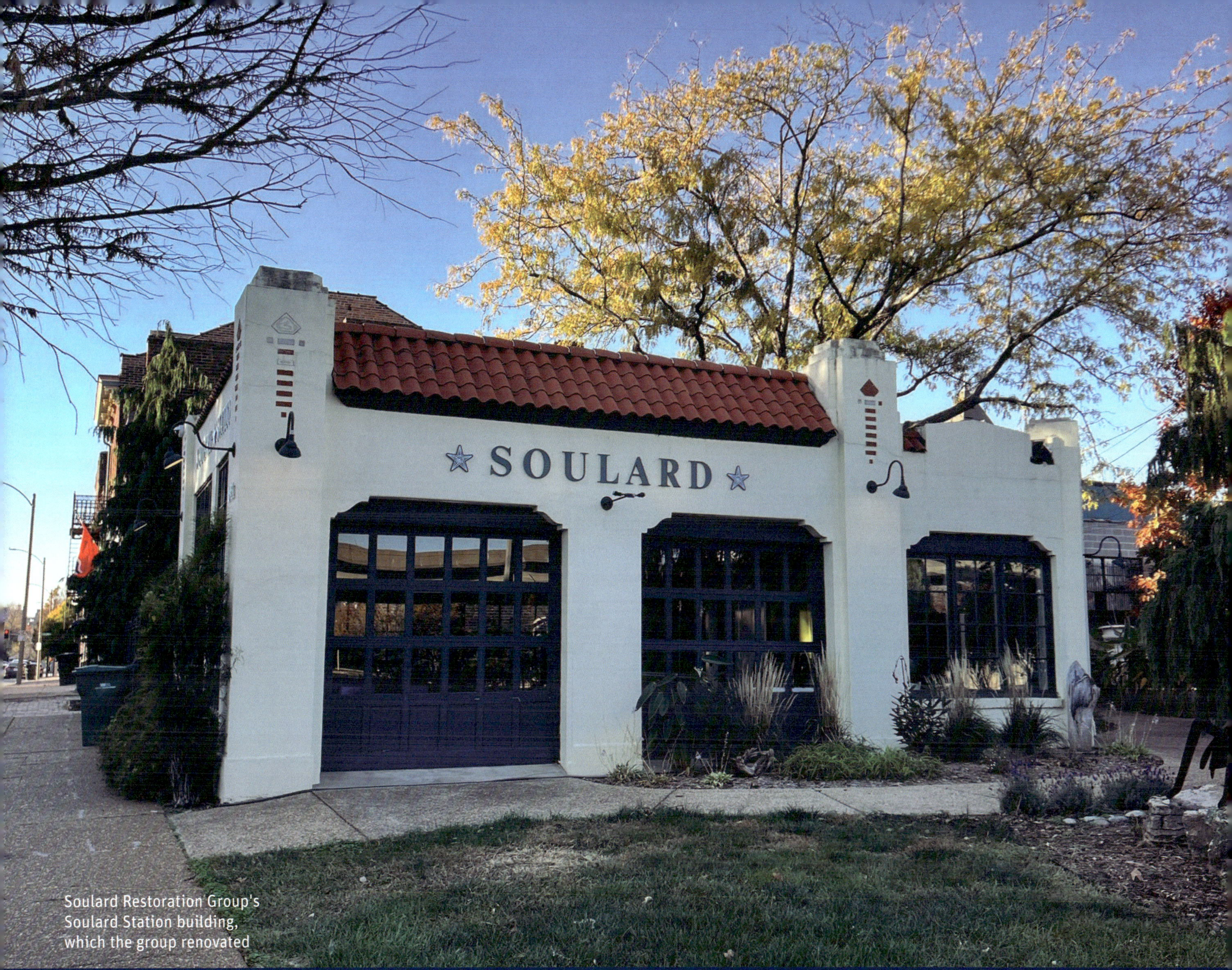

Soulard Restoration Group's Soulard Station building, which the group renovated

Resolution from the St. Louis Board of Aldermen honoring the SBAC for its 125 years

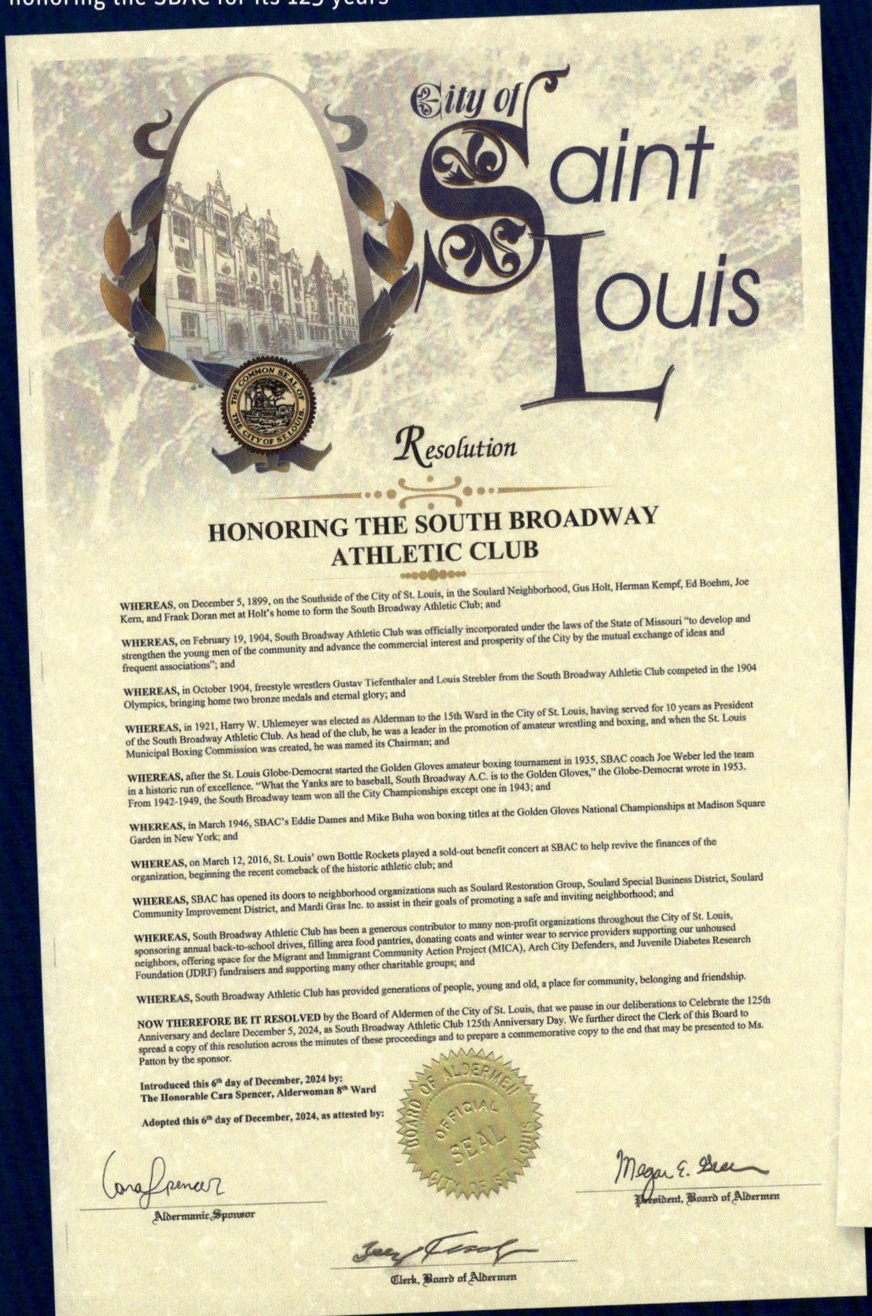

City of Saint Louis

Resolution

HONORING THE SOUTH BROADWAY ATHLETIC CLUB

WHEREAS, on December 5, 1899, on the Southside of the City of St. Louis, in the Soulard Neighborhood, Gus Holt, Herman Kempf, Ed Boehm, Joe Kern, and Frank Doran met at Holt's home to form the South Broadway Athletic Club; and

WHEREAS, on February 19, 1904, South Broadway Athletic Club was officially incorporated under the laws of the State of Missouri "to develop and strengthen the young men of the community and advance the commercial interest and prosperity of the City by the mutual exchange of ideas and frequent associations"; and

WHEREAS, in October 1904, freestyle wrestlers Gustav Tiefenthaler and Louis Strebler from the South Broadway Athletic Club competed in the 1904 Olympics, bringing home two bronze medals and eternal glory; and

WHEREAS, in 1921, Harry W. Uhlemeyer was elected as Alderman to the 15th Ward in the City of St. Louis, having served for 10 years as President of the South Broadway Athletic Club. As head of the club, he was a leader in the promotion of amateur wrestling and boxing, and when the St. Louis Municipal Boxing Commission was created, he was named its Chairman; and

WHEREAS, after the St. Louis Globe-Democrat started the Golden Gloves amateur boxing tournament in 1935, SBAC coach Joe Weber led the team in a historic run of excellence. "What the Yanks are to baseball, South Broadway A.C. is to the Golden Gloves," the Globe-Democrat wrote in 1953. From 1942-1949, the South Broadway team won all the City Championships except one in 1943; and

WHEREAS, in March 1946, SBAC's Eddie Dames and Mike Buha won boxing titles at the Golden Gloves National Championships at Madison Square Garden in New York; and

WHEREAS, on March 12, 2016, St. Louis' own Bottle Rockets played a sold-out benefit concert at SBAC to help revive the finances of the organization, beginning the recent comeback of the historic athletic club; and

WHEREAS, SBAC has opened its doors to neighborhood organizations such as Soulard Restoration Group, Soulard Special Business District, Soulard Community Improvement District, and Mardi Gras Inc. to assist in their goals of promoting a safe and inviting neighborhood; and

WHEREAS, South Broadway Athletic Club has been a generous contributor to many non-profit organizations throughout the City of St. Louis, sponsoring annual back-to-school drives, filling area food pantries, donating coats and winter wear to service providers supporting our unhoused neighbors, offering space for the Migrant and Immigrant Community Action Project (MICA), Arch City Defenders, and Juvenile Diabetes Research Foundation (JDRF) fundraisers and supporting many other charitable groups; and

WHEREAS, South Broadway Athletic Club has provided generations of people, young and old, a place for community, belonging and friendship.

NOW THEREFORE BE IT RESOLVED by the Board of Aldermen of the City of St. Louis, that we pause in our deliberations to Celebrate the 125th Anniversary and declare December 5, 2024, as South Broadway Athletic Club 125th Anniversary Day. We further direct the Clerk of this Board to spread a copy of this resolution across the minutes of these proceedings and to prepare a commemorative copy to the end that may be presented to Ms. Patton by the sponsor.

Introduced this 6th day of December, 2024 by:
The Honorable Cara Spencer, Alderwoman 8th Ward

Adopted this 6th day of December, 2024, as attested by:

Board of Aldermen Official Seal City of St. Louis

Aldermanic Sponsor

President, Board of Aldermen

Clerk, Board of Aldermen

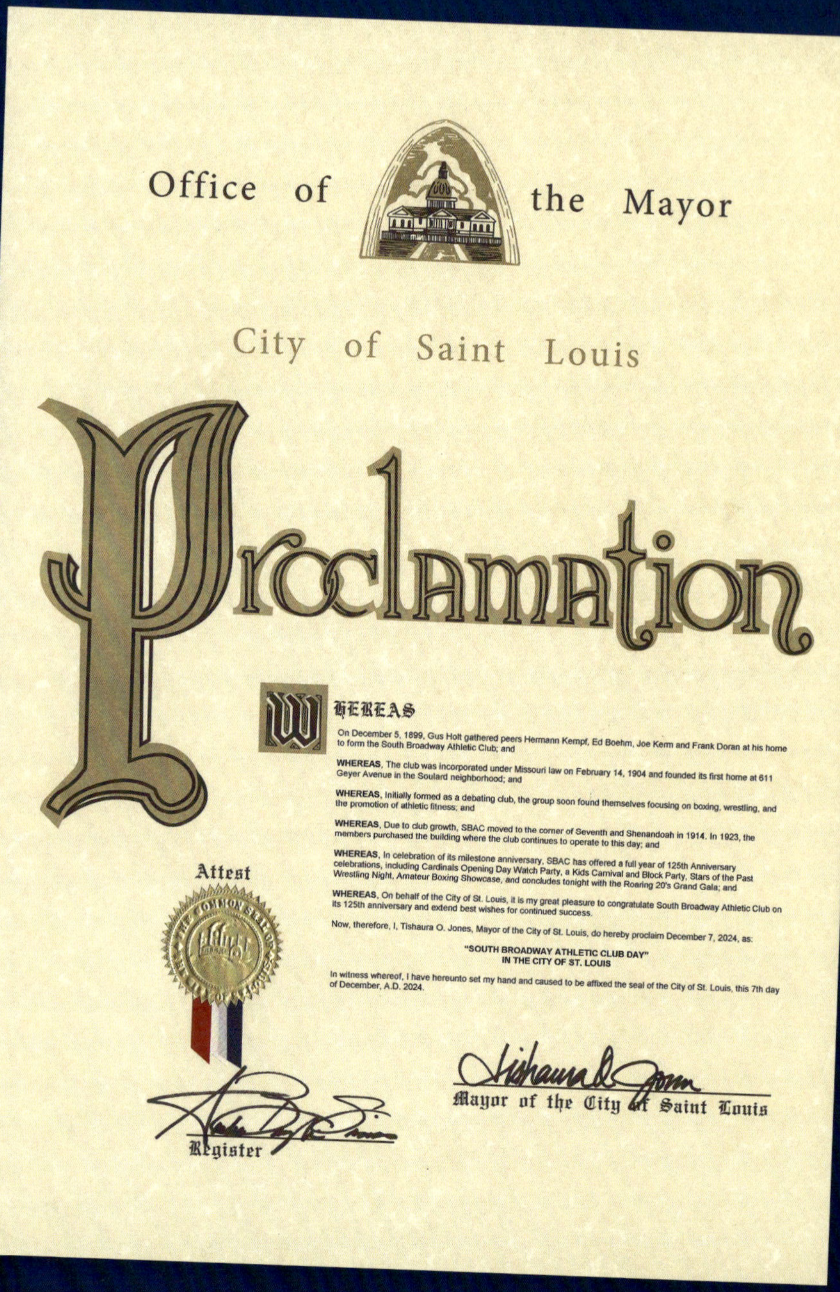

Office of the Mayor

City of Saint Louis

Proclamation

WHEREAS

On December 5, 1899, Gus Holt gathered peers Hermann Kempf, Ed Boehm, Joe Kern and Frank Doran at his home to form the South Broadway Athletic Club; and

WHEREAS, The club was incorporated under Missouri law on February 14, 1904 and founded its first home at 611 Geyer Avenue in the Soulard neighborhood; and

WHEREAS, Initially formed as a debating club, the group soon found themselves focusing on boxing, wrestling, and the promotion of athletic fitness; and

WHEREAS, Due to club growth, SBAC moved to the corner of Seventh and Shenandoah in 1914. In 1923, the members purchased the building where the club continues to operate to this day; and

WHEREAS, In celebration of its milestone anniversary, SBAC has offered a full year of 125th Anniversary celebrations, including Cardinals Opening Day Watch Party, a Kids Carnival and Block Party, Stars of the Past Wrestling Night, Amateur Boxing Showcase, and concludes tonight with the Roaring 20's Grand Gala; and

WHEREAS, On behalf of the City of St. Louis, it is my great pleasure to congratulate South Broadway Athletic Club on its 125th anniversary and extend best wishes for continued success.

Now, therefore, I, Tishaura O. Jones, Mayor of the City of St. Louis, do hereby proclaim December 7, 2024, as:

"SOUTH BROADWAY ATHLETIC CLUB DAY"
IN THE CITY OF ST. LOUIS

In witness whereof, I have hereunto set my hand and caused to be affixed the seal of the City of St. Louis, this 7th day of December, A.D. 2024.

Attest

Register

Mayor of the City of Saint Louis

City of St. Louis proclamation commemorating SBAC's 125th anniversary in 2024

A letter from St. Louis Mayor Fred M. Darst celebrating the 50th anniversary of the club in 1949

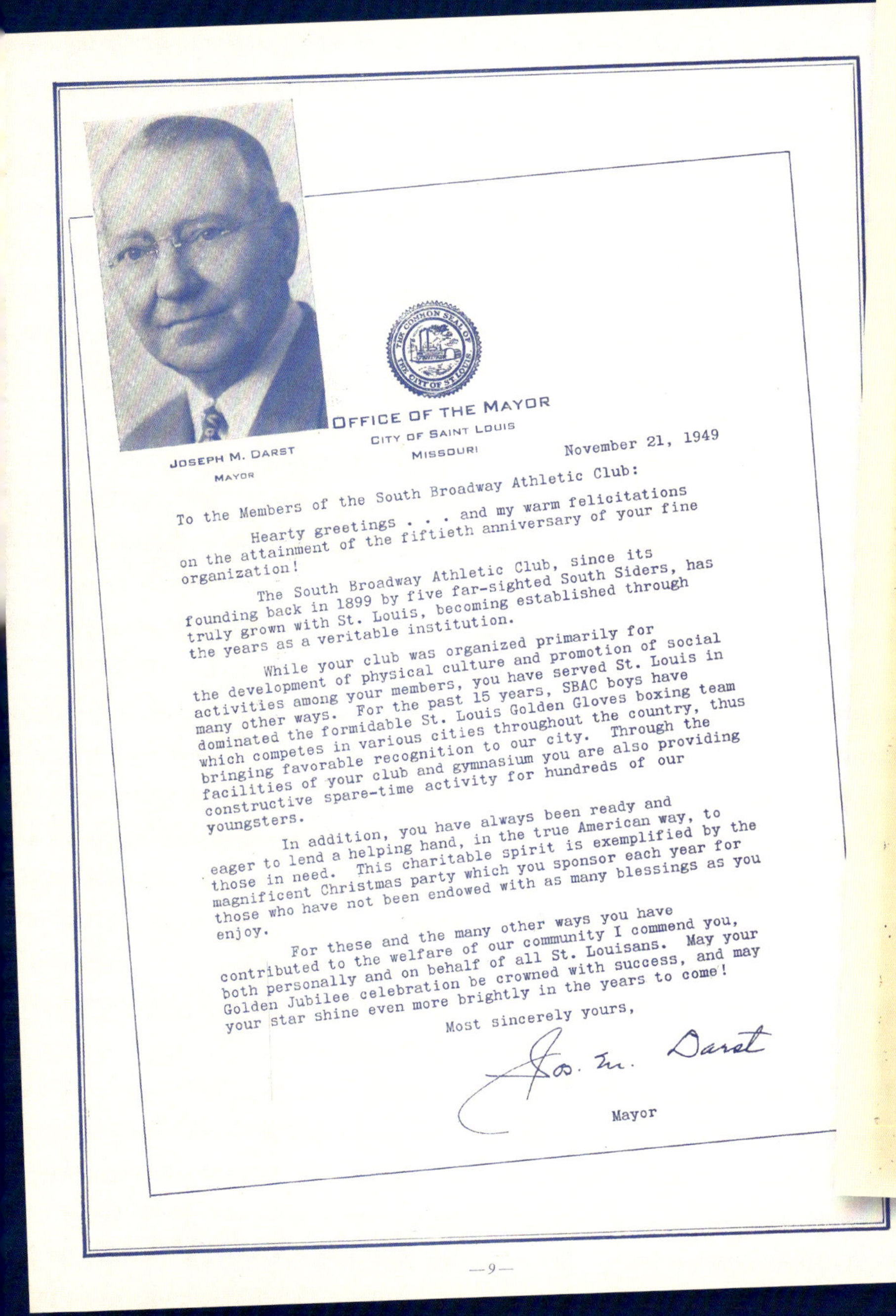

JOSEPH M. DARST
MAYOR

OFFICE OF THE MAYOR
CITY OF SAINT LOUIS
MISSOURI

November 21, 1949

To the Members of the South Broadway Athletic Club:

Hearty greetings . . . and my warm felicitations on the attainment of the fiftieth anniversary of your fine organization!

The South Broadway Athletic Club, since its founding back in 1899 by five far-sighted South Siders, has truly grown with St. Louis, becoming established through the years as a veritable institution.

While your club was organized primarily for the development of physical culture and promotion of social activities among your members, you have served St. Louis in many other ways. For the past 15 years, SBAC boys have dominated the formidable St. Louis Golden Gloves boxing team which competes in various cities throughout the country, thus bringing favorable recognition to our city. Through the facilities of your club and gymnasium you are also providing constructive spare-time activity for hundreds of our youngsters.

In addition, you have always been ready and eager to lend a helping hand, in the true American way, to those in need. This charitable spirit is exemplified by the magnificent Christmas party which you sponsor each year for those who have not been endowed with as many blessings as you enjoy.

For these and the many other ways you have contributed to the welfare of our community I commend you, both personally and on behalf of all St. Louisans. May your Golden Jubilee celebration be crowned with success, and may your star shine even more brightly in the years to come!

Most sincerely yours,

Jos. M. Darst

Mayor

—9—

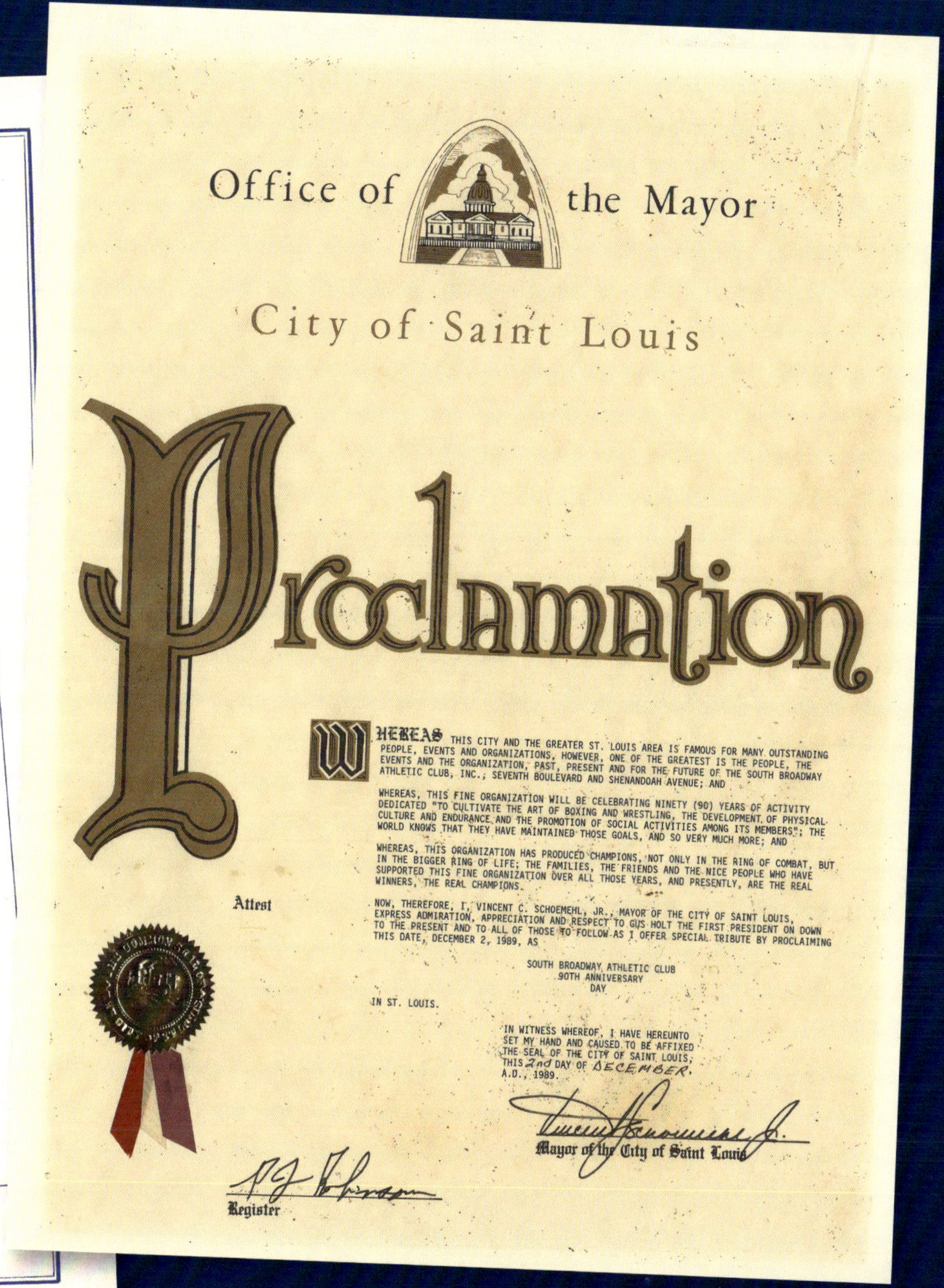

Office of the Mayor

City of Saint Louis

Proclamation

WHEREAS THIS CITY AND THE GREATER ST. LOUIS AREA IS FAMOUS FOR MANY OUTSTANDING PEOPLE, EVENTS AND ORGANIZATIONS, HOWEVER, ONE OF THE GREATEST IS THE PEOPLE, THE EVENTS AND THE ORGANIZATION, PAST, PRESENT AND FOR THE FUTURE OF THE SOUTH BROADWAY ATHLETIC CLUB, INC.; SEVENTH BOULEVARD AND SHENANDOAH AVENUE; AND

WHEREAS, THIS FINE ORGANIZATION WILL BE CELEBRATING NINETY (90) YEARS OF ACTIVITY DEDICATED "TO CULTIVATE THE ART OF BOXING AND WRESTLING, THE DEVELOPMENT OF PHYSICAL CULTURE AND ENDURANCE AND THE PROMOTION OF SOCIAL ACTIVITIES AMONG ITS MEMBERS"; THE WORLD KNOWS THAT THEY HAVE MAINTAINED THOSE GOALS, AND SO VERY MUCH MORE; AND

WHEREAS, THIS ORGANIZATION HAS PRODUCED CHAMPIONS, NOT ONLY IN THE RING OF COMBAT, BUT IN THE BIGGER RING OF LIFE; THE FAMILIES, THE FRIENDS AND THE NICE PEOPLE WHO HAVE SUPPORTED THIS FINE ORGANIZATION OVER ALL THOSE YEARS, AND PRESENTLY, ARE THE REAL WINNERS, THE REAL CHAMPIONS.

NOW, THEREFORE, I, VINCENT C. SCHOEMEHL, JR., MAYOR OF THE CITY OF SAINT LOUIS, EXPRESS ADMIRATION, APPRECIATION AND RESPECT TO GUS HOLT THE FIRST PRESIDENT ON DOWN TO THE PRESENT AND TO ALL OF THOSE TO FOLLOW AS I OFFER SPECIAL TRIBUTE BY PROCLAIMING THIS DATE, DECEMBER 2, 1989, AS

SOUTH BROADWAY ATHLETIC CLUB
90TH ANNIVERSARY
DAY

IN ST. LOUIS.

Attest

IN WITNESS WHEREOF, I HAVE HEREUNTO SET MY HAND AND CAUSED TO BE AFFIXED THE SEAL OF THE CITY OF SAINT LOUIS, THIS 2nd DAY OF DECEMBER, A.D., 1989.

Mayor of the City of Saint Louis

Register

The SBAC 90th anniversary proclamation by Mayor Vince Schoemehl in 1989

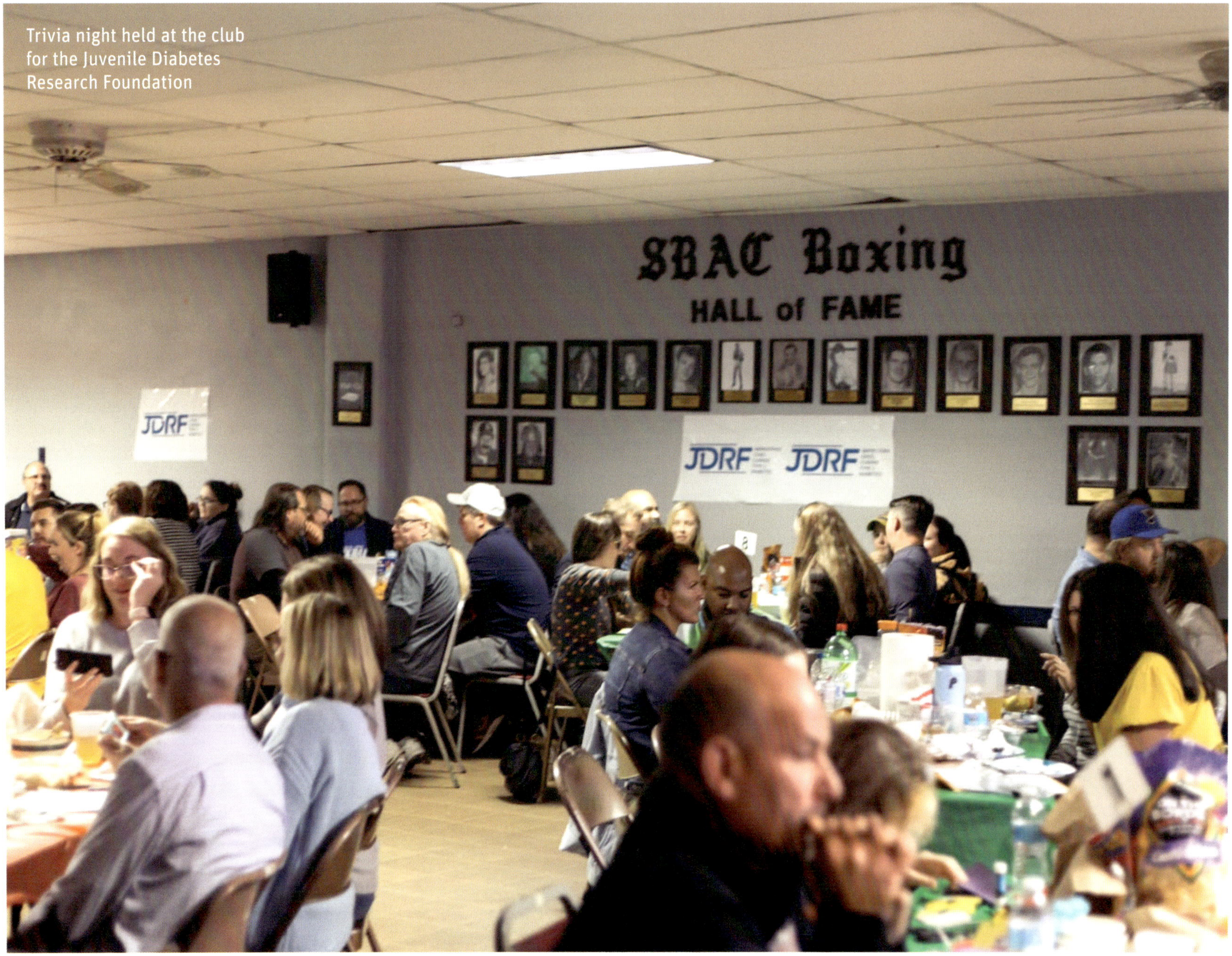

Trivia night held at the club for the Juvenile Diabetes Research Foundation

and CareSTL, a St. Louis animal shelter with an "adopt-a-stray" event during the holiday season.

The SBAC has donated hall and event space to many leading city organizations. In recent years, trivia nights have become popular fundraising events. The SBAC, with its large hall, has donated space to the Migrant and Immigrant Community Action Project (MICA), Arch City Defenders, and Juvenile Diabetes Research Foundation (JDRF) alongside the Theresa J. Winkler Memorial Foundation. These charity events offer members an opportunity to assist thousands of neighbors during their times of need.

For 125 years, the SBAC has been a fixture of the Soulard neighborhood, and with our recent revival, giving back to Soulard has been one of our main objectives.

—Dan Guenther

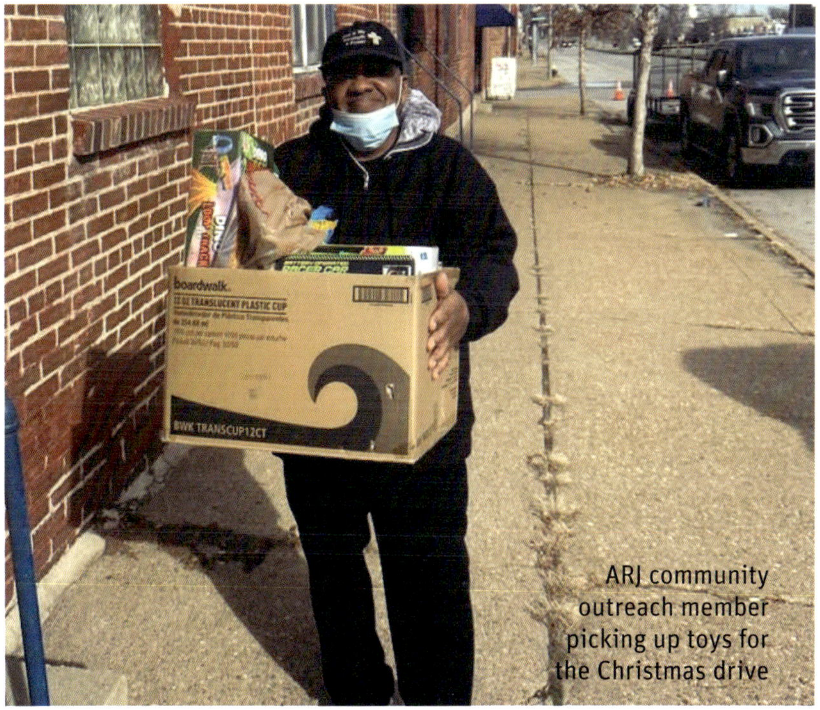

ARJ community outreach member picking up toys for the Christmas drive

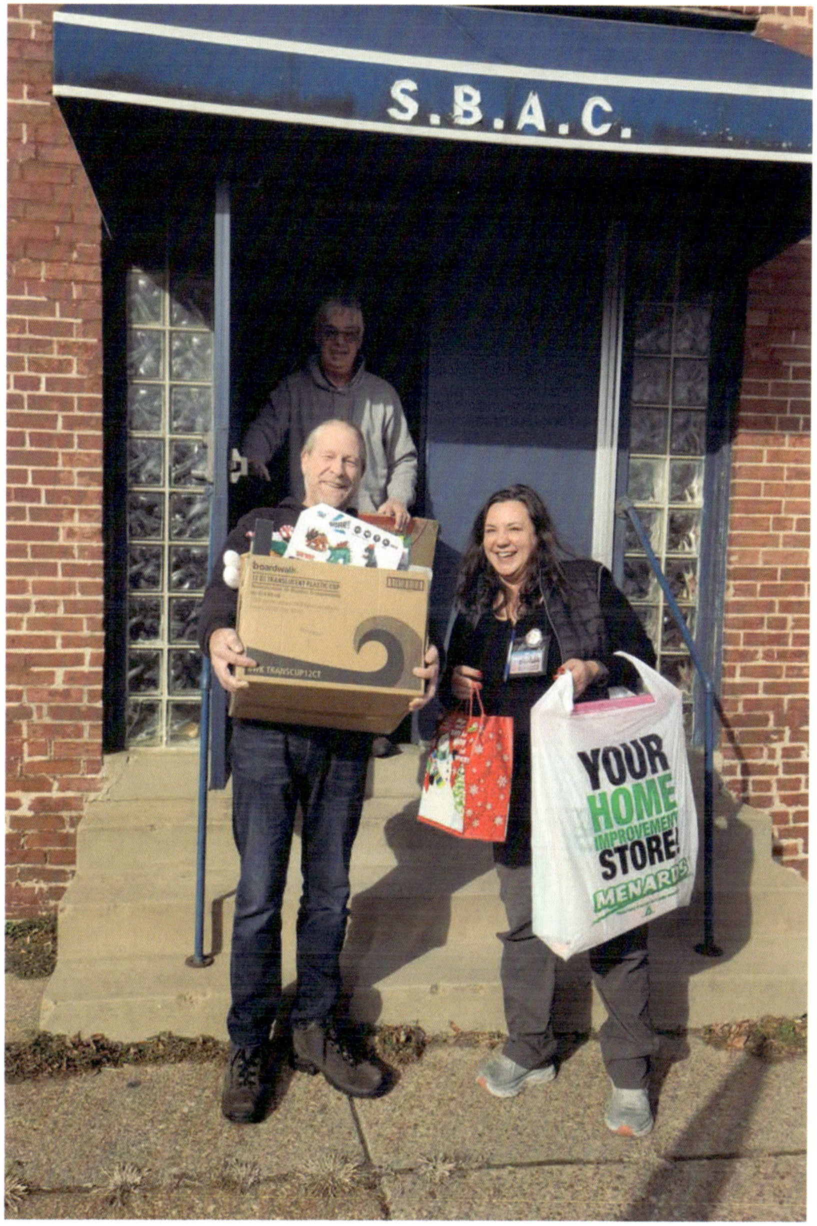

Members pitch in at the ARJ community outreach gift drive: Bob Moynihan (back), Dan Guenther, Sarah Folkemer

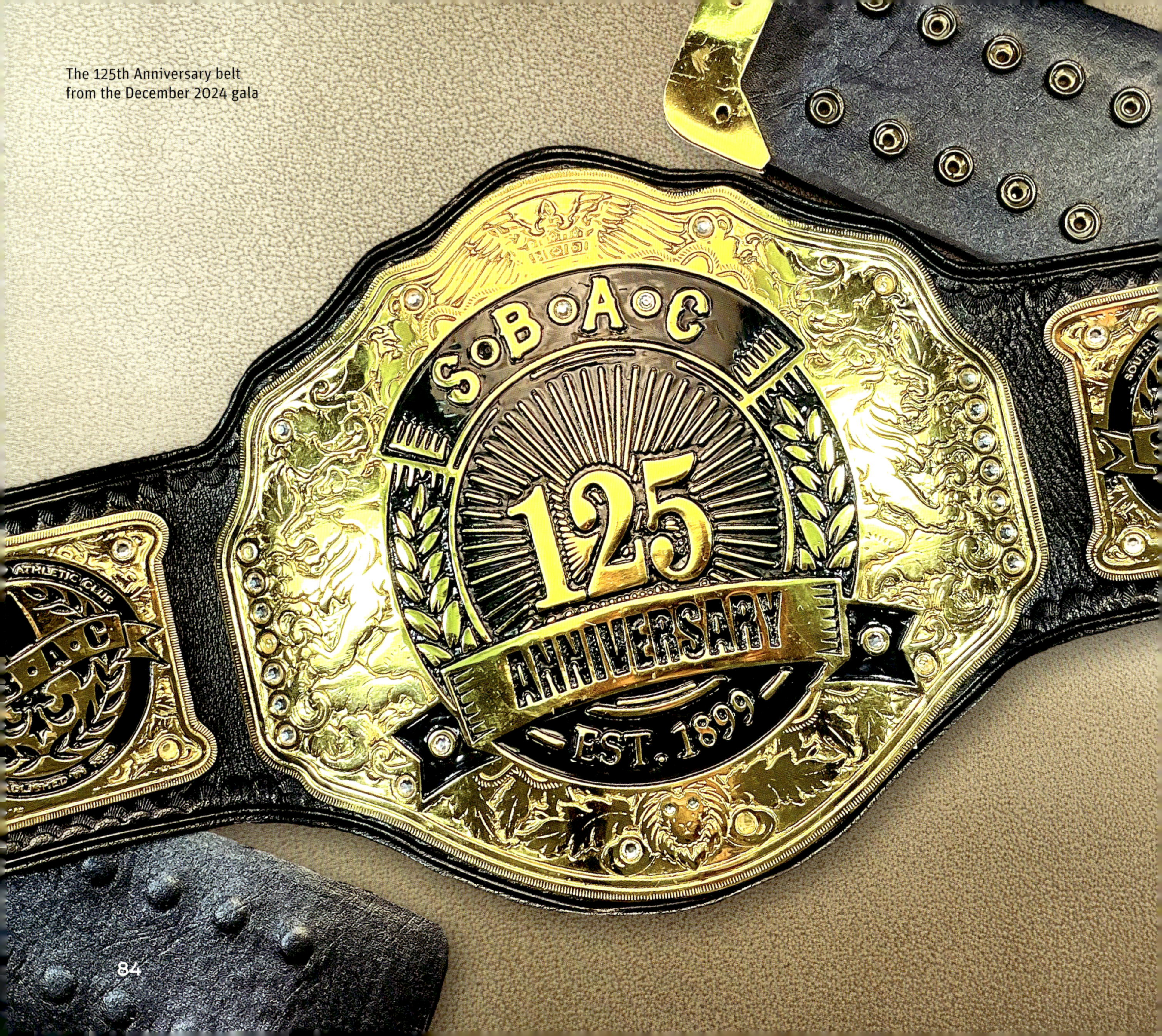

The 125th Anniversary belt from the December 2024 gala

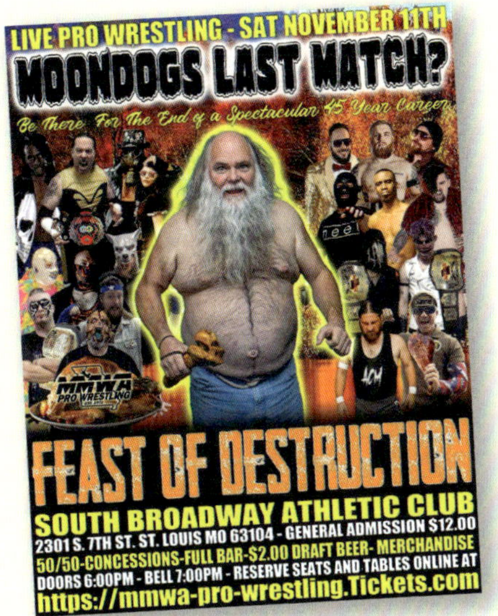

Poster from the 2023 Mid-Missouri Wrestling Alliance event

Chapter 5

The Comeback

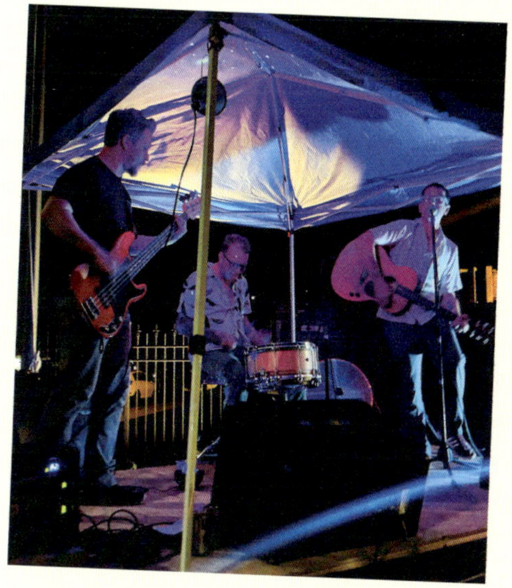

Ryan Buckley (left), Jeff Lehmann, and Steve Whetstone played at the Punk Rock Pig Roast in 2023.

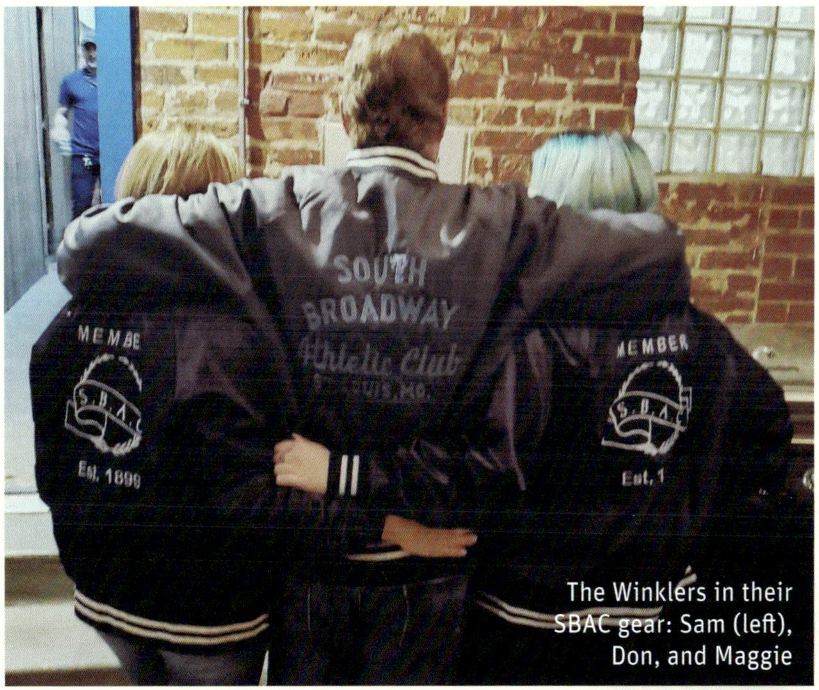

The Winklers in their SBAC gear: Sam (left), Don, and Maggie

The Decline of Glory

IN THE 1980S AND 1990S, the SBAC was riding high. Membership was strong at more than 300 members, and the club's calendar was filled with boxing matches, wrestling events, and community gatherings such as weekly bingo that helped fill the club's coffers. However, as the decades rolled on, the glow began to fade.

By the early 2010s, the SBAC was in dire straits. Years of declining revenues, financial mismanagement, and a dwindling membership of fewer than 50 people had left the club strapped for cash. Both the red-brick building on 7th Street and the nearby boxing gym showed visible signs of age; leaky roofs, ragged HVAC systems, and peeling paint told a story of neglect. The club owed three years of back taxes on the buildings, and the city was on the verge of forcing its sale on the courthouse steps.

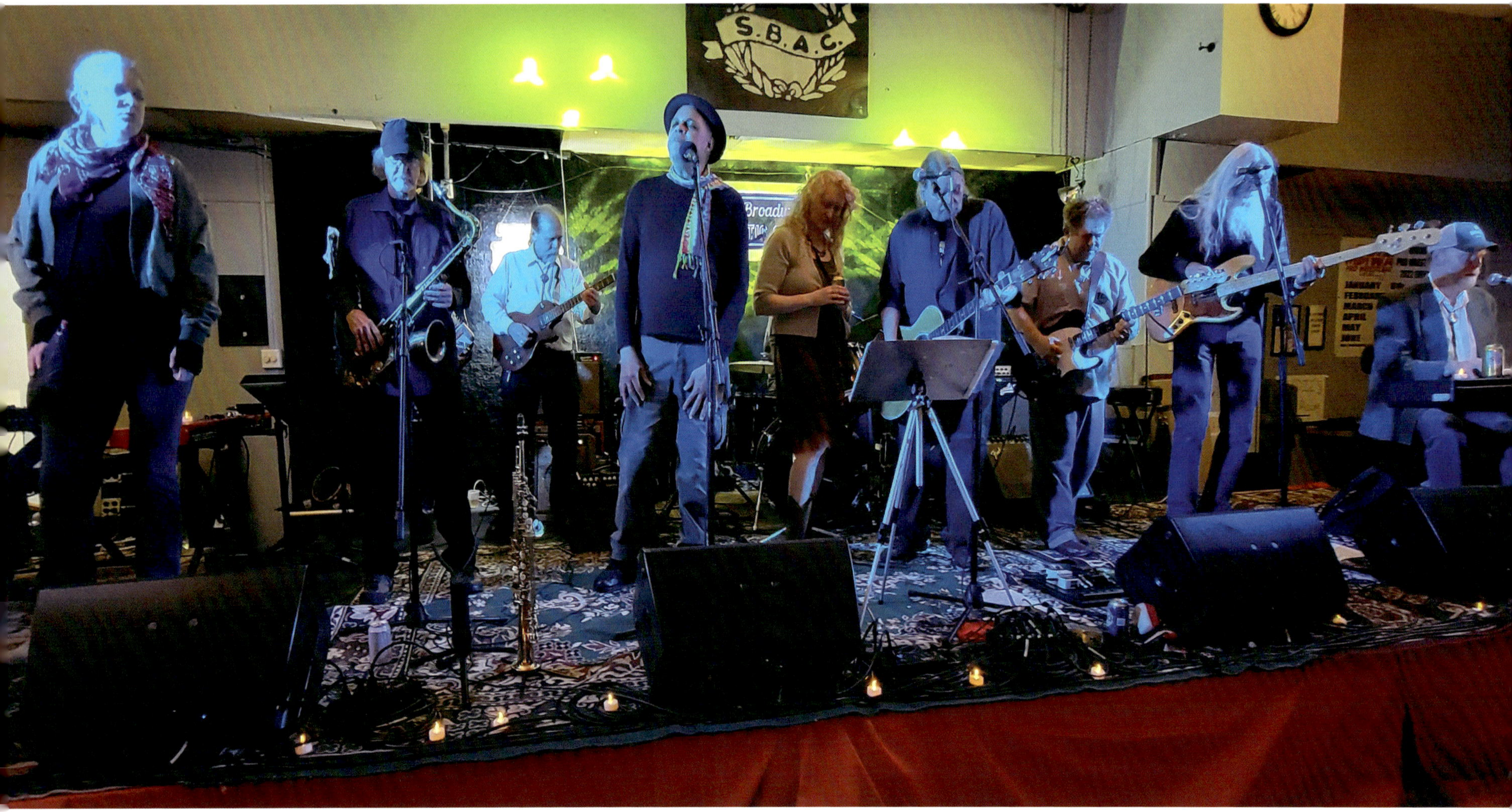

Some of the major players in the annual Stag Nite All-Stars Thanksgiving eve *Last Waltz* show; *from left*: Irene Allen, Randy Reece, Thom Pallozola, Tom Wood, Maureen Sullivan, Mark Moynihan, T. O. Lucas, David Henry Spangler, and Tim Sullivan

The Resurgence

RUNNING OUT OF OPTIONS, in early 2015, the Club launched a Kickstarter campaign to raise funds and reached out to local news outlets to help rally support. Fox 2 News and the *Riverfront Times* both ran stories about the club's struggles. While the Kickstarter campaign ultimately failed, raising under $500, the news stories caught the attention of a small group of friends and residents who were eager to get involved and help.

Historical Note

Early Booster of SBAC

As a local businessman, Billy Westhus rallied the community to support the SBAC. Born in Missouri in the wake of the Civil War, this ingenious businessman showcased the latest in home amenities at his furniture store in the early 20th century. During the Teens, he became a dealer for Columbia Records at his store located at 2001 South Broadway. When housewives were using scrubboards and brooms, he displayed revolutionary electric washing machines and vacuum cleaners.

Westhus was a fan of all sporting activities. He served on the Athletic Committee of the SBAC and backed some of the best amateur boxers in St. Louis.

Along with his promotion of the SBAC, he was a leader of the Western Rowing Club, encouraged bicycling, and promoted a five-mile river swim. He was best known in his Dutchtown neighborhood, where he and his wife moved to a bungalow on Meramec Street, for his fascination with pigeons. His pigeon loft boasted international champions.

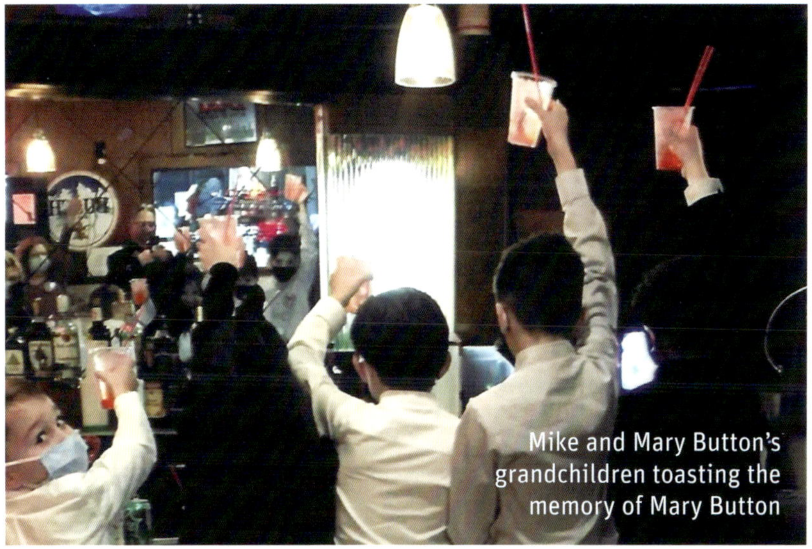

Mike and Mary Button's grandchildren toasting the memory of Mary Button

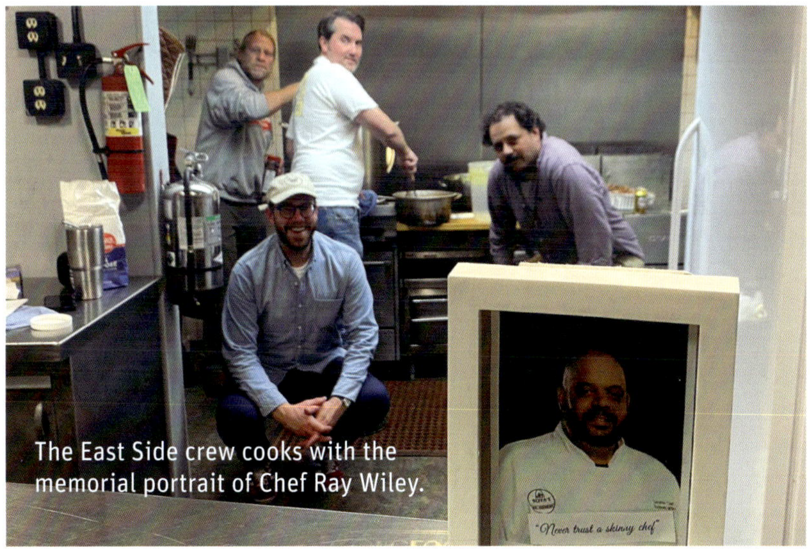

The East Side crew cooks with the memorial portrait of Chef Ray Wiley.

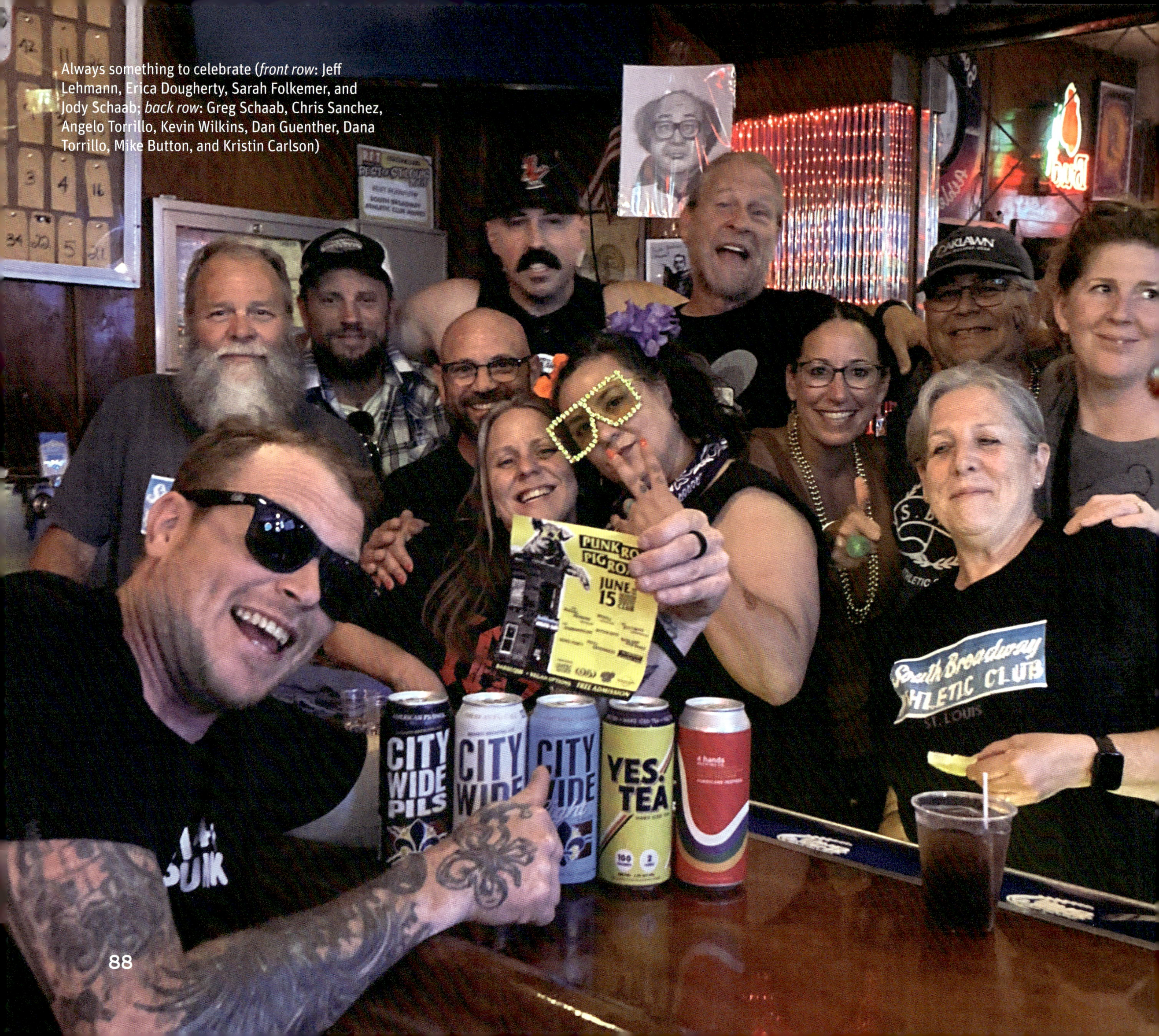

Always something to celebrate (*front row*: Jeff Lehmann, Erica Dougherty, Sarah Folkemer, and Jody Schaab; *back row*: Greg Schaab, Chris Sanchez, Angelo Torrillo, Kevin Wilkins, Dan Guenther, Dana Torrillo, Mike Button, and Kristin Carlson)

Longtime fans of the wrestling events Kevin Wilkins and Evan Bolesta joined in March 2015, and their friends Jim Gehrs and Patrick McEvilly came on board soon after. They were welcomed with open arms, and within months Wilkins was appointed to the Board of Directors. When elections rolled around in December 2015, the club's president, Al Bauman, asked Wilkins to take the reins as president. The group soon began recruiting a flurry of new members and finding ways to generate revenue and cut expenses.

Wilkins saw the club's potential as a concert venue and tapped local legends The Bottle Rockets to play a benefit concert that raised more than $20,000. Then he brought in the Whiskey War

Dan Guenther and Sharon Tyus worked during an aldermanic Intergovernmental Affairs Committee in 2019. SBAC member Guenther served as a two-term alderman for St. Louis's 9th Ward.
Courtesy of Mark Shlinkman/St. Louis Post-Dispatch/*Polaris*

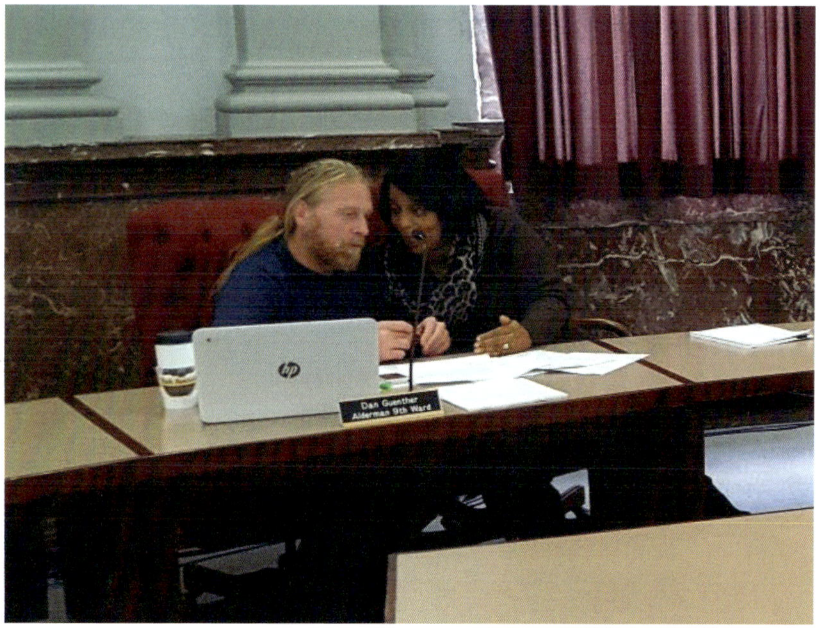

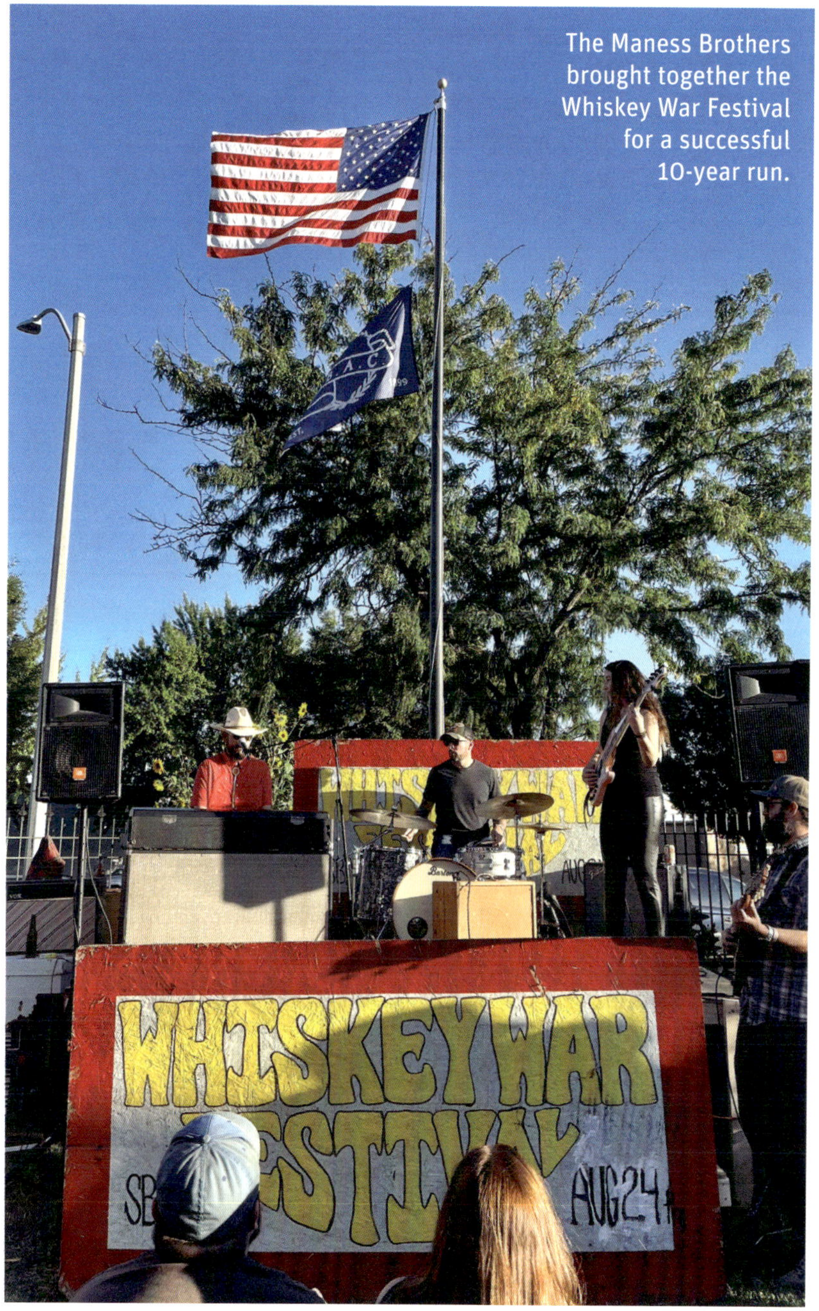

The Maness Brothers brought together the Whiskey War Festival for a successful 10-year run.

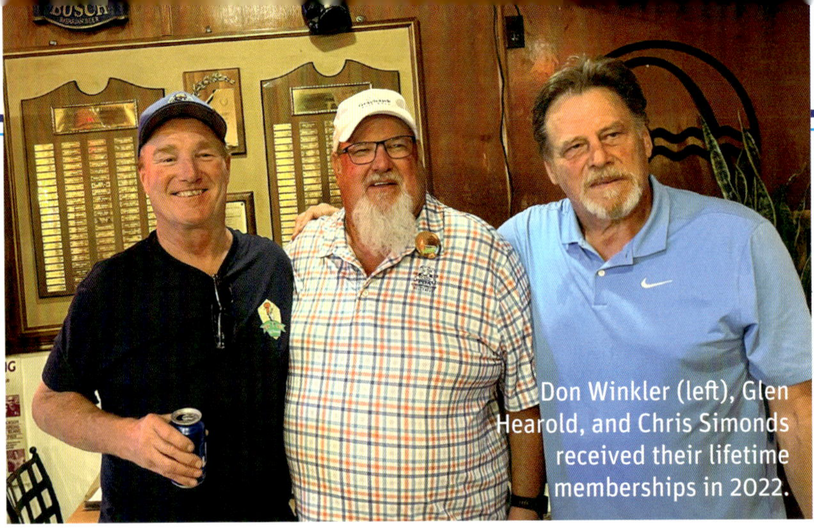

Don Winkler (left), Glen Hearold, and Chris Simonds received their lifetime memberships in 2022.

Festival, an annual all-day music festival that had previously been held in St. Charles. St. Louis's annual *Last Waltz* concert, a tribute to The Band and their farewell concert filmed by Martin Scorsese, was the next major music event that switched venues and made SBAC its annual home.

The club saw its membership grow as more and more people became excited about getting involved and volunteering. Old members came back to help—many of whom hadn't set foot in the

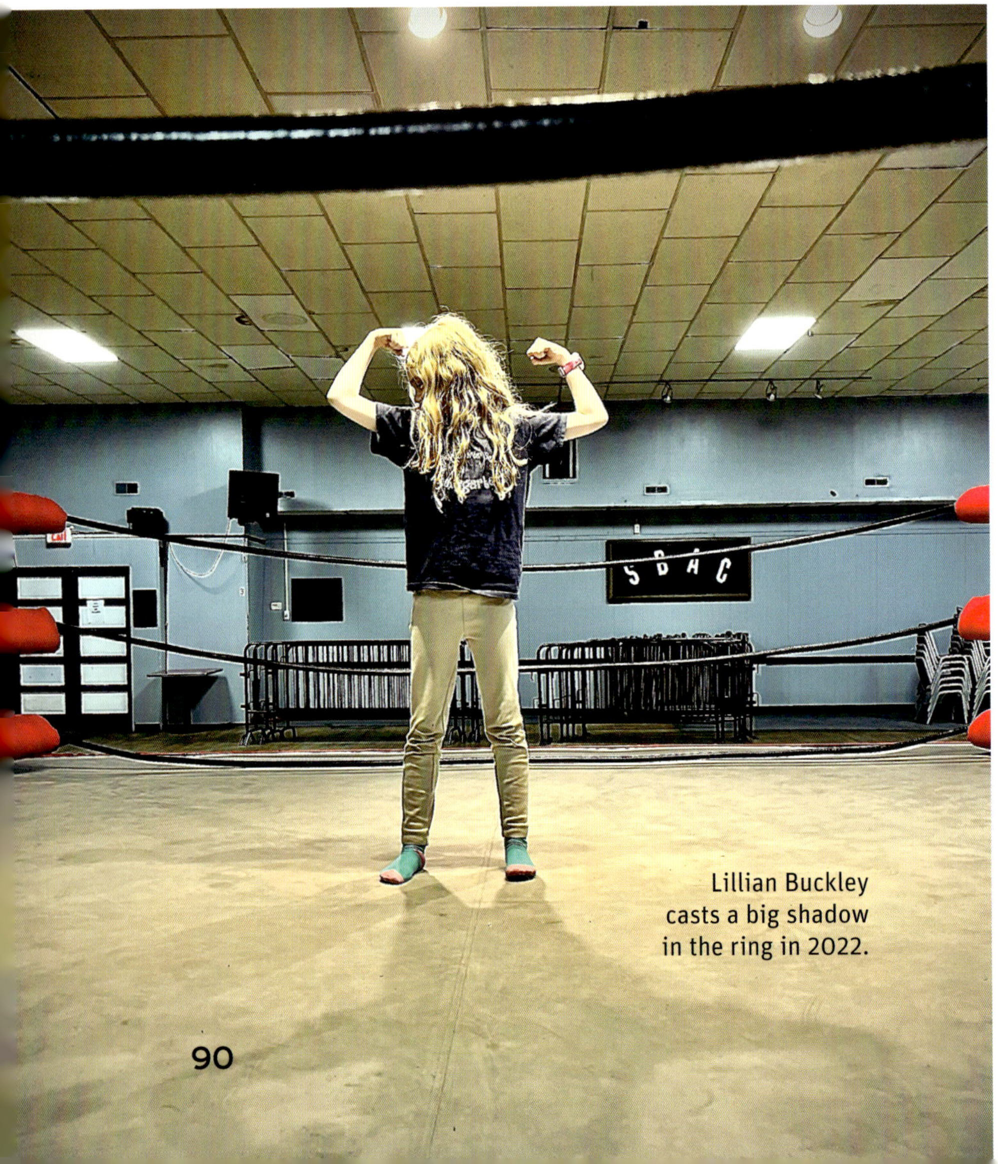

Lillian Buckley casts a big shadow in the ring in 2022.

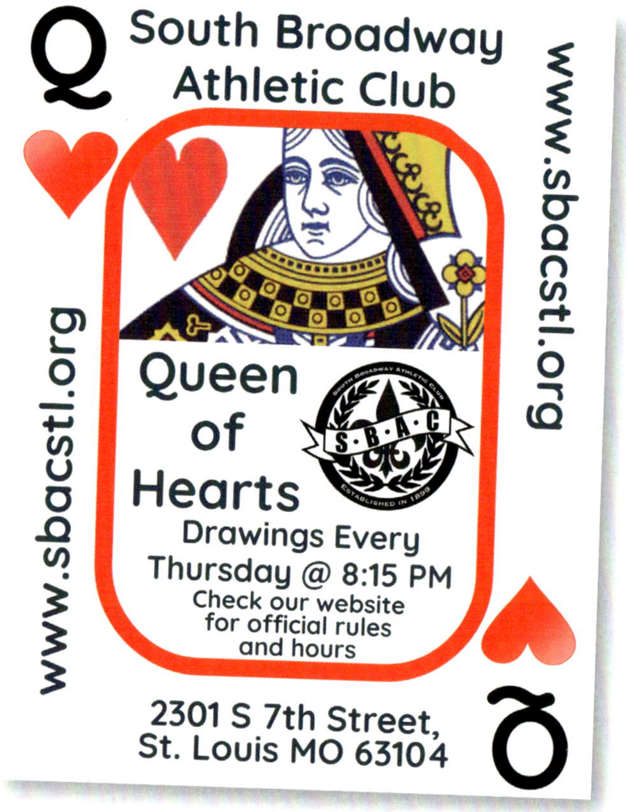

The Queen of Hearts progressive raffle takes place every Thursday night. The fundraiser was launched to fund the new roof, built in 2024, and has continued to draw crowds.

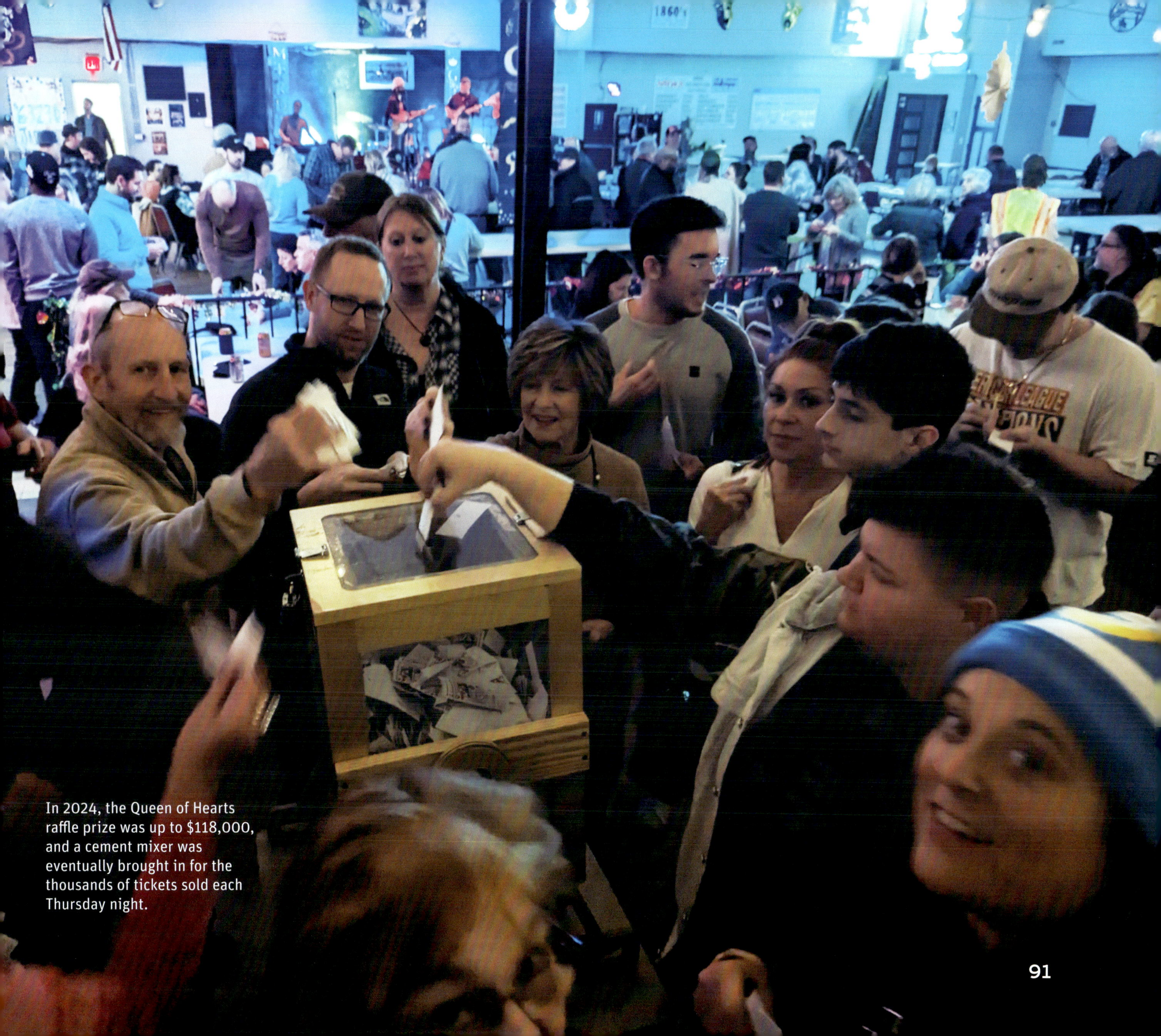

In 2024, the Queen of Hearts raffle prize was up to $118,000, and a cement mixer was eventually brought in for the thousands of tickets sold each Thursday night.

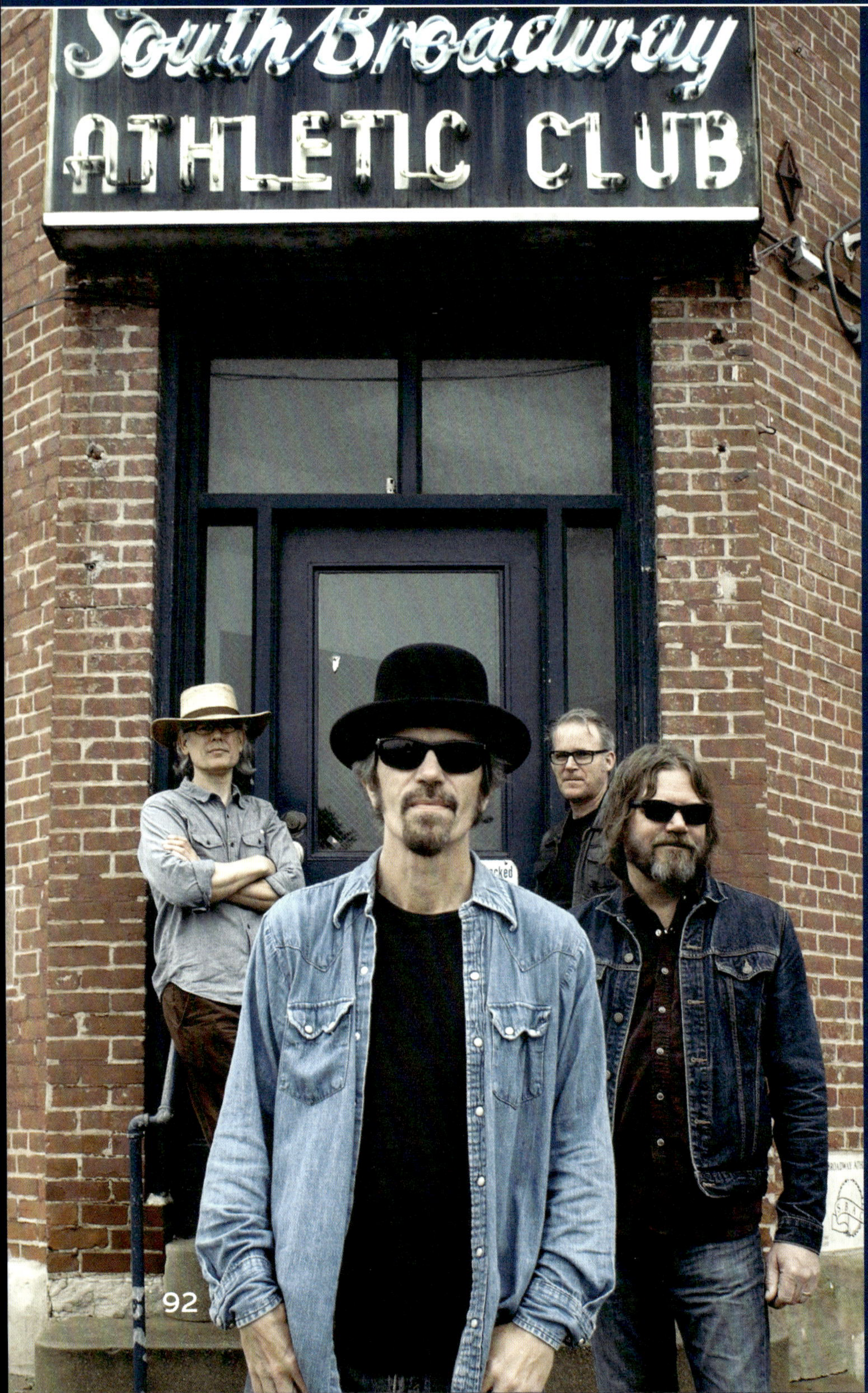

BOTTLE ROCKETS SHOW

THE NIGHT of March 12, 2016, was one to remember at the SBAC. Fans began gathering early, and by showtime the venue was packed with almost 500 people, the crowd buzzing with anticipation. For many, this was a homecoming; the Bottle Rockets were one of St. Louis's own. The historic venue, usually known for wrestling and boxing, transformed into a raucous haven of rock 'n' roll when the band took the stage.

Six months earlier, in a stroke of serendipity, the Bottle Rockets had released a new album named *South Broadway Athletic Club*. Legend has it that the band had been out taking publicity photos and stopped to take one in front of the club's famous neon sign. They liked it so much they decided to use it for their album cover.

At the time, the SBAC was in the throes of its financial difficulties. Looking for ways to turn things around, its newly elected president, Kevin Wilkins, reached out to the Bottle Rockets with the idea of playing a benefit concert. The band graciously agreed and donated the entirety of their ticket sales to help the club.

When the Bottle Rockets finally hit the stage, the roar from the crowd was electric. The band kicked off with "Welfare Music," a track that had become something of an anthem of Midwestern resilience. The first chords sent a ripple through the room. The lyrics about hard times and small-town struggles hit close to home, a reminder of the blue-collar grit of the region and the SBAC itself.

The set list was a perfect mix of classics and deeper cuts, giving longtime fans what they wanted while showcasing the band's range.

The Bottle Rockets (*front*: Brian Henneman; *right*: Keith Voegle; *back left*: Mark Ortmann; *back right*: John Horton) shot some promotional photos in front of the club before deciding to name their new album after it.
Todd Fox photo

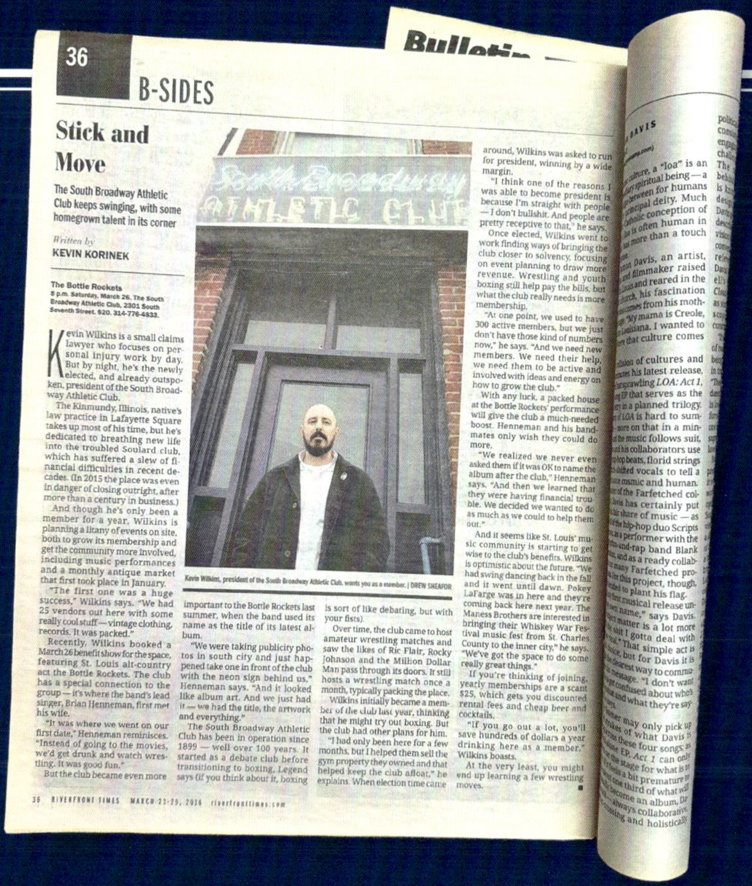

36 B-SIDES

Stick and Move

The South Broadway Athletic Club keeps swinging, with some homegrown talent in its corner

Written by KEVIN KORINEK

A *Riverfront Times* article describes the club's financial troubles and the problem-solving that went into fixing it.

Songs like "Radar Gun" had the crowd singing along, fists pumping in the air, while slower tracks like "Dog" offered moments of reflection, with frontman Brian Henneman's voice carrying a raw, emotional weight.

As the night went on, the band played tracks from their latest album, *South Broadway Athletic Club*. Henneman joked about the "full circle" feeling of debuting these songs in the very place that inspired the album's name. It felt like a celebration of all the ups and downs, a band and a place that had seen its fair share of struggles and somehow kept going. The crowd knew they'd shared something special that night.

"We were glad to do it," said Bottle Rockets guitarist John Horton, who now is with Son Volt. "We wanted to help."

And for the SBAC, it was a turning point: the show had raised more than $20,000. The SBAC wasn't out of the woods, but the Bottle Rockets had given it a jolt and helped set the course for one of the greatest comebacks in history.

—Kevin Wilkins

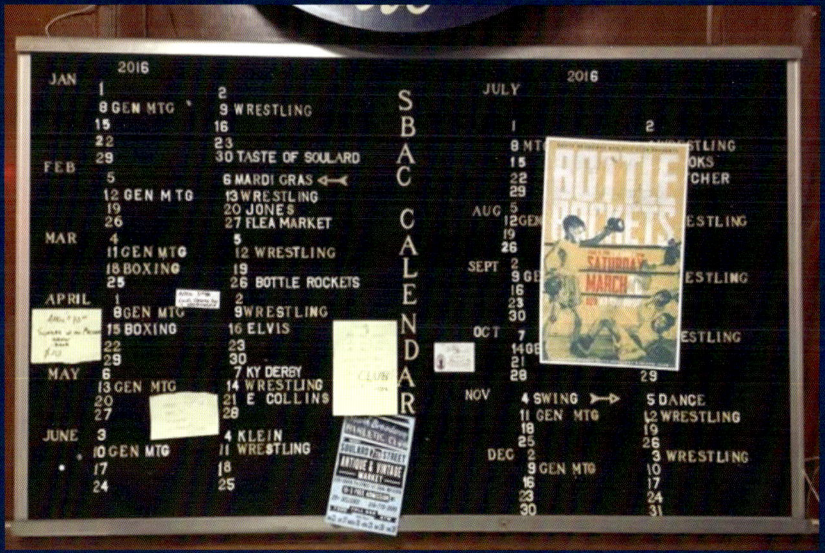

Bottle Rockets show poster

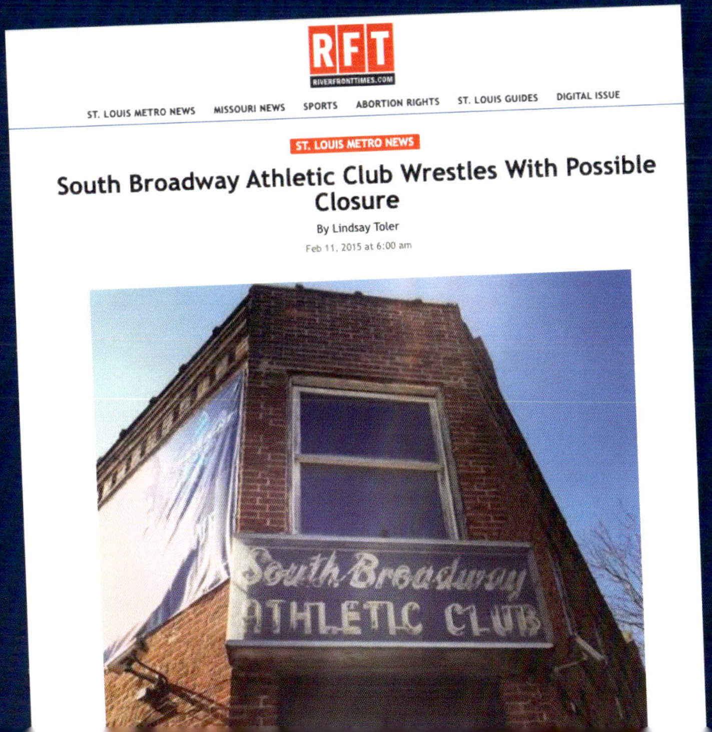

RFT

RIVERFRONTTIMES.COM

ST. LOUIS METRO NEWS MISSOURI NEWS SPORTS ABORTION RIGHTS ST. LOUIS GUIDES DIGITAL ISSUE

ST. LOUIS METRO NEWS

South Broadway Athletic Club Wrestles With Possible Closure

By Lindsay Toler

Feb 11, 2015 at 6:00 am

Riverfront Times article about how the South Broadway Athletic Club wrestled with possible closure

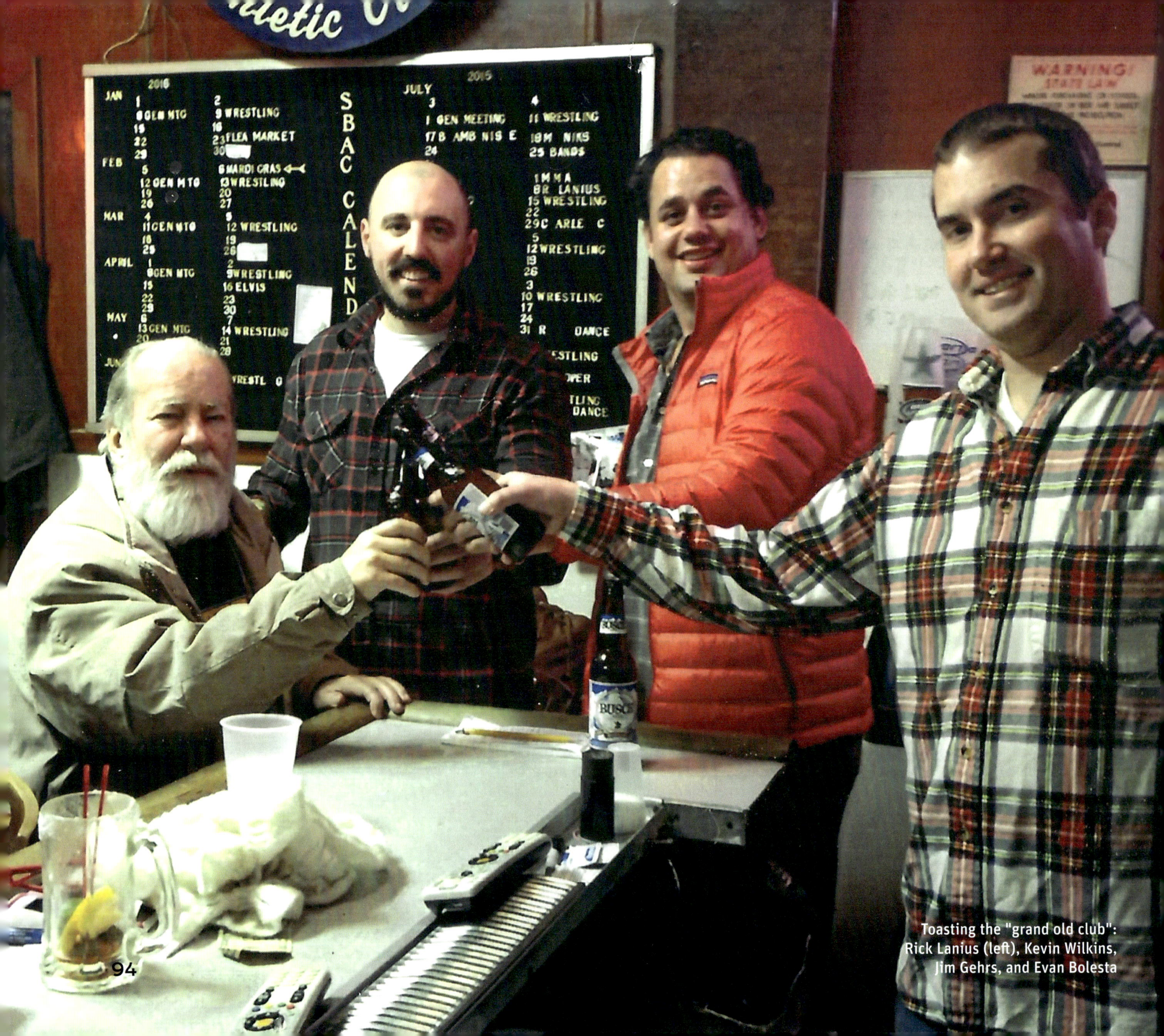

Toasting the "grand old club": Rick Lanius (left), Kevin Wilkins, Jim Gehrs, and Evan Bolesta

club for years. Eventually, the club was able to pay off $30,000 in back taxes and more than $20,000 in past due loans that members had given in the early 2000s.

The decision was made that major events such as Mardi Gras and club-sponsored concerts would be staffed entirely by volunteers, with the bar tips being donated back to the club. Soon, opportunities arose outside of the club to work events such as the Soulard Oktoberfest and the Music at the Intersection festival, which provided additional revenue. The weekly Queen

"Big Poppa Pump" Scott Steiner made a special appearance at a 2021 wrestling show.

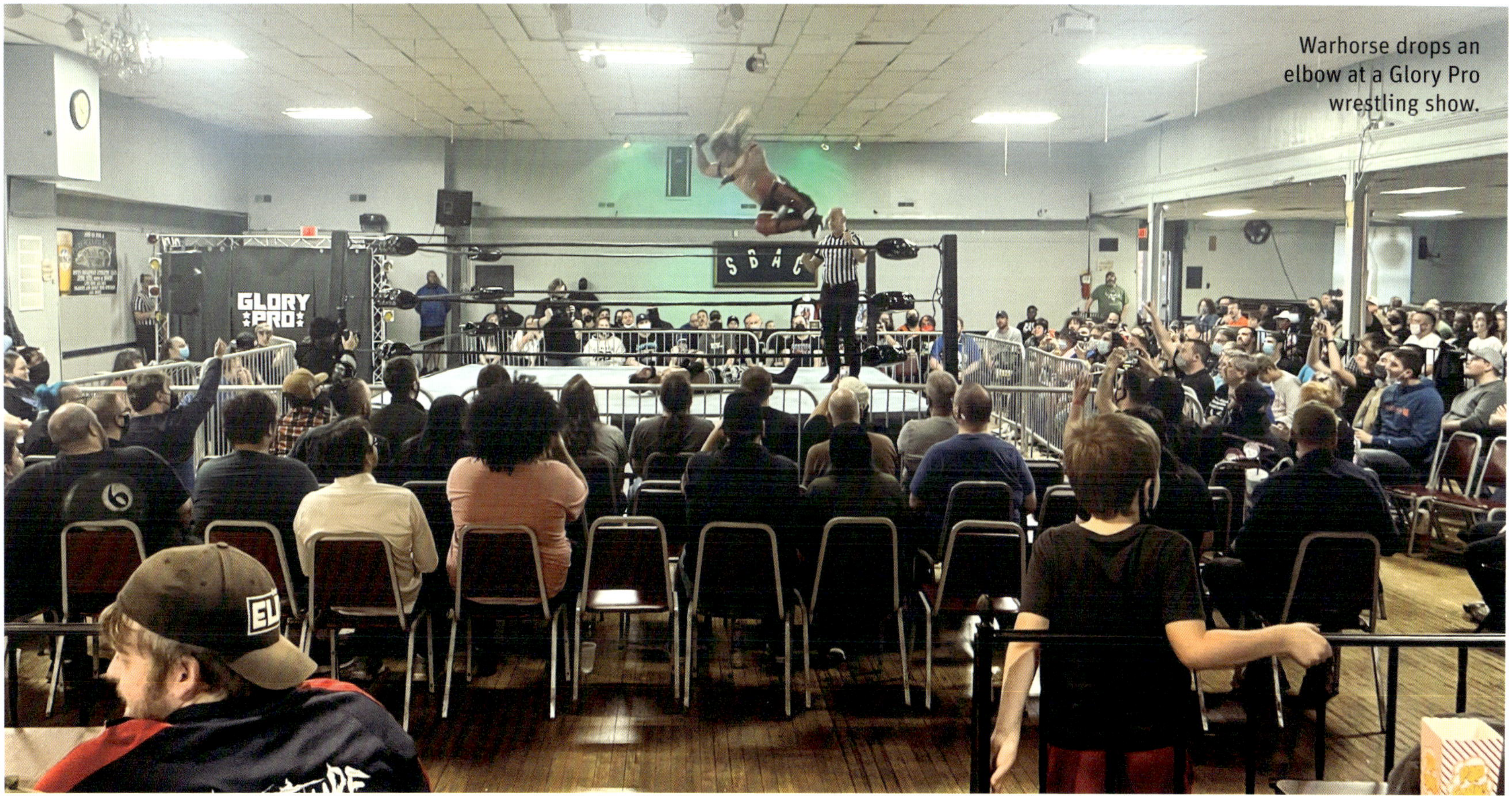

Warhorse drops an elbow at a Glory Pro wrestling show.

S·B·A·C·
125
ANNIVERSARY
EST. 1899

ON DECEMBER 7, 2024, the club celebrated the 125th anniversary of its founding with a 1920s-themed gala. More than 400 people attended, many dressed in Roaring '20s flapper dresses, tuxedos, period suits, or other finery. Numerous catered food stations and themed cocktails helped drive the celebration.

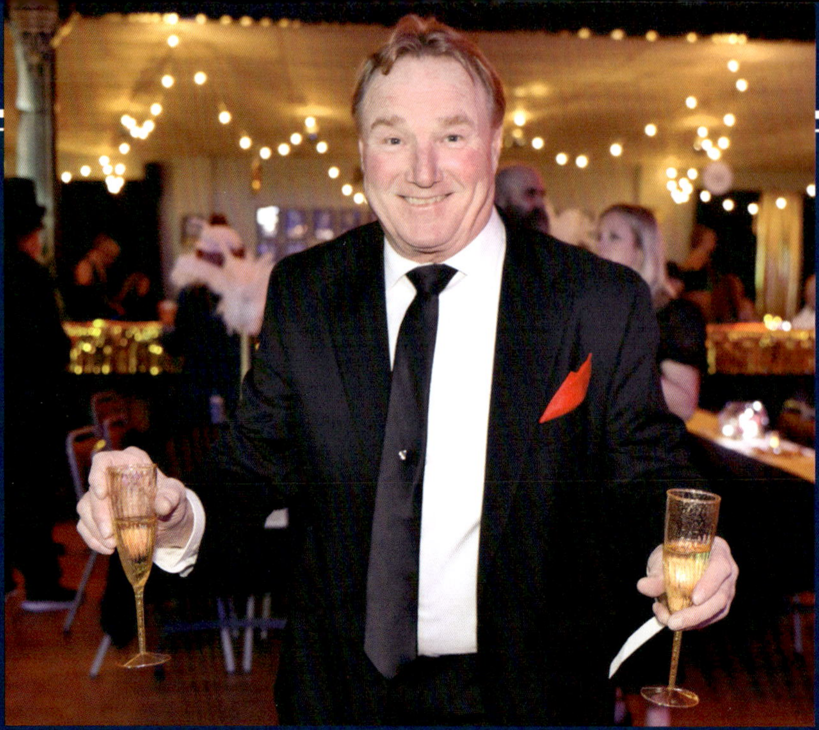

Lifetime member Don Winkler toasts 125 years of South Broadway.

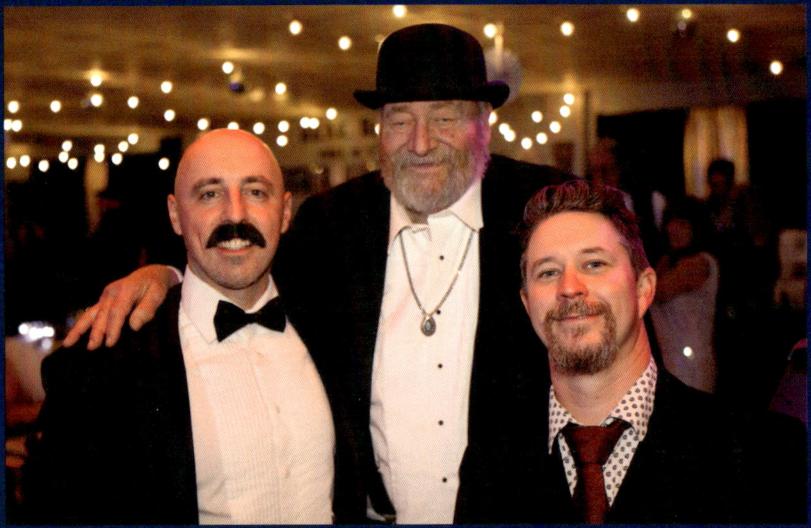

Club officers Kevin Wilkins (left) and Ryan Buckley (right) with longtime member Jules Sardo

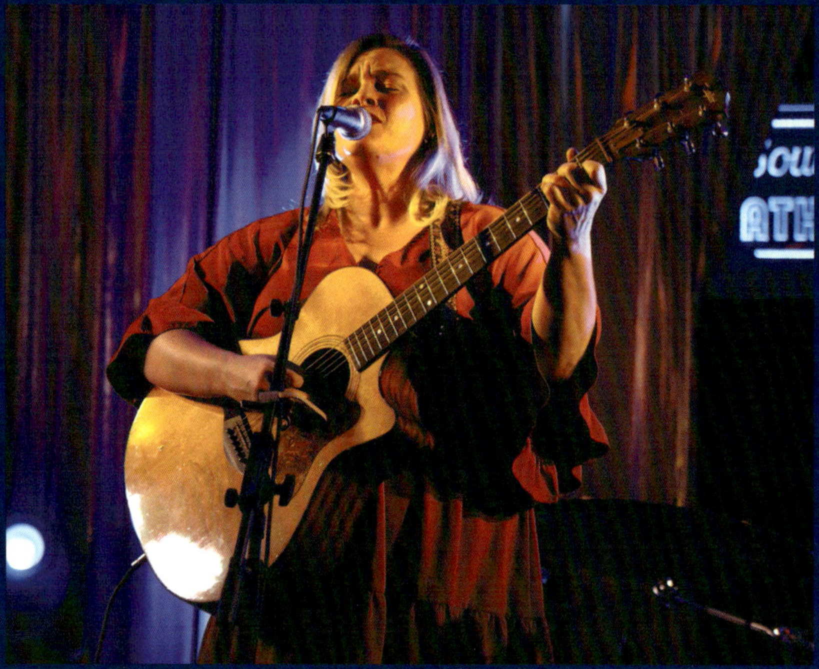

Emily Wallace serenades club members at 125th Anniversary Gala.

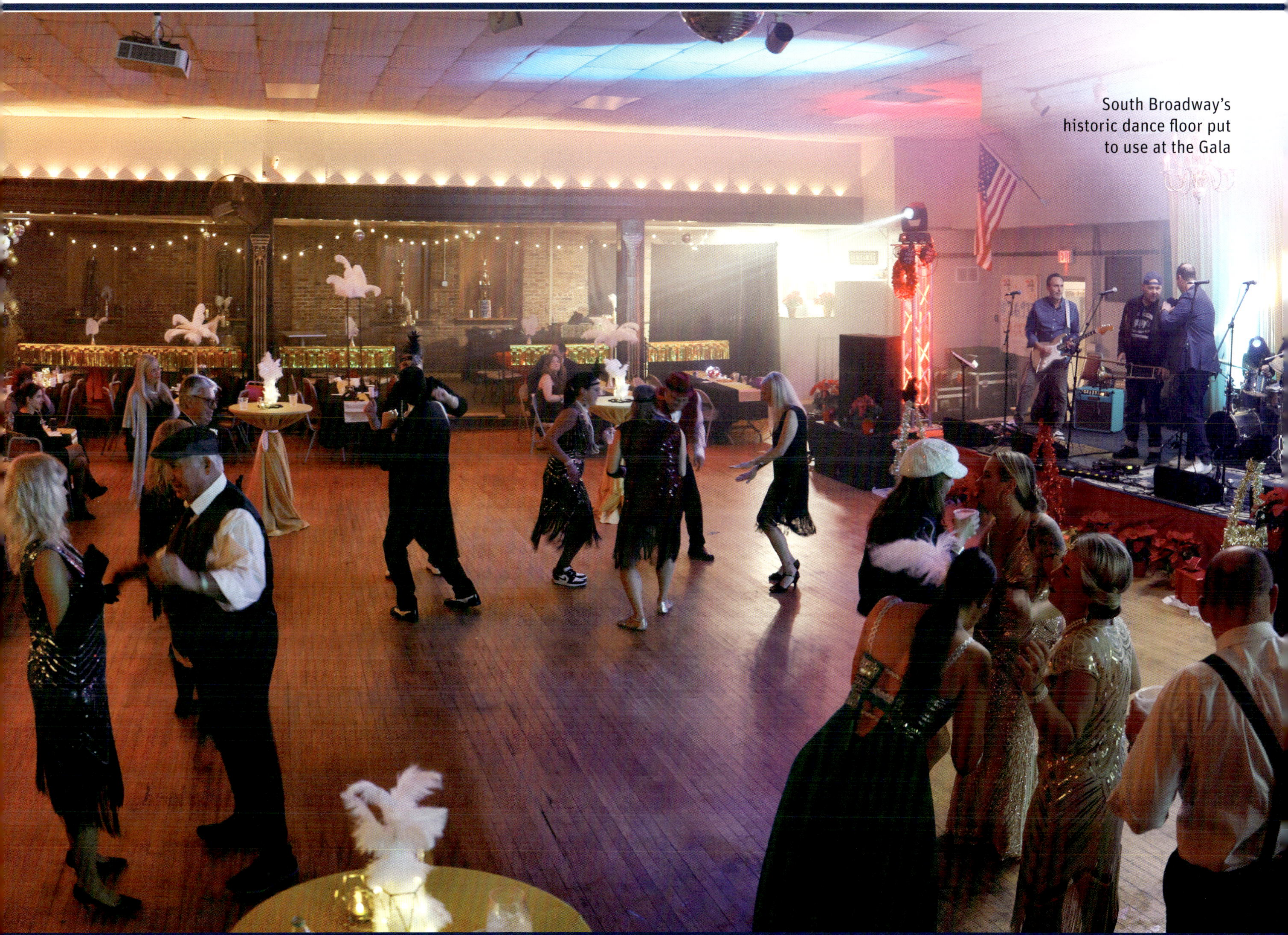

South Broadway's historic dance floor put to use at the Gala

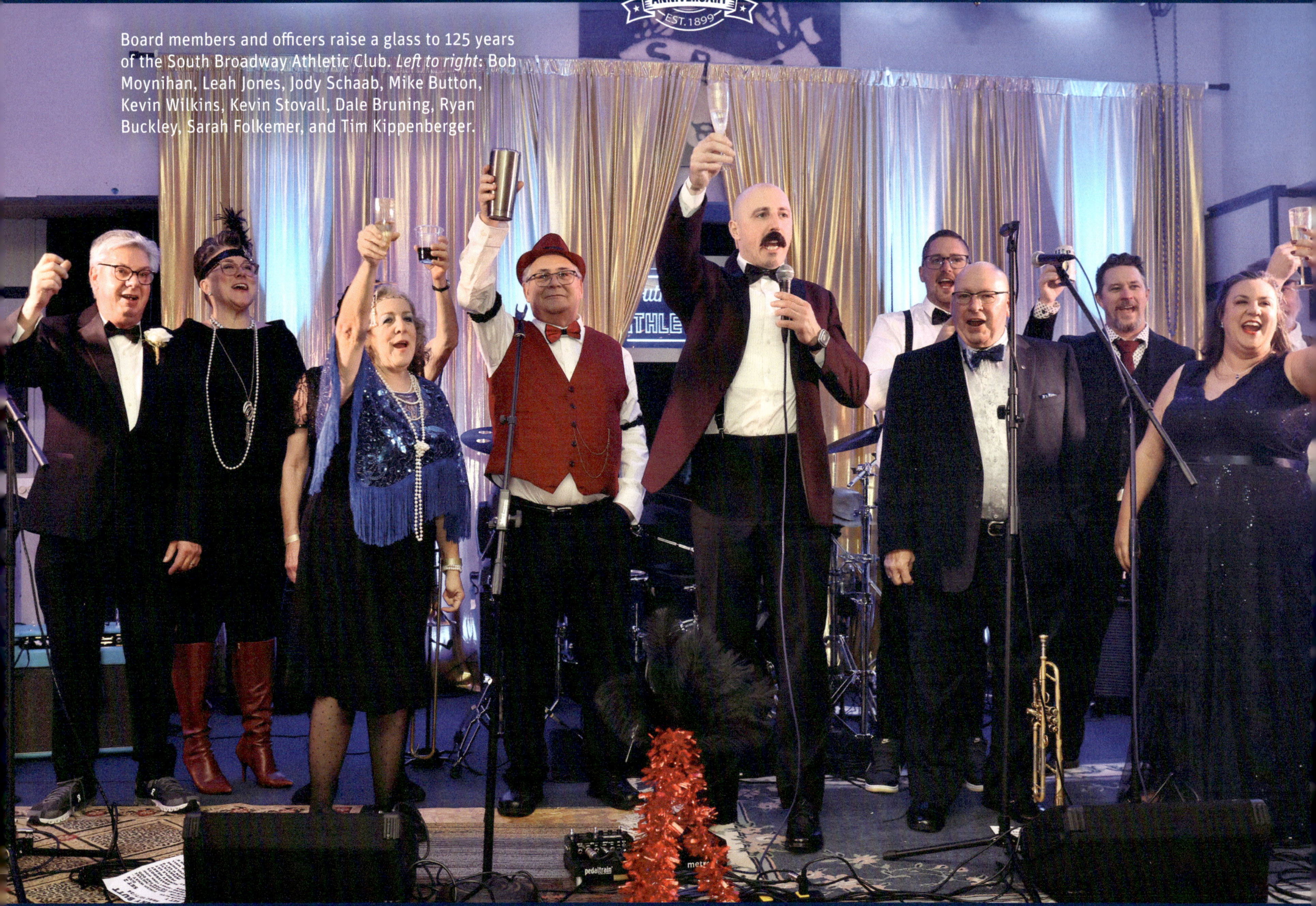

Board members and officers raise a glass to 125 years of the South Broadway Athletic Club. *Left to right*: Bob Moynihan, Leah Jones, Jody Schaab, Mike Button, Kevin Wilkins, Kevin Stovall, Dale Bruning, Ryan Buckley, Sarah Folkemer, and Tim Kippenberger.

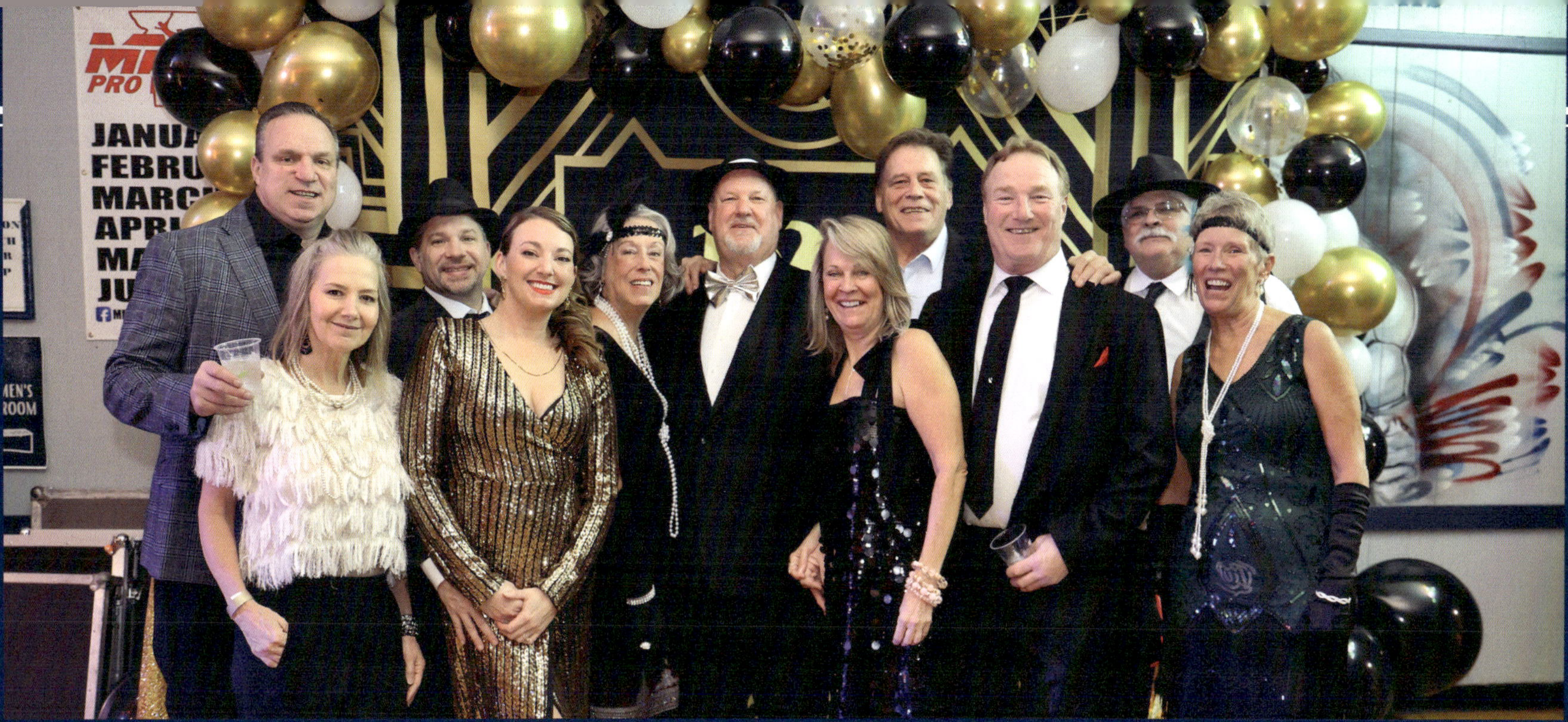

Jerry Winkler, Sue Meyer, Zach Mertens, Sam Mertens, Ruth Hearold, Glen Hearold, Liz MacDonald, Chris Simonds, Don Winkler, Mike Hearold, and Jane Hearold

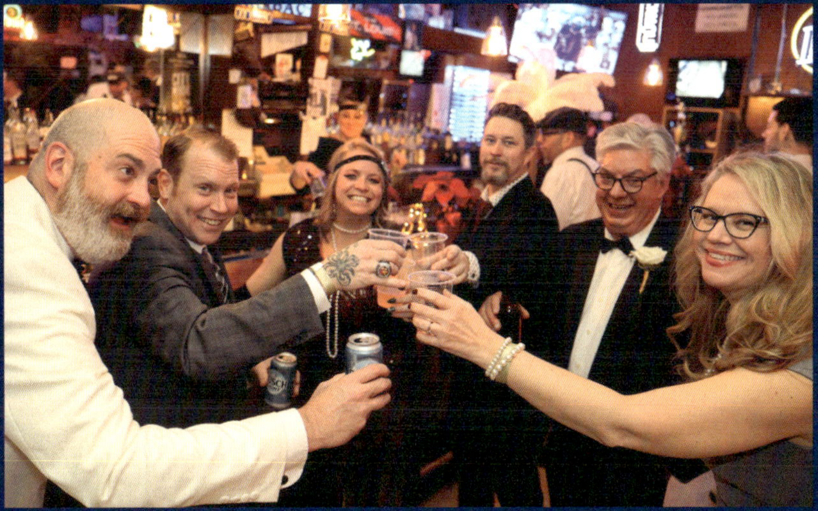

James Lay, Jeff Lehmann, Abigail Manwarren, Ryan Buckley, Bob Moynihan, and Christina Buckley

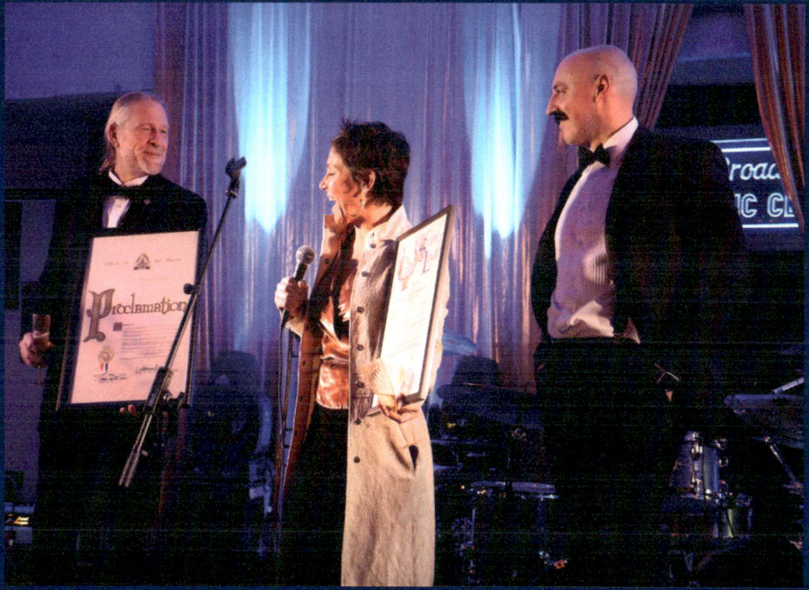

Dan Guenther, Alderwoman Cara Spencer, and Kevin Wilkins present Gala attendees with St. Louis City proclamations declaring South Broadway Athletic Club Day.

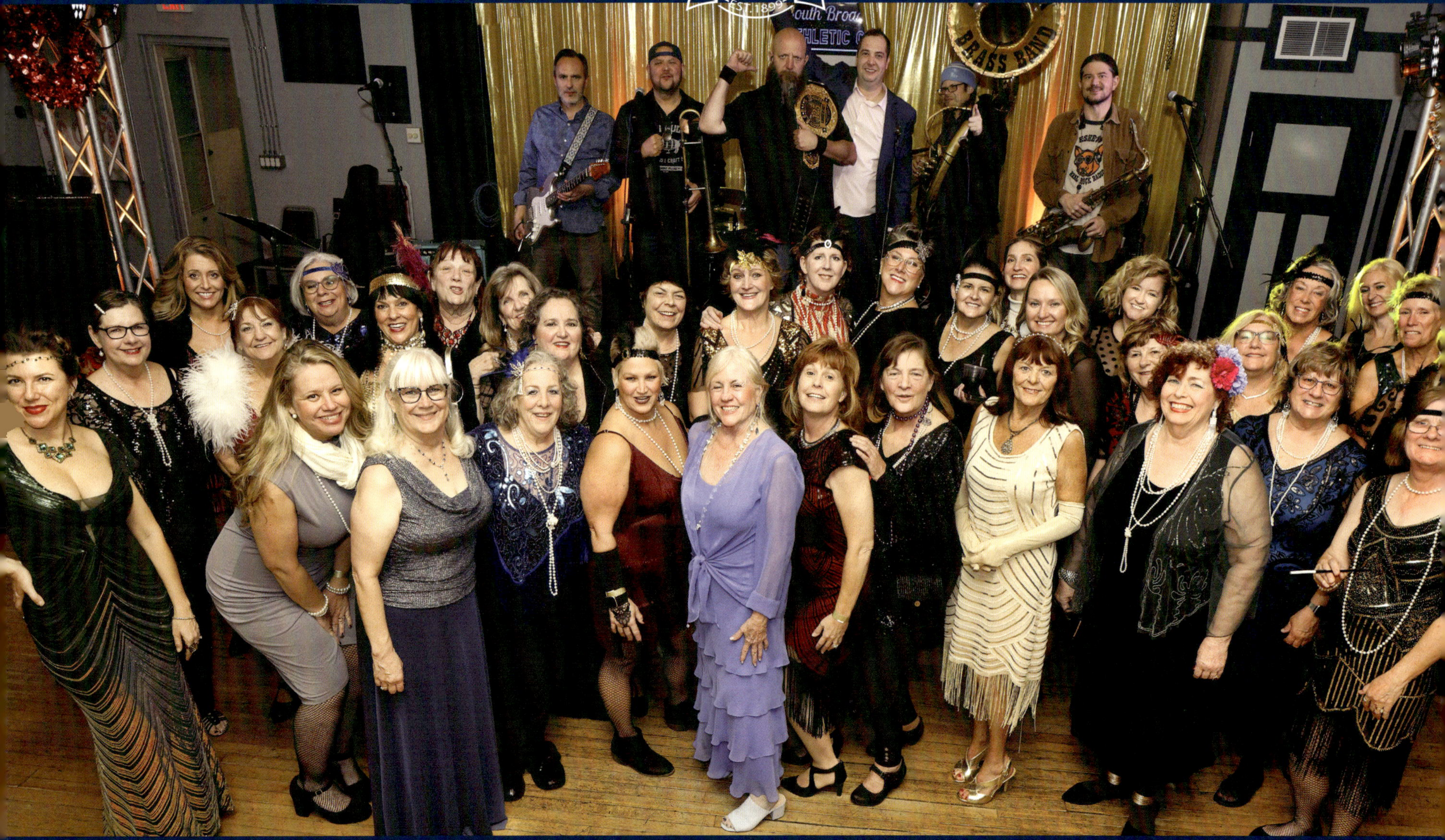

On stage, left to right: The Funky Butt Brass Band members Jim Peters, Aaron Chandler, Ron Sikes, Adam Hucke, Cody Henry, and Charlie Cerpa. *Front row, left to right:* Christina Buckley, Connie Bafaro, Jody Schaab, Johanna Mertensmeyer, Maura Nagel, Tracy Laxton, Margaret Bianchetta, Brookie Blake, unknown, Brenda Cash, and Cheryl Bauman

Back row, left to right: Shina Dill, Stephanie Amen, unknown, Patti Crites, Cathy Bruning, Julie Price, Michelle Northington, Mary Tabacchi, Marcia Craig, Marcia Tolcou, Jackie Harris, Kristin Carlson, Leah Jones, unknown, Abbey Willen, Amy Stovall, Denise Naughton, Shirley Button, Mary Moynihan, Ruth Hearold, Renee Becker, Jane Hearold, and Lisa Mullins

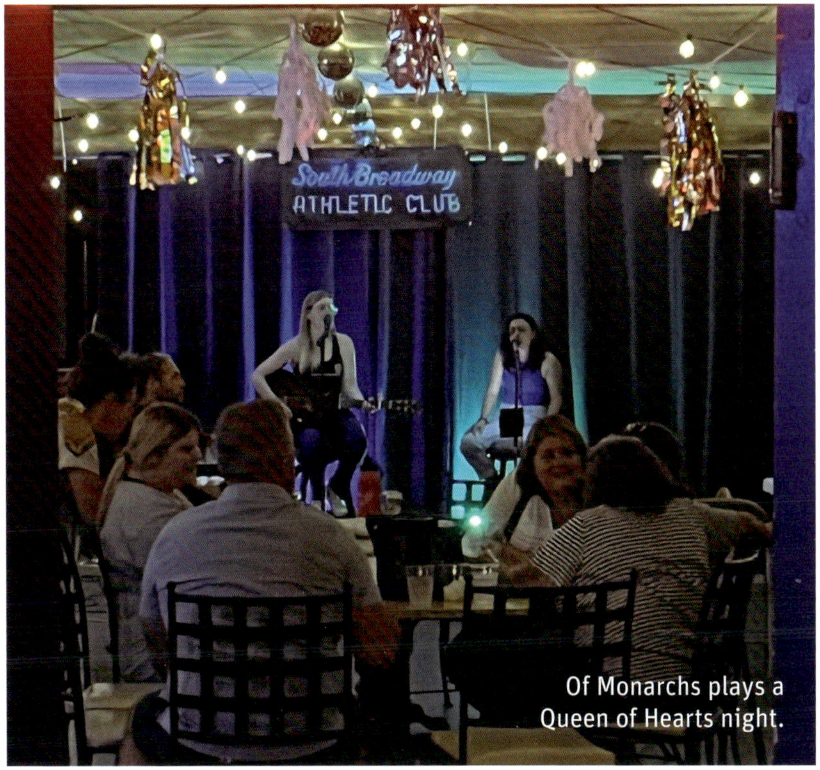

Of Monarchs plays a Queen of Hearts night.

Historical Note

Membership Booms at SBAC

The membership grew to 500 during the early years. Every club member had to be 21 years of age. They enjoyed a game of cards (pinochle was the favored game among the South Side Germans) and a local brew before the fight. The members could get 24 chips for a dollar, which paid for 24 beers or their equivalent.

of Hearts raffle has now become of a staple of the Soulard community and allowed the SBAC to welcome its neighbors on a weekly basis. The club recently put a new roof on the building with funds raised entirely from donated tips and revenue from working outside events.

Legacy of Survival

TODAY, THE SOUTH BROADWAY ATHLETIC CLUB boasts more than 300 members and stands as a testament to perseverance and community spirit. Its comeback from near collapse is a celebration of resilience, driven by the passion of its members and the love for a place that has become their community.

The revival of the South Broadway Athletic Club was more than just a business success; it was proof of the power of community and the enduring appeal of a space where people could come together and be part of something bigger.

From the brink of closure, it has reemerged stronger, adapting to the needs of a changing community while staying true to its roots. The South Broadway Athletic Club has reclaimed its place as a pillar of the Soulard community, ensuring that its legacy will continue for generations to come.

—Kevin Wilkins

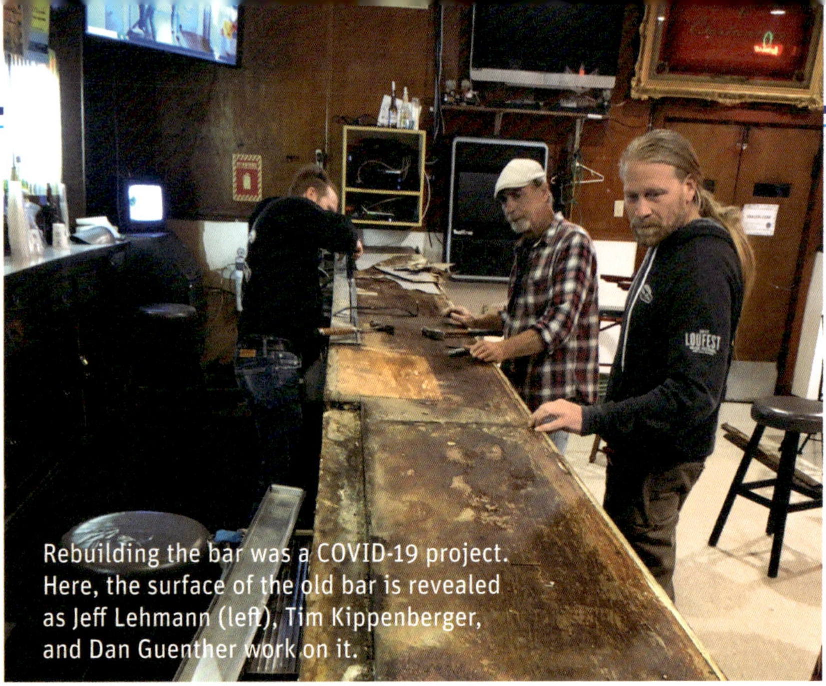

Rebuilding the bar was a COVID-19 project. Here, the surface of the old bar is revealed as Jeff Lehmann (left), Tim Kippenberger, and Dan Guenther work on it.

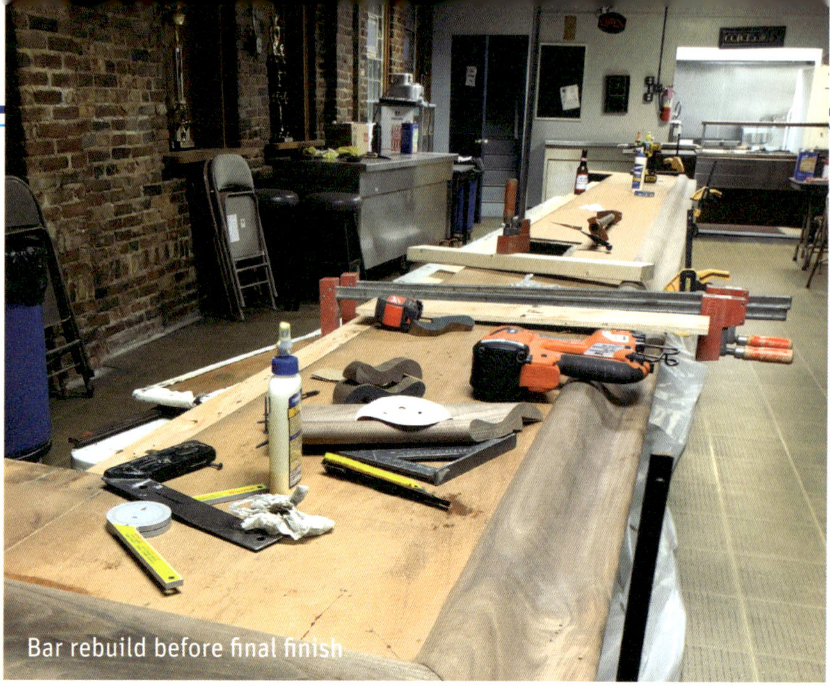

Bar rebuild before final finish

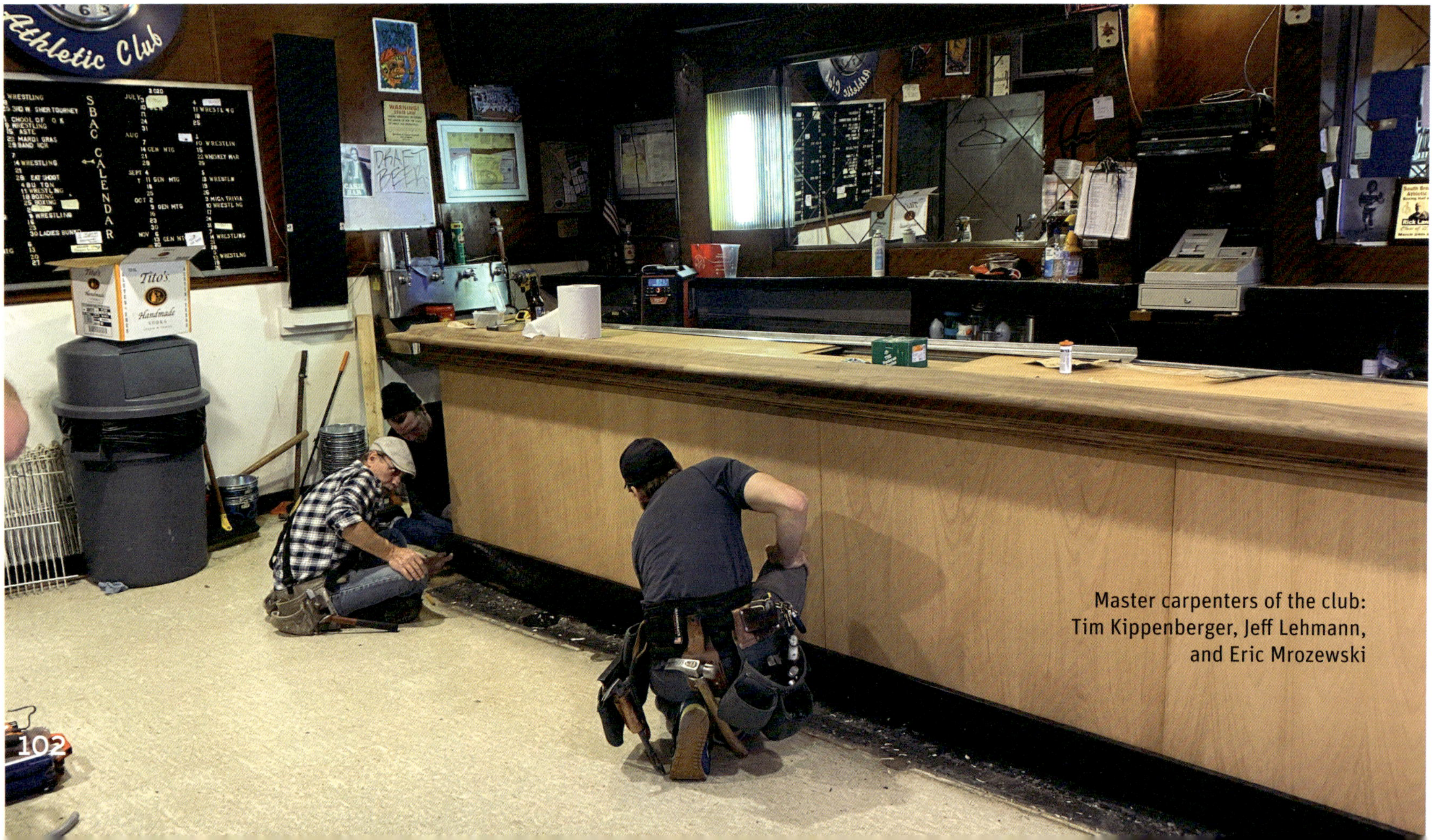

Master carpenters of the club: Tim Kippenberger, Jeff Lehmann, and Eric Mrozewski

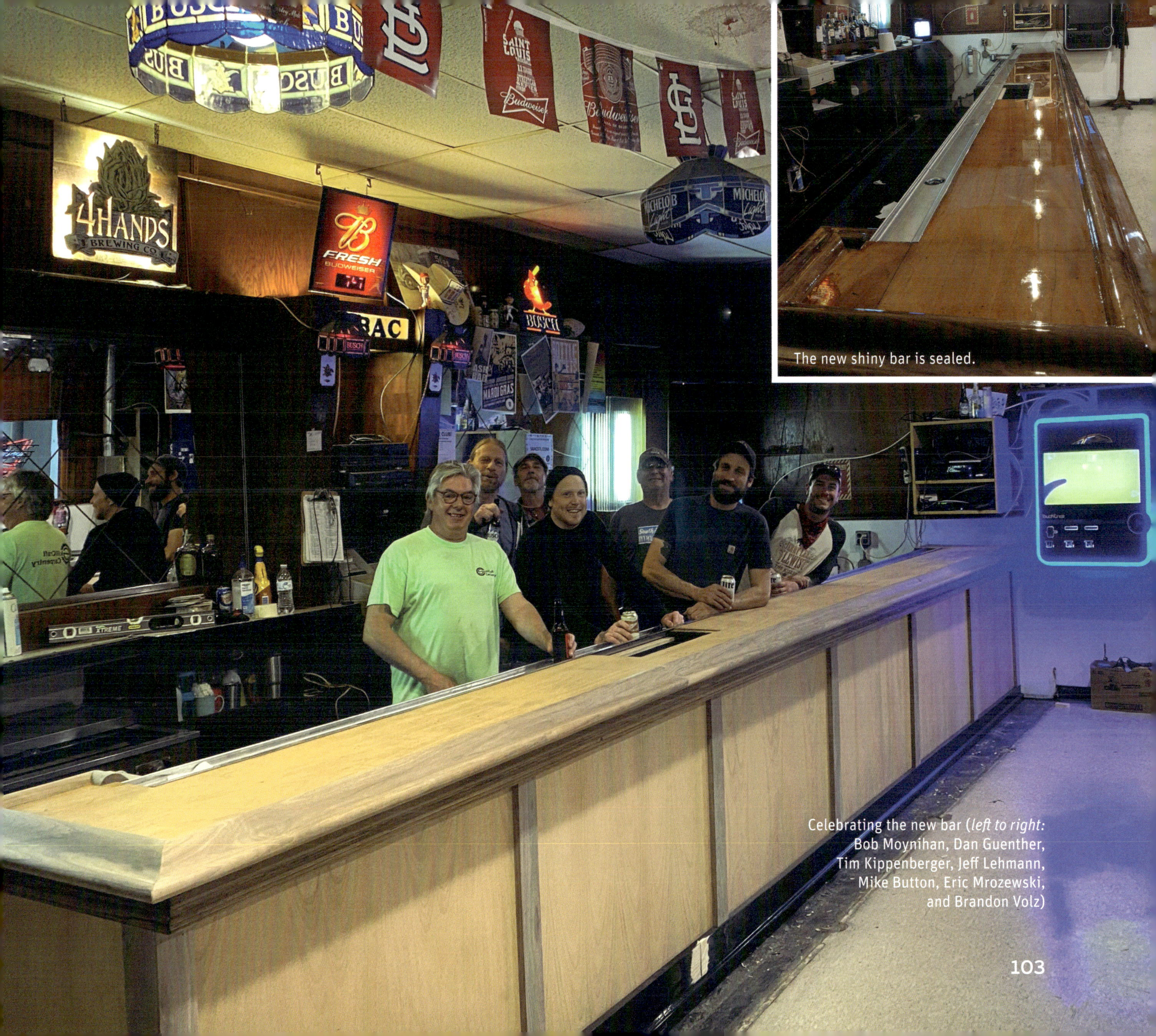

The new shiny bar is sealed.

Celebrating the new bar (*left to right:* Bob Moynihan, Dan Guenther, Tim Kippenberger, Jeff Lehmann, Mike Button, Eric Mrozewski, and Brandon Volz)

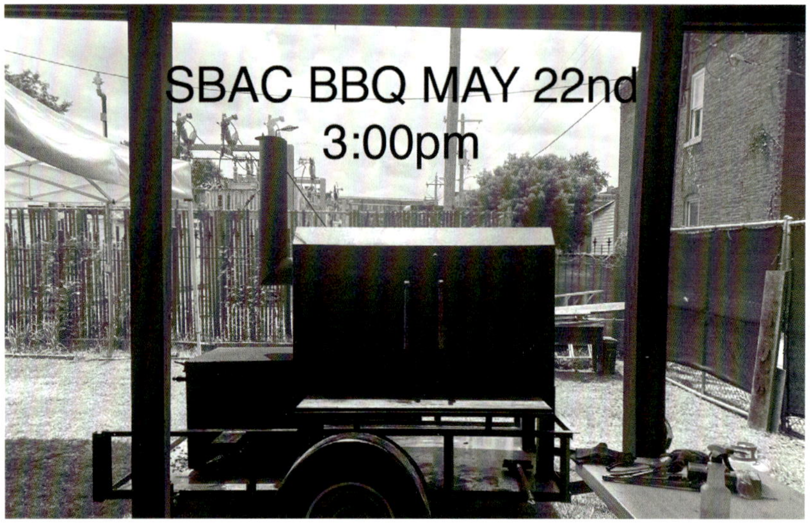

The Sooner Or Later crew's custom-made barbecue smoker is shown in this flier. The rig lives at the club permanently.

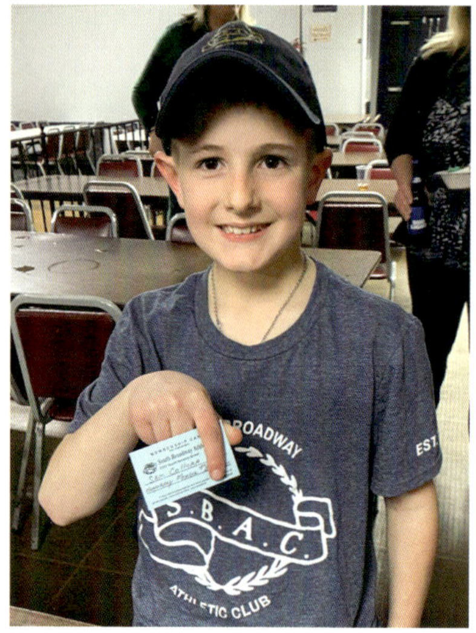

Sam Collora joins the club as an honorary member.

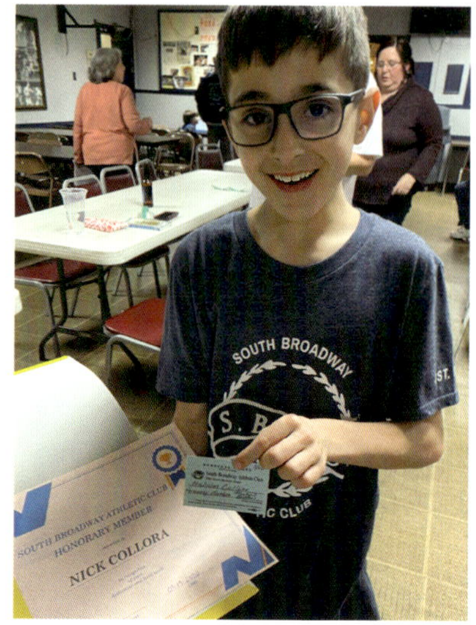

Nick Collora joins the club as an honorary member.

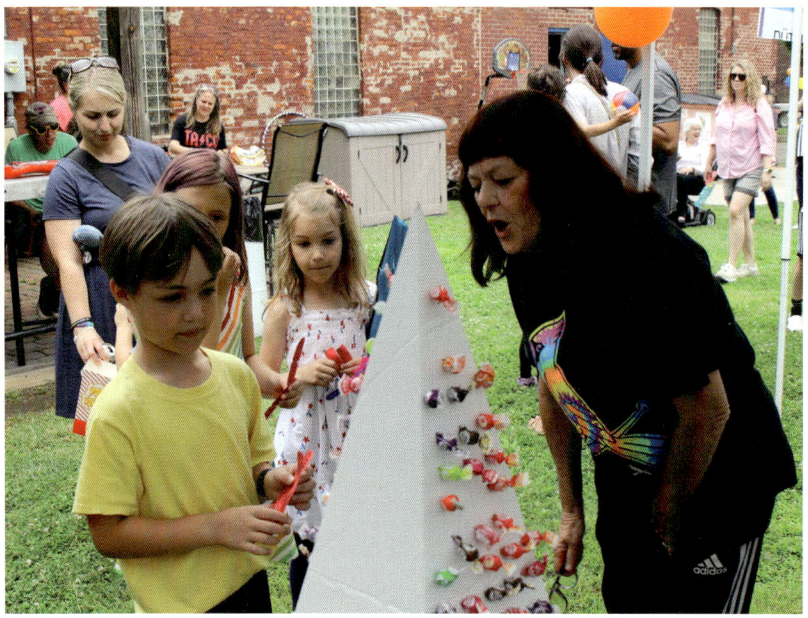

Brookie Blake entertaining kids at the Homecoming Carnival

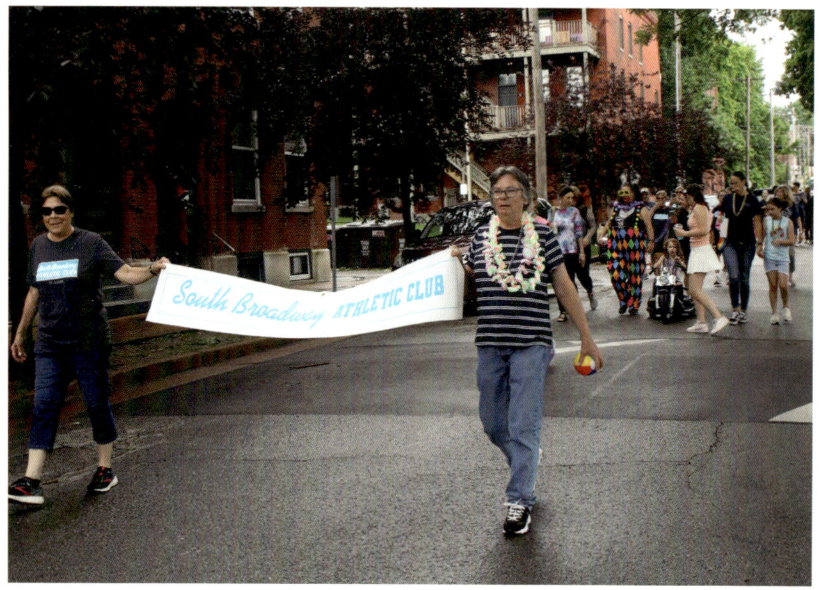

Club treasurer Marcia Tolcou (left) leads the parade down Shenandoah to kick off the carnival.

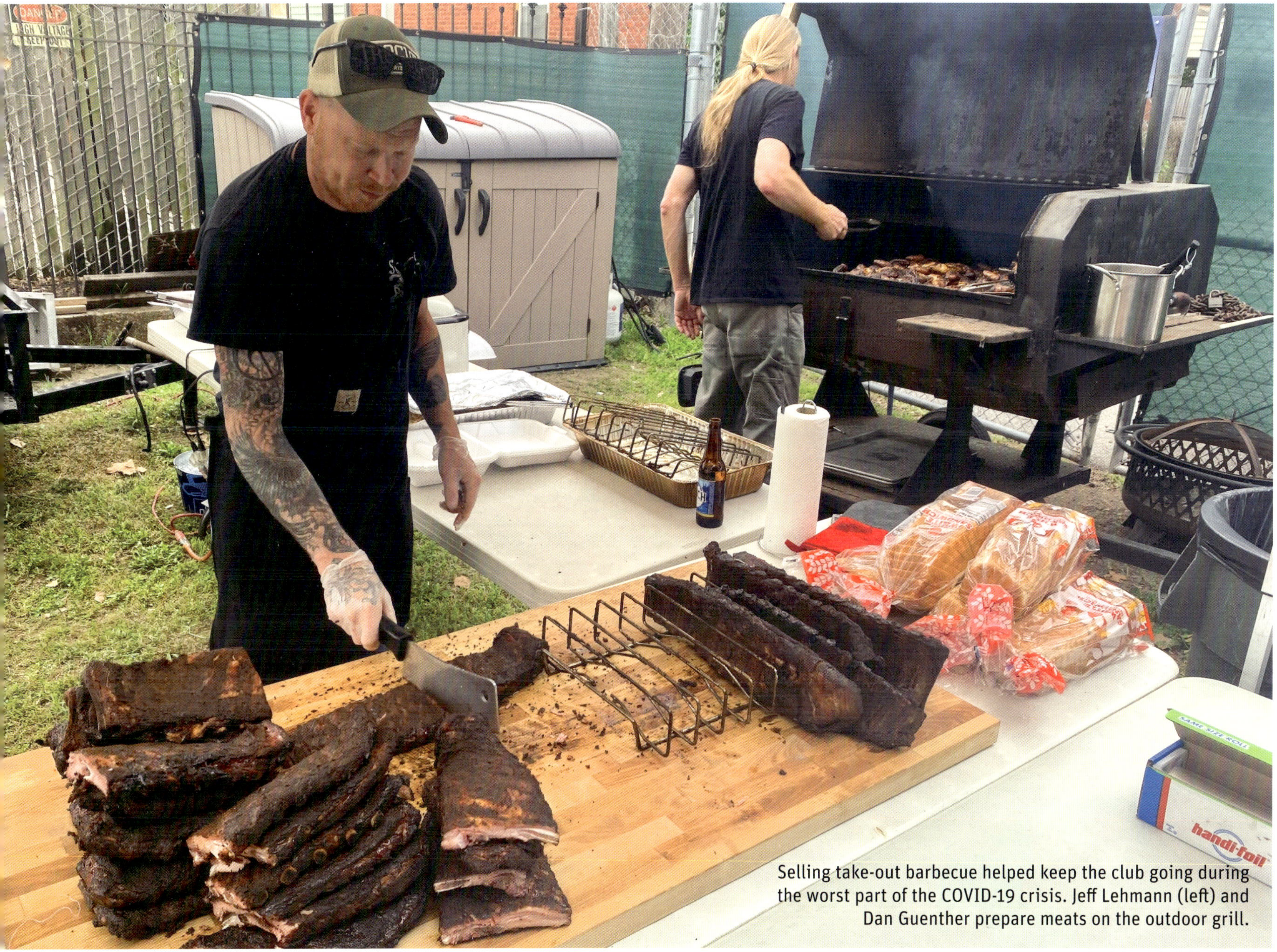

Selling take-out barbecue helped keep the club going during the worst part of the COVID-19 crisis. Jeff Lehmann (left) and Dan Guenther prepare meats on the outdoor grill.

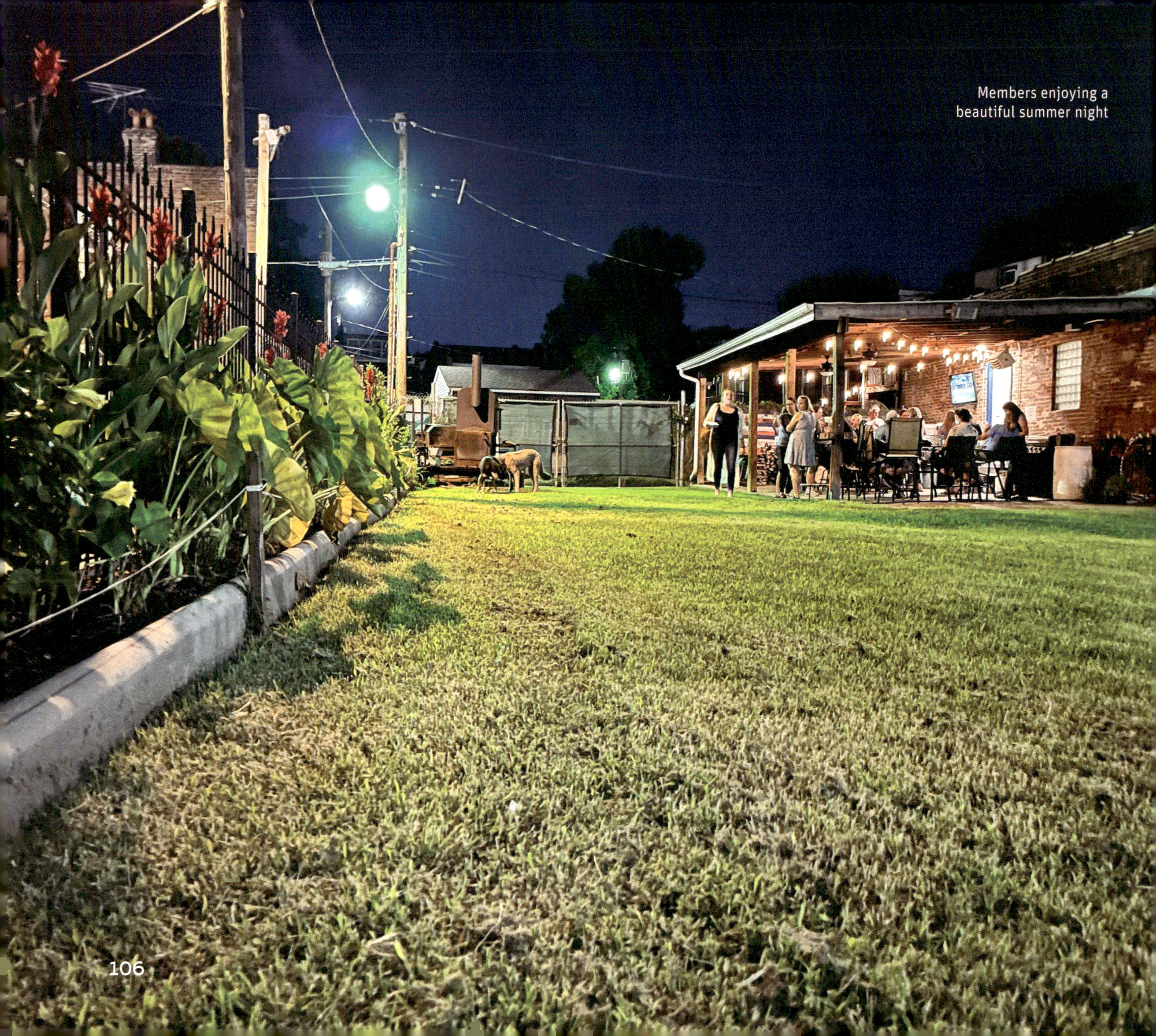

Members enjoying a
beautiful summer night

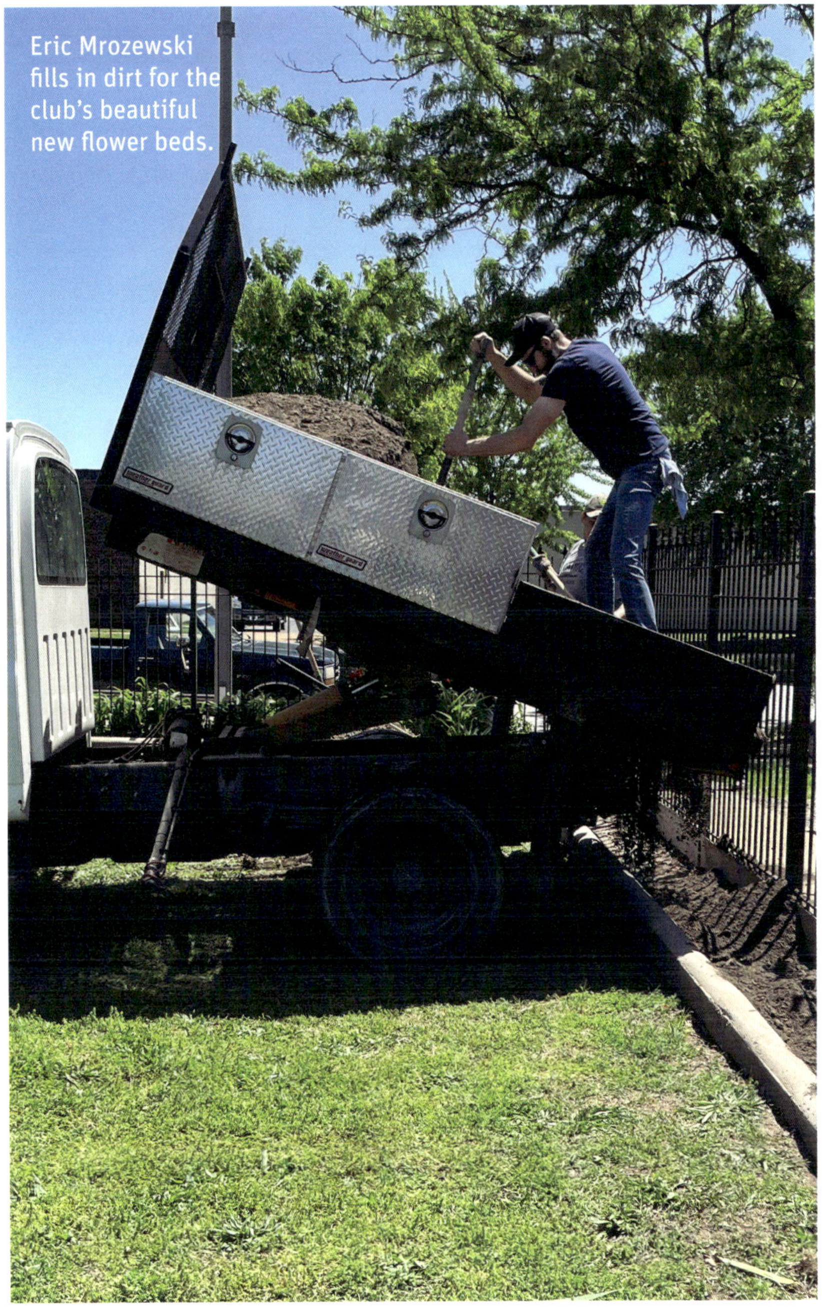

Eric Mrozewski fills in dirt for the club's beautiful new flower beds.

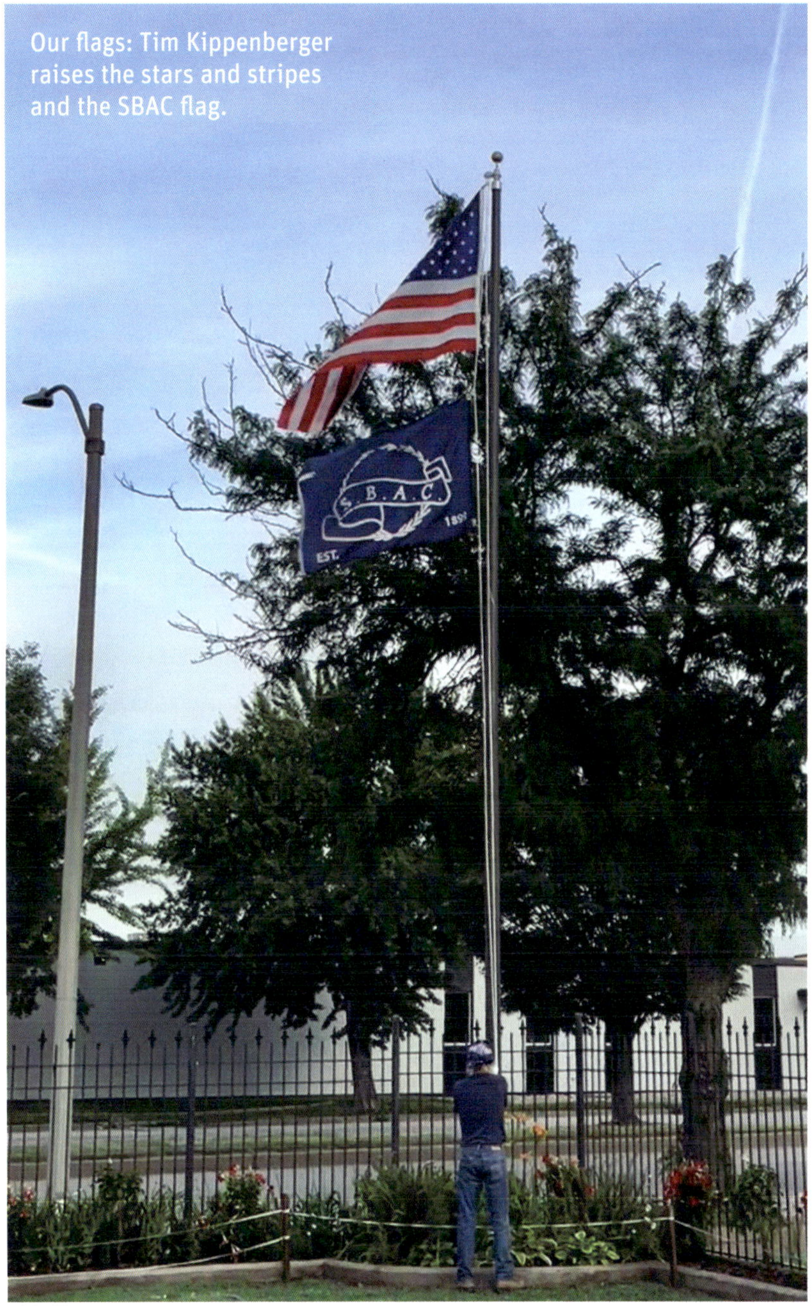

Our flags: Tim Kippenberger raises the stars and stripes and the SBAC flag.

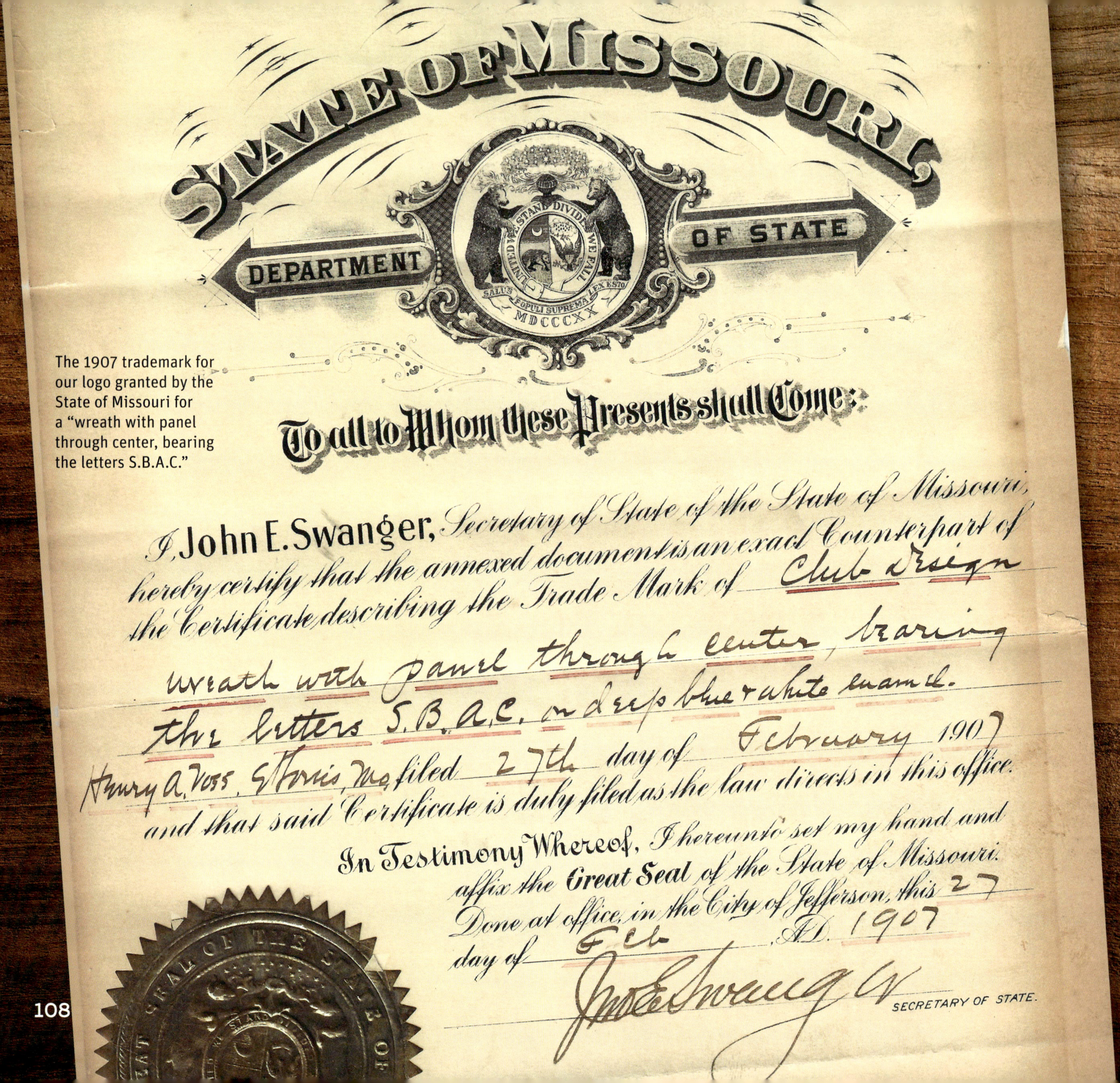

STATE OF MISSOURI,

DEPARTMENT OF STATE

SALUS POPULI SUPREMA LEX ESTO

MDCCCXX

To all to Whom these Presents shall Come:

I, John E. Swanger, Secretary of State of the State of Missouri, hereby certify that the annexed document is an exact Counterpart of the Certificate describing the Trade Mark of Club Design wreath with panel through center, bearing the letters S.B.A.C. on deep blue & white enamel. Henry A. Voss, St Louis, Mo. filed 27th day of February 1907 and that said Certificate is duly filed as the law directs in this office.

In Testimony Whereof, I hereunto set my hand and affix the Great Seal of the State of Missouri. Done at office, in the City of Jefferson, this 27 day of Feb A.D. 1907

Jno E Swanger

SECRETARY OF STATE.

The 1907 trademark for our logo granted by the State of Missouri for a "wreath with panel through center, bearing the letters S.B.A.C."

Acknowledgments

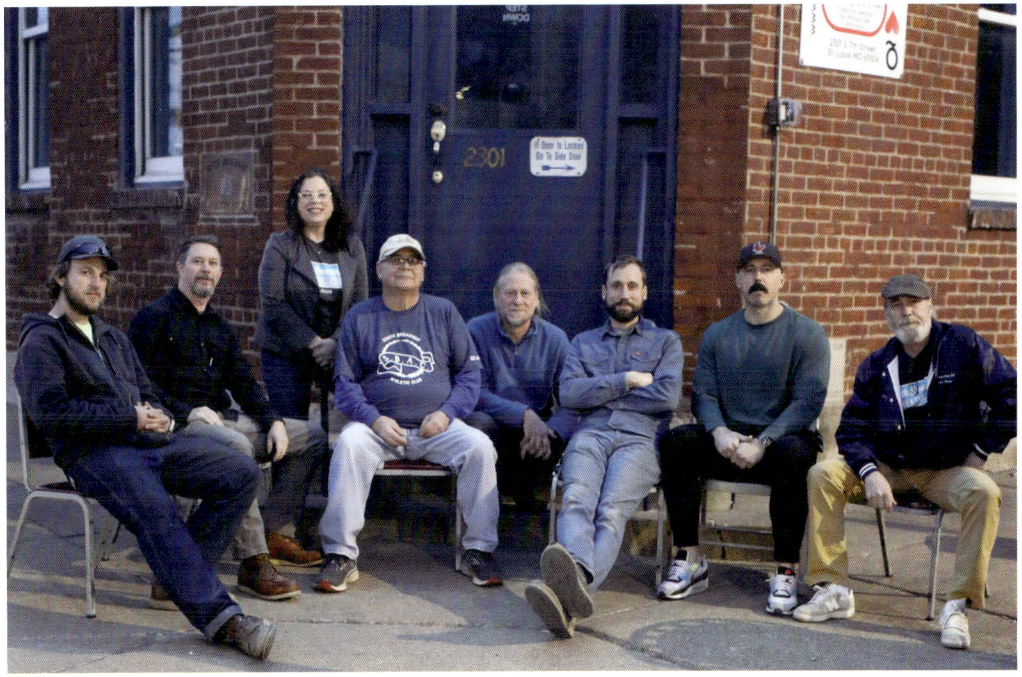

The SBAC 125th Anniversary Archive Committee, the volunteers who spent hundreds of hours and more than a year researching, writing, compiling, and curating this book: *from left to right*, Mitchell Goist, Ryan Buckley, Miriam Moynihan, Mike Button, Dan Guenther, Eric Mrozewski, Kevin Wilkins, and Tim Kippenberger (not shown: Tim Wescovich)
Kit Kellison photo

We would like to thank Katie Graebe at Landmarks Association of St. Louis, Tom Gullickson at 1860 Saloon, Charles Brown at the St. Louis Mercantile Library at the University of Missouri–St. Louis, Maureen McMillan, the late Rick Lanius for his work preserving the story of the club, Cheryl Bauman, Sharon Holloman from the City of St. Louis Comptroller's Office, and the Bottle Rockets.

Boosters

Throughout its 125 years, the SBAC has been sustained and operated by its members and their volunteer efforts. With more than a century of commitment to promoting community and social events in the heart of the Soulard neighborhood, "South Broadway Boosters" have always played an integral part.

Boosters are community members, local businesses, sports clubs, and other groups that purchased advertisements or gave other kinds of financial support for boxing/wrestling fight bills, dance programs, bingo cards, newsletters and concerts.

With a long history of community support, we are continuing that tradition with this book. The people and businesses listed on these pages have provided support in bringing the SBAC's storied history to print. The Club thanks and commends these Boosters.

It's a grand old club.

- Michael & Mary Button
- It's a Grand Old Club!—Glen & Ruth Hearold
- Al & Cheryl Bauman
- Dale Bruning
- Bill Christman
- Don Winkler
- Austin and Evan Brown
- Chris Simonds
- Soulard Business Association
- Mary & Parker Carlson
- Elizabeth A. Turpin
- Brenda Cash & Jeff Taylor
- Jasa & Preston
- The Stovall Family—Kevin, Amy, Brody & Blake
- Steve & Dana Grosch
- Daniel Button, Shirley Button & Kevin Button
- Jeff & Connie Bafaro
- Brent & Leah Jones
- Mary Tabacchi
- Steve & Terri Maddux
- Barry & Vicki Guiot
- Kristin Carlson
- Brookie Blake
- Michelle Stuckey & Jeremy Faust
- Linda & Mike Berry
- Joe Dorsey
- Jules Sardo
- Michelle Landy Northington
- Marcia Tolcou
- Donna Regh Braswell
- Ken & Lisa Mullins
- Bo & Lori Proffitt
- Julie Price & Scotty Fielder
- Kevin Wilkins
- Gabby & Nick Moynihan
- Sarah Folkemer
- Jim Gehrs & Lauren Choate
- Greg & Jody Schaab
- Denise Naughton
- Frank Mudro
- Brian "Dog" Thomason
- Abigail Buckley
- Nicholas Kanter
- Zach & Sam Mertens
- Jackie Harris
- Jo Jo Mertensmeyer
- Joe Moore
- Matthew Smith & Rebecca Rio
- Vincent Becker
- Michael Mudro
- Leisa L. Marshall
- James H Marshall
- "Soulardians Forever!" SBA has been a cornerstone of the neighborhood through good and bad times. Thanks to all the volunteers over the years for their hard work and dedication. May you always hear the echo of the ring-side bell.
  John Wallace
  Neal Thompson
- Mark Burroughs Moynihan
- Kerry O'Reilly Moynihan
- Joe & Karen Tyler
- In Memory of Kenny & Lori Nienhaus
- Scott Sturm
- Joshua Venverloh
- Angelo, Yvonne, Angelo & Margie Torrillo
- Jason Stuhlmann
- John Pendergast & Miriam Moynihan
- Bob & Mary Moynihan
- Tim Kippenberger
- Mitchell Goist & Amanda Ramcharan
- In Memory of Stephen "Wilk" Wilkins
- Stephanie Blackwelder
- Johnny Moynihan
- Dan Guenther & Megan Bennett: Thanks for giving up two years of Mondays for "Book Club"
- Tim Wescovich
- Guenther & Mosley Family: Bob, Dixie, Jennifer, Jessie and Jessie
- Christina and Lillian Buckley
- Lauren Casper-Mrozewski
- David Hill
- The SOL Club:
  - Ryan Buckley
  - Eric Mrozewski
  - Jeff Lehmann
  - Angelo Torrillo
  - Matt Berra
  - Matt Martin
  - Jason Orsega
  - Tom Ryan
  - Gabe Murr
  - Josh Fajkowski
  - John Wright
  - Jessie Weitzel
  - Ronnie Lipp

Sponsors

CONSTRUCTORS 911
ROOFING & CONSTRUCTION

Together
CREDIT UNION

LOHR
DISTRIBUTING CO.

REALTY EXECUTIVES
OF ST. LOUIS
Marybeth Wallace

SkillCraft Carpentry
What can we build for you?
www.skillcraftstl.com

Kippenberger Woodworking

WILKINS SCHNELLER LAW

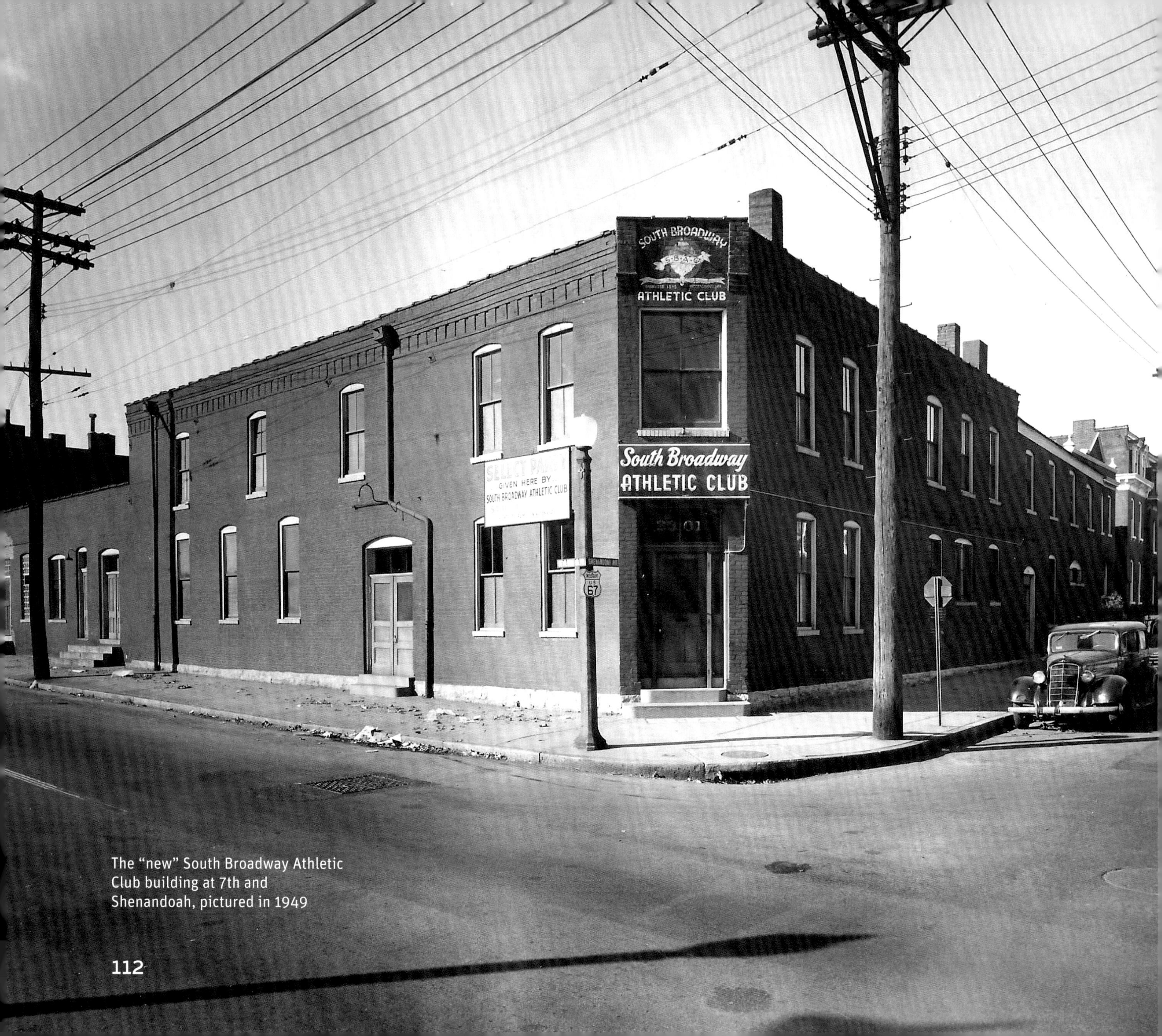

The "new" South Broadway Athletic Club building at 7th and Shenandoah, pictured in 1949

Index

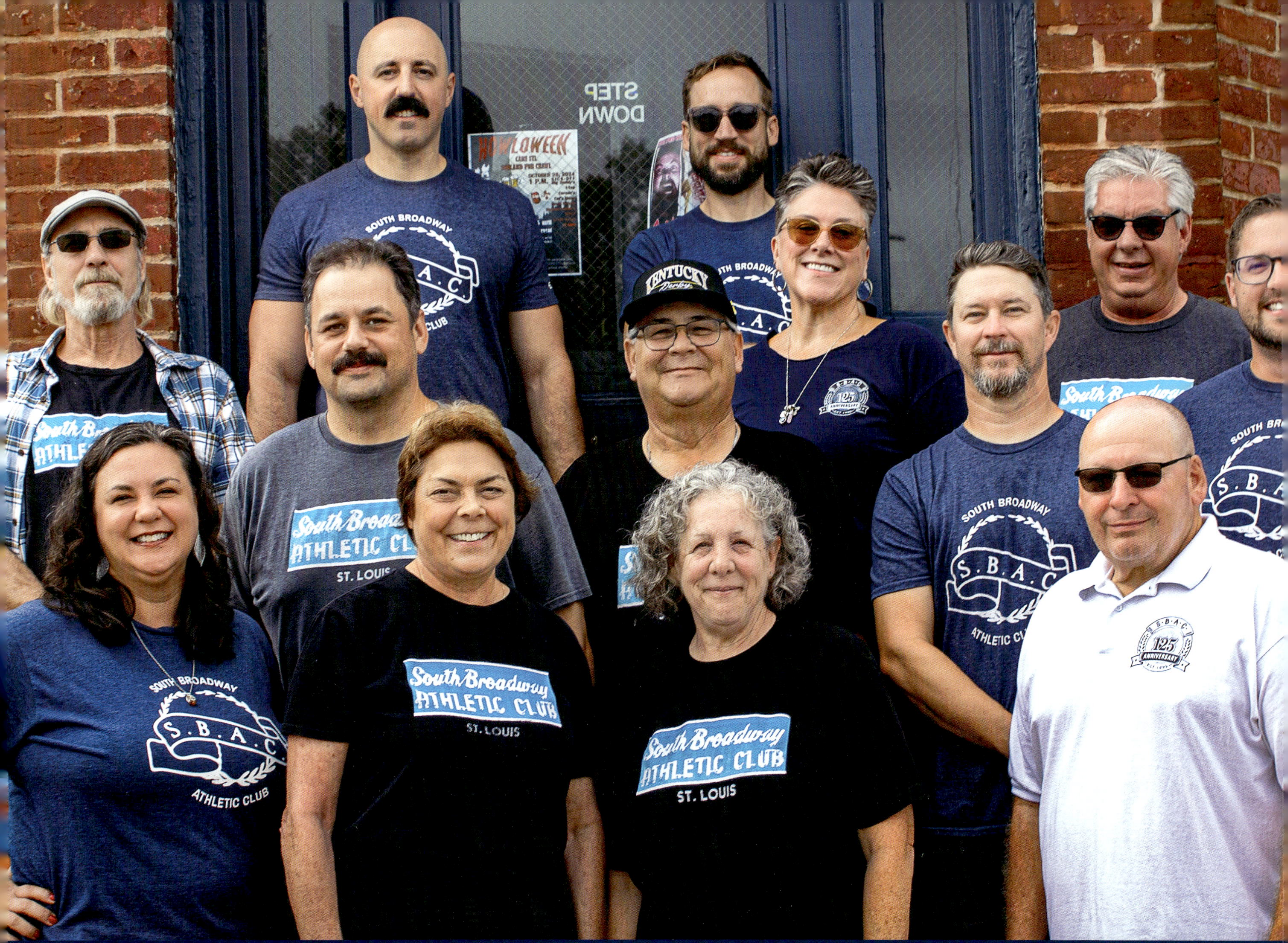

SOUTH BROADWAY ATHLETIC CLUB BOARD AND OFFICERS, 2024

Front row: Sarah Folkemer, sergeant at arms; Marcia Tolcou, treasurer; Jody Schaab, vice president; Dale Bruning, financial secretary

Middle row: Tim Kippenberger, board member; Jim Gehrs, board member; Mike Button, vice treasurer; Leah Jones, recording secretary; Ryan Buckley, board member; Bob Moynihan, board member; Kevin Stovall, board member

Back row: Kevin Wilkins, president; Eric Mrozewski, board member

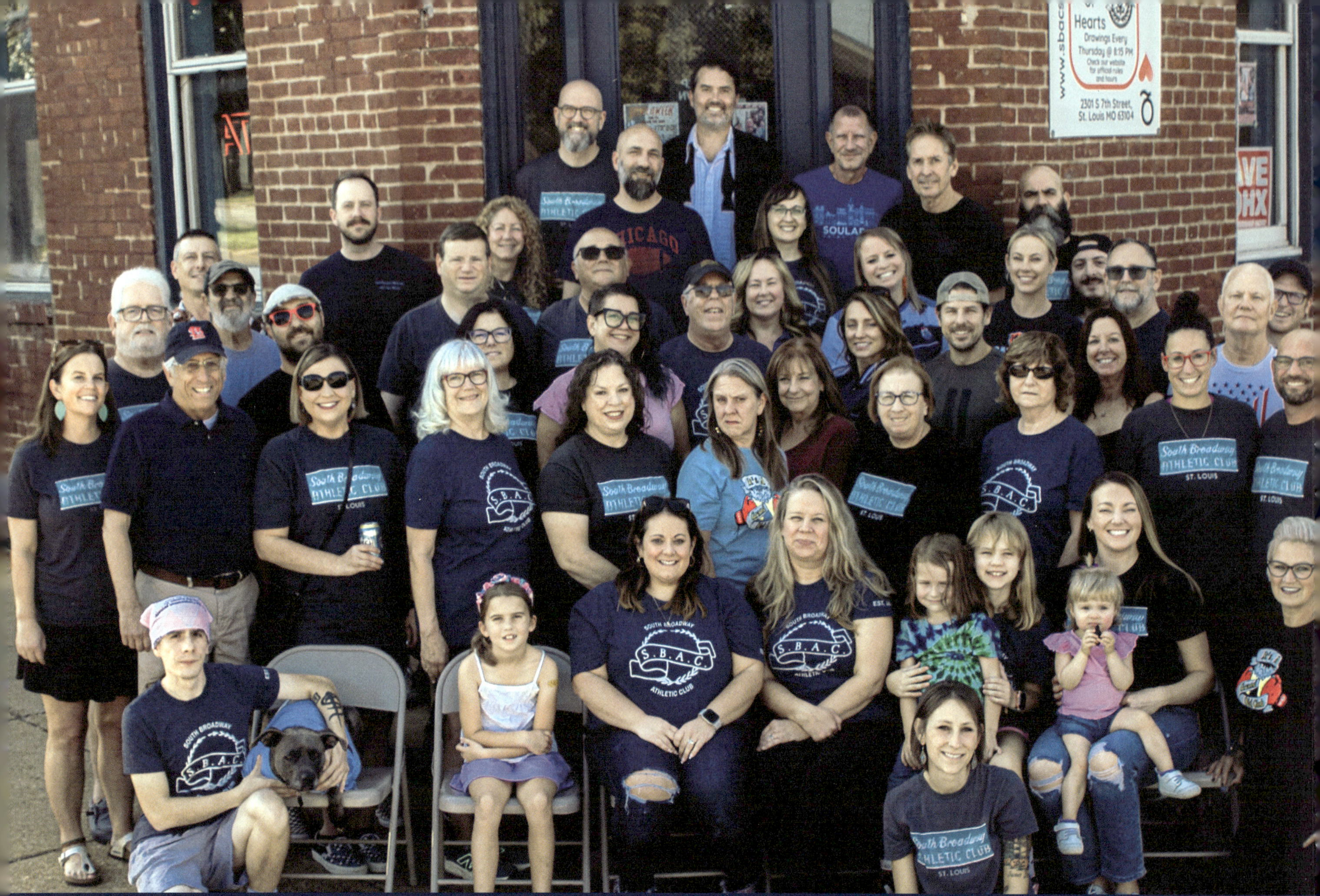

Hearts
Drawings Every Thursday @ 8:15 PM
Check our website for official rules and hours
2301 S 7th Street, St. Louis MO 63104
South Broadway
ATHLETIC CLUB
ST. LOUIS
SOUTH BROADWAY
S.B.A.C.
ATHLETIC CLUB
CHICAGO
SOULARD